How To Live A Long Life

By
Betty Yülin Ho, MIOF, IOM

Juvenescent Research Corporation
New York

HOW TO LIVE A LONG LIFE
COPYRIGHT 2003 By Betty Yulin Ho
Cover drawing by Arthur Skowron, Copyright 2003
All Rights Reserved
First Edition
Juvenescent Research Corporation
New York, New York
Graphics and Typeset by Wall-to-Wall Press
Manufactured in the United States of America

Library of Congress Cataloging-in-Publication Data
Ho, Betty Yu-Lin, date-
    How to live a long life / by Betty Yulin Ho.
      p. cm. – (The system of government in the living body)
    Includes bibliographical references and index.
    ISBN 1-884996-01-9
    1.   Health. 2. Human biology. 3. Longevity. I. Title.

RA776 .H6738 2003
613—dc21

Library of Congress Control Number   00-069479

First Edition
First Printing

Dedication

To all the scientists who have made this book possible

Credo

May this book fulfill the credo so beautifully expressed by Claude Bernard in the following passage:

Je supporte l'ignorance: c'est là ma philosophie. J'ai la tranquillité de l'ignorance et la foi de la science. Les autres ne peuvent vivre sans foi, sans croyance, sans théorie. Moi je m'en passe. Je dors sur l'oreiller de l'ignorance. Je ne sais pas et je ne saurai jamais, je l'accepte sans me tourmenter, j'attends. Je ne tombe pas pour cela dans le nihilisme, je cherche a connaître les rapports.

I can bear ignorance: it is my philosophy. I have the serenity of ignorance and the faith of science. Others cannot live without faith, creed or theory. I do without them. I sleep upon the pillow of ignorance. I don't know and shall never know I accept without tormenting myself. I wait. I do not fall thereby into nothingness. I seek to know relations.

From "Introduction à l'Etude de la Médecine Expérimentale" by Claude Bernard. Translated by B. Y. Ho.

THE SYSTEM OF GOVERNMENT IN THE LIVING BODY
OTHER BOOKS BY Betty Yulin Ho, NUMBERED IN ORDER WRITTEN
UNDER THE SAME IMPRINT

1. The Living Function of Sleep, Life and Aging, 1967.
2. The Origin of Variation of Races of Mankind and the Cause of Evolution, 1969.
3. A Scientific Guide to Peaceful Living, 1972.
8. How to Stay Healthy a Lifetime Without Medicines, 1979.
9. A Chinese and Western Daily Practical Health Guide, 1982.
12. Immediate Hints to Health Problems, 1992.
13. One Hundred and One Ways to Live 150 Years Young and Healthy, 1992.
14. Una Guía Unica Para la Salud, la Juventud y la Longevidad, 1992.
15. A Unique Health Guide for Young People, 1994.

BY PILOT BOOKS
4. A Chinese and Western Guide to Better Health and Longer Life, 1974.

UNPUBLISHED MANUSCRIPTS
5. Answers to over 200 Questions About the Living Body, 1975.
6. The Six Systems of the Body and their Manifestations, 1976.
7. Healing with your Blood: A Message from the East, 1977.
10. Your Living Body, 800 pp., 1981-1989.
11. Vive Napoléon, 1991.
16. Understanding your Living Body, 400 pages, 1993.

Acknowledgements

The author wishes to thank the following for permission to use the illustrations in her book.

Fig. 13, p. 41: Preparations from vitally injected muscles from guinea pig. Optical transverse sections. From **Anatomy and Physiology of Capillaries**, revised edition, copyright 1929, by August Krogh. Reprinted by permission of Yale University Press.

Fig. 2, p. 8: The muscle capillaries of guinea pig injected during life with India ink showing different degrees of constriction. From **Anatomy and Physiology of Capillaries**, revised edition, copyright 1929, by August Krogh. Reprinted by permission of Yale University Press.

Fig. 49, p. 289: The Female Beetle Phengodes, from **Living Light**, by E. Newton Harvey, copyright 1940, renewed 1968 by Princeton University Press. reprinted by permission of Princeton University Press.

About the Author

Born in China, Ms. Ho spent her early years in Shanghai where she attended the Lycée Français de Shanghai. Later, she obtained a B.S. in Biology at Columbia University. While attending medical school at Lausanne University in Switzerland, Ms Ho also studied piano and was inspired by many scientific ideas. These ideas eventually led her to abandon medical school and devote herself to piano studies. Applying her scientific ideas to her newborn infants, from her first born to the last, Ms. Ho developed an infant feeding method and later obtained both U.S. and Canadian patents for her invention.

Upon returning to the U.S. in 1963, Ms. Ho began researching to prove her scientific ideas and wrote a series of 16 books of which 10 are published and available in print.

It is her hope that this 17th book provides great insight into the living body that Ms. Ho has tried to convey.

A resident of New York City, Ms. Ho is an accomplished pianist and is fluent in six languages.

Why this book was written

In the December 1999 issue of the Reader's Digest, author Paul Johnson said that though mankind has conquered many scourges, he has not conquered death. This century man has gained great power over inorganic matter. Man has reached the moon and space, yet knows little about life and death. Physicians perform organ transplants, use body parts of the dead to revive the living, but are helpless with a terminally ill patient who must resign himself to approaching death.

Medical science is very daring: pregnancy is fearlessly induced by fertility drugs, resulting in multiple births of as many as seven infants. Female implantation of an in vitro fertilized egg is another example.

Medical science also has the power to separate Siamese twins, often maiming the infants. Some drugs deemed dangerous one year is later found to be beneficial. Some people's medicine cabinets are full of different pills with dubious curative powers. Recently milk has been found to cause cancer. Prepared foods contain ingredients dangerous to health: preservatives, coloring, this acid, that fat. For istance, a gamut of ingredients are in potato chips, yet they can easily be made with salt, oil and potatoes.

Restaurants are hazardous to health; workers do not wash hands after blowing the nose or using the toilet. Many people experience diarrhea after eating in a restaurant. One young man turned black and died. Mistakes are often made in hospitals; removing a healthy organ instead of a diseased, leaving sponges, towels, instruments in a patient's abdomen after an operation.

This indicates a lack of respect for human life. Working quarters have no circulating fresh air. In many schools, windows are hermetically sealed. Apartments have no balconies; and in some high rises, stepping onto a balcony is a frightening experience. Skyscrapers tower over three-story brownstones, apartments facing the street get sunshine coupled with noise whereas back apartments are always in the dark yet so quiet one can hear a pin drop. Some apartments face eight lanes of cars. Others face a rumbling, noisy highway or an elevated subway.

The West should begin to rebuild their cities for a city is not simply a place to contain people but to allow families to have sunshine, peace and happiness in this short stay on earth. Our life is but minutes in eternity, said Napoleon. Houses should have a garden in front and a yard behind. A large glass window on the roof would allow the sun's rays to heat the house all year round. A six-foot brick or bamboo wall should wrap around a house and separate from the neighbor. Enclave of houses should be enclosed in a lane, separated from the rumble of moving vehicles. Ambulances, police cars should use a lower, beeping sound and cars should tinkle a bell. This would make life friendlier in an inhospitable atmosphere of an asphalt jungle.

Most important is to stop building skyscrapers. Towering buildings stir fear in the onlooker. When stimulated by fear one becomes angry. An angry person can easily commit crime. Buildings should not be higher than a tall tree whose leafy top is soft and friendly to man's eyes.

In New York City an acquaintance quickly becomes an enemy. True friendship is most difficult to find; a close family relationship is possible, resulting in a lonely life for most city people. Whereas in country places, distance often prevents country folk from having close friends. This situation must change. Though the U.S. is modeled after the great European cities, Paris, Venice, Florence, etc. the latter have retained their charm. It is time for cities in the U.S. to develop greater charm.

Table of Contents

Chapter 1
A SCIENTIFIC AXIOM FOR EVERY HUMAN BEING 1
Blood vessels are controlled by nerve endings of the nerve center. What happens to red cells after passing through open blood vessels? What happens to blood in a closed circuit of blood vessels? Assessing the amount of blood flowing to the many organ-systems. Ensure a constant optimum blood-flow to the regulatory organs.

Chapter 2
CONCEPTION WITHOUT ARTIFICIAL MEANS 7
Understanding female reproductive organs. Female puberty. Male reproductive organs. Male puberty. Fertilization of an egg. To ensure fertilization. Spontaneous abortion of an embryo. Conceive an embryo without fail.

Chapter 3
IMPROVE PRENATAL CONDITIONS FOR A DEVELOPING EMBRYO 12
The kind of work and tests to avoid during pregnancy. Fluctuation of blood to the growing embryo. Damaging activities to avoid during pregnancy. Activities to avoid during pregnancy. Some examples from the medical library. Saving the lives of Siamese twins. Do not induce labor. Dwarf uterus.

Chapter 4
A PEACEFUL CHILDBIRTH LEADS TO LONGEVITY 16
Current means used to reduce labor pains. Tests performed on the infant at delivery. Preparatory surgical means used on laboring mothers. Reduce pain naturally and hasten pelvic expansion at labor. No hand insertions please! We delivered our grandson. Do not turn an infant at childbirth. Why pelvic insertions, perineum cutting are senseless procedures. Damaging effects of circumcision. Abolish circumcision and prolong men's lives.

Chapter 5
FORM A BEAUTIFUL BABY AND ENSURE LONGEVITY 22
Diet of premature infants. Problems of intravenous feeding. Improve a premature infant's growth. Our daughter breastfed her infant. We developed an infant feeding method. Breasts. Things to watch out for in a newborn infant. Eradicate autism and epilepsy by improving the feeding method during the first year of life. Understand epilepsy. Help for autistic and epileptic children. How to prevent birthmarks.

Chapter 6
Form a beautiful child during 20 years and ensure a long life 31

When should a child begin to walk? Should we expose baby to direct sunlight? A child's skin should be very clean. Daily bath. Grooming a child's hair. Should boys and men wear long or short hair? Girls should wear their hair long, Clothing for health. Wear clothes for good health. Footgear for growing children. Daily care of teeth. To preserve teeth for a lifetime, What to do when a nerve is dying. Immediate action to take upon loss of teeth. To remove tartar from roots of teeth. Remove earwax from the ear canal. Care of the navel. Serious infectious diseases. Inflammation of tonsils and adenoids. To remove pus from acne pustules. Do not play around with skin. Adorning with jewelry Prepare a child for immunization shots Work for a growing child. Choose foods for better growth and improve adult formation. Select foods according to the theory of evolution. Choose foods according to determinism. Vegetable oils are indigestible. Some criteria to observe in cooking.

Chapter 7
Preserve the skeletal system to ensure a long life 42

Walk healthfully. Running and/or jogging. Skate, ski, climb and swim. Calisthenics and bicycling. Why is creative work tiresome. Dangers of vigorous exercise. Why exercise with force? Preserve energy when seated. The detrimental effects of constant standing. How to carry weights. Physical fitness. A sleeping limb.

Chapter 8
The use of vocal activities to ensure a long life 50

Our voice box. The larynx when speaking. Effect of the spoken language on longevity. Detect illness by the voice's sound. Work using voice forcefully is a danger to life. Singing. Laughter and its effects. The danger of crying. Humming, whistling. The thymus: gland of muscles and bones. Location and structure of thymus.

Chapter 9
The three important nervous centers 56

The brain's external appearance and between arachnoid and pia. The brain: its internal appearance and fissures on the brain's surface. Nervous structures leading to the spinal cord. Brain ventricles. The brain: its blood supply. The spinal cord's enveloping membranes. Cerebrospinal fluid. The spinal cord: its internal configuration. Nervous tissue: general information. The cranial nerves. Direction of spinal nerves after leaving the cord. Voluntary action: its nervous control. Reflex action. The number of brain cells. Processing information. A

How to Live a Long Life   v

necessary condition of nerve cells: oxygen in the atmosphere. Speed of nerve impulses. How nerve fibers obtain a myelin sheath. The conduction of nerve impulses. The sympathetic ganglia. The parasympathetic ganglia. How to assess human behavior. Dying explained. Approaching death. The death agony. Accumulated wastes. Sudden death. Extreme terminal state. Remove poisons rapidly. Poisons must be removed.

CHAPTER 10
CONTROL EXTERNAL STIMULI AND LIVE LONG 70

The eyes. How eyes are protected. The eye: its external formation. The eyeball's three layers. The lens of the eye. When light strikes the eye. When an object is perceived. How an object is seen. Vision: the ill effects of faulty nutrition. The best lighting to maintain youthful eyesight and ensure longevity. Take immediate action. Maintain perfect eyesight for a long life. Noise - Medication. The external ear & the three divisions of the ear. How sound is heard. What happens when one hears sounds. Music: its beneficial effect on health. How to preserve hearing. The sense organs of equilibrium: their exact location. The sense organs of equilibrium. Macular organs: their purpose. Maintain optimum spatial position without feeling dizzy. The location of taste buds. The exact position of taste buds. How food elicits taste sensation; taste protects. Immediate action after swallowing poisonous substances. Different taste sensations perceived. Taste perception and disease. The sense of smell: its exact location. Sense organs of smell: their cellular structure. How smell is perceived. Odors: their danger. Breath odor may indicate certain diseases. Advancing age and the sense of smell. The various sense organs of touch. How touch sensation is transmitted. Blood flow through skin. Importance during growth, sense organ stimulation. Beneficial effect of touch, massage. Stimulation of skin's sense organs invigorates health. Sense organs of touch in later life. Safeguard all sense organs.

CHAPTER 11
CONTROL FATIGUE, EMOTION, PAIN AND LIVE A LONG LIFE 86

Different types of fatigue. Factors causing fatigue. Combating fatigue. Powerful emotions affect the organism. Dangerous effects of powerful emotion. Beneficial effects of music. Anxiety and fear affect the organism. Healthful feeling to fear death. Jealousy and envy affect the organism. Pain can be understood as capillary distension.1. Pain when the body performs an action. 2. Pain from something done to the body. a. Coping with a sudden deep bruise. b. A sudden burn. c. Coping with a cut. d. Coping with a burn on mucous membrane. e Coping with back pain. f. Pain when hit on the head. 3. Pain experienced when something penetrates the body. a. Pain from blood poisoning. b. Coping with appendicitis. 4. Pain when something desires to leave the body. a. A painful tooth. b. Immediate action when several teeth are painful. c. A fecal impact. Coping with an excruciating headache. Coping with pain from abnormal regeneration of cells. How to be rid of a cramp. The present theory of pain is in accordance with all previous theories of pain.

Chapter 12
SLEEP DEEPLY, PREVENT AGING AND PROLONG LIFE **98**
The sleep mechanism: an ancient physician's impression. The mechanism of sleep revealed through research. Why does blood fill up the regulatory organs during sleep? Causes of insomnia. Ensure a good night's sleep. What if despite all previous precautions one yet cannot fall asleep?. If I awaken in the middle of the night and can no longer sleep. Awaken someone healthfully. Understanding a nervous breakdown. What recourse when one has slept badly? Required sleep. Required hours of sleep. Understanding coma. Daily regulations to follow upon awakening. Understand the threefold aging process. Combat the first aging action: never perform two actions simultaneously. Combat the second aging action: balance actions. Combat the third aging action: avoid all strenuous movements. Cold floors can age you prematurely. Wearing fur, leather and wool can prolong lives. An apartment can cause aging. Excess food and aging - processed foods

CHAPTER 13
STEER AROUND DIGESTIVE DISTURBANCES AND LIVE A LONG LIFE **107**
Hunger explained. Deep hunger pangs. Appetite explained. Understand thirst. The loss of hunger pangs. Teeth: their growth and maintenance. Temporary and permanent teeth. Tooth structure. A long section through a tooth. Chemical composition of a tooth. Preparation and growth of a tooth. The difference in man's chewing power. How food should be chewed. The mouth: its external appearance. The mouth: its salivary glands. Function of saliva. Saliva: its chemical composition. The pharynx: its description. The pharynx: its three parts. How food is swallowed. How food should be swallowed. The esophagus: its description. Food descends the esophagus. The stomach: its position and make-up. Gastric glands: their location. Stomach varies in size. How food is digested. Digestion: factors affecting its rate. Gastric juice produced. The digestive tract: its most common diseases. Good digestion. Hydrochloric acid is formed. The small intestine and its various coats. The small intestine. The duodenum. The jejunum. The ileum. Digestion in the small intestine. Other secretions aiding digestion. Effects of excessive bile pigments. The small intestine. Food absorption. Diffusion and osmosis. The large intestine. The caecum: The large intestine, its internal structure. The large intestine: its solitary glands. The anal canal: a general view. Blood supply of the large intestine.

The large intestine: its food masses. The colon. Its six sections. The colon: its main function. Stool evacuation. Feces and what they represent. Importance of defecation. Constipation: its causes. Some tips to promote good elimination. Some artificial stimuli used to induce regularity. The digestive system: its large glands. a. The liver. The substance of the liver. Functions of the liver. Composition of bile. Jaundice. b. The pancreas. The internal structure of the pancreas. Pancreatic juice. External signs of a lack of pancreatic secretion.

CHAPTER 14
SOME NOTIONS ABOUT FOODS AND HOW TO ASSESS NUTRITIONAL REQUIREMENTS FOR A LONG LIFE 130
Better preparation of foods stirs longevity. Food digestion. Additional tips in preparing foods for health. Nutritional requirements: Carbohydrates, Fats, Proteins, Water, Calcium, Salt, Phosphorus, Magnesium, Potassium, Iron, Fluorine, Iodine, Copper, Vitamins: the Fat-soluble vitamins, the Water-soluble vitamins

CHAPTER 15
HOW TO COPE WITH EXTERNAL SIGNS OF ILLNESS 142
Detect illness by pulse and breathing rates. How to cope with changes in breathing rate. How air is brought to blood. What happens to air before it reaches the lungs. Preserve good breathing. Cope with snoring. Cope with coughing. Cope with changes in heartbeat. Avoid a heart attack. The myth of high blood pressure. External signs indicative of weak kidney function. What one should know about kidneys. The path taken by sieved blood. Principal functions of kidneys. Other functions of kidneys. What affects kidney filtration rate. Some causes of kidney disease. The diet to follow in kidney malfunction. Skin sensitivity. What skin reflects. General structure of skin. The epidermis. The skin's components. The dermis. The hypodermis. Mucous membranes. The chemical composition of skin. Hair. How hair is formed. Dark and curly hair. Loss of hair. Nails. Painful toenails. Sebacious glands. Sweat glands. Blood flow through skin. Deal with aging skin. To maintain youthful skin. How to deal with warts, moles, wens, excrescences, wrinkles. The various functions of skin.

CHAPTER 16
COPE WITH PROBLEMS OF ENDOCRINE GLANDS 164
The thyroid in and the hormone. Iodine in the body. Thyroid gland utilizes iodine to form thyroxine. Thyroxine: its function. Thyroxine deficiency: its effects. Over-secretion of thyroxine. Hypo and hyperthyroidism, external manifestations. Other factors preventing formation of thyroxine by the gland.

What to do about bulging eyes and goiters. The parathyroid gland: the gland and the hormone. Calcium and phosphate in blood. Insufficient parathyroid secretion. Parathyroid gland, signs of hyper-secretion. Calcium regulation is affected by parathormone. The thyroid and parathyroid glands, surgical operations. The pituitary gland: origin of anterior and posterior lobes. Functions of the pituitary gland. Dwarfism or gigantism. To ensure normal growth processes. The reproductive hormones: their actions. Changes at puberty. Enhance reproductive powers without artificial hormones. The pancreas, the islets of Langerhans. Hormones of alpha and beta cells. Insulin: its functions. Ketone bodies. Glucagon, its functions. Diabetes and how to control its ravaging effects. Secretions of the adrenal glands. The most important functions of adrenal glands. Adrenal cortex disease. The function of the pineal gland.

CHAPTER 17
HOW TO COPE WITH PROBLEMS OF BLOOD AND LYMPH 177
Blood: its composition. Plasma's composition. 1. Water in blood. 2. Blood plasma proteins. How proteins are formed in the body. 3. Inorganic constituents. 4. Organic constituents. 5: Respiratory gases in blood plasma. 6. Internal secretions. Substances to be excreted from plasma. Homeostasis is a basic requirement for normal cellular function. Types of cells in blood: the red blood cells and where they are formed. Red cells alter shape and structure. Life span of red cells. Function of red blood cells. White blood cells: 1) Granulocytes. 2) Lymphocytes: The site of production of lymphocytes. 3) Monocytes. The function of white blood cells. Some abnormal white blood cell counts. Blood platelets: thrombocytes. The laking of blood: hemolysis. How blood clots. The external appearance of the spleen. The spleen stores blood cells. Functions of the spleen. The lymphatic system. Where lymph vessels are found. The right lymphatic duct, the thoracic duct. Lymph nodes or glands. Lymph: its chemical composition. Lymph: its cellular composition.

CHAPTER 20
HOW BLOOD IS DISTRIBUTED TO ALL BODY PARTS 191
Arteries - description. Circulation through the heart. a. The pulmonary circulation. b. The systemic circulation. 1. The ascending aorta. 2.The aortic arch and its branches. Head and neck arteries. 3. The descending aorta. a. The thoracic aorta. b. The abdominal aorta. The external iliac artery. The internal iliac artery. Circulation of capillaries. Veins in general. The systemic veins. Sinuses. Two groups of systemic veins. 1.Veins emptying into the superior vena cava. 2.Veins emptying into the inferior vena cava.

Chapter 19
A GOOD SEXUAL RELATIONSHIP AND A LONG LIFE **197**
Love: the different degrees. Conditions of deep love. Seeking deep love. Despair in an unrequited love. Essentials in sexual parts. The erectile organ, in women. Fall in love and engage in sex. Enjoy love and sex. The orgasm, the climax. The climax - some beneficial after-effects. The orgasm, some dangerous after-effects. Masturbation- its dangerous effects. Living without sexual intercourse. Disturbance during the sex act. Advancing age and sexual activity. For those engaging frequently in intercourse: some general advice. How to care for the vaginal entrance, the uterus, etc.

Chapter 20
ALCOHOLISM, SMOKING, INTEMPERANCE VIOLENCE **204**
Alcoholism. Alcohol, a product of slow burning or digestion. Alcohol rate of absorption. Danger of alcohol to replace food. An alcoholic deprived of alcohol. Origin of tobacco-smoking. Tobacco inhalation and its deleterious effects. Tobacco: its chemical contents. Dangerous effects of smoke inhalation. Intemperance causes. A warning from 1745. Huge structures: their effect on man's mind. Buildings. Violence. Essentials of normal behavior. Factors preventing normal blood flow to the brain.

Chapter 21
HAPPINESS AND SUCCESS CONTRIBUTE TO LONGEVITY **209**
Happiness: the essentials. How education affects life and health. Results of a good education. Problems facing young people. Look for the proper mate. Raising a family. How to acquire personality. Industry, the number of hours. In search of happiness. The years of maturity.

Chapter 22
PROLONG LIFE WHEN THE END APPROACHES **213**
Conditions for living organisms to live perpetually. Normal cellular regeneration: necessary conditions. Help for the dying. Signs to watch out for approaching death. Importance of a desire to live. Longevity program. Great scientists' thoughts on death. A diet for the terminally ill patient. 1. A one-dish meal in broth. 2. String beans. 3. Meat in strips. 4. Serve a one dish meal. 5 Meat Balls. Ingredients. 6. Potato and rice Balls. 7. Delicious fish recipe. 8 Pancakes. 9. Pot roast of pork neck bones. 10. Dim Sim Dough. 11. Gelatin. 12 Desserts: Fruit Pie. 13 Apple Betty. 14 Mistress or wife's cakes. 15 Amanda's Chocolate cookies. 16 Cakes. 17 Custard. Miscellaneous. Another alternative to prolong life. A medical annals case. Daily schedule for a patient with a life-threatening condition or terminally-ill. Recipe for the very

sick. Clothing for the terminally-ill patient. Signs of fast-approaching death.

CHAPTER 23
LIVE A LONG LIFE DESPITE INFECTION WITH VIRULENT BACTERIA OR VIRUSES 224
Bacteria and Viruses: a description. Virulent bacteria in the body. A better approach in dealing with virulent bacteria: white blood cells. Curing syphilis. Curing gonorrhea. Curing leprosy. A.I.D.S. Chemical make-up of a virus. Viruses: multiplication and effect on the organism. The HIV patient and diseases. A natural means to suppress A.I.D.S.

CHAPTER 24
LIVE A LONG LIFE DESPITE PARKINSON'S, ALZHEIMER'S, MUSCULAR DYSTROPHY 229
Parkinson's Disease. Alzheimer's. Cancer. Muscular Dystrophy.

CONCLUSION 230

List of Illustrations

Fig. 1 Preparation from vitally injected muscles from guinea pig.
Optical transverse sections (From Krogh). 2
Fig. 2 Muscle capillaries of guinea pig injected during life with
India ink, showing different degrees of constriction. (From Krogh) 2
Fig. 3 Left cerebral hemisphere of a human brain (author's drawing) 2
Figs. 4, 5 The involuntary nervous system.
(author's drawing after Best and Taylor) 2
Fig. 6 Systemic circulation (Exterofective-muscles and bones.)
Parasympathetic = digestive and sex organs
Sympathetic = regulatory = reproductive organs
(author's drawing) 3
Fig. 7 Diagramatic representations of the three great systems at work.
a. in heavy work, b. after a meal, c. during sleep (author's drawing) ...3
Fig. 8 The pearly butterfly. Pattern variation in Python, Female larva
of the beetle Phengodes. (drawn by the author and Amanda
after E. Newton Harvey, Living Light) 5
Fig. 9 Schematic representation of the six systems with
five systems at work (author's drawing) 5

Tables

1. The expenditure of energy in calories per hour 49
2. Sleep required at different ages 103
3. Carbohydrate content in 100 g of various food groups 140
4. Alcohol content and caloric value in 100 g of
common alcoholic beverages 140
5. Lipid content and caloric value per 100g of
some commonly used fats 141
6. Some pathological conditions due to increased concentration
of some blood constituents 181
7. Some pathological conditions due to decreased concentration
of some blood constituents 182

Chapter 1
A Scientific Axiom For Every Human Being

A beating heart or normal breathing demonstrates life, but human beings are unaware of what occurs in an organ when speaking, singing, hearing music, chewing food, etc. We owe the Danish physiologist August Krogh who received the Nobel Prize for his discovery that in an active organ, the tiny blood vessels are open, but when the organ is inactive, many small blood vessels close (Fig. 1). The increased metabolism of an active organ requires a greater exchange of nutrients between blood and body tissues.

According to Krogh, we can see that blood vessels open up; let us visualize them expanding: when speaking blood vessels in vocal cords expand; when the ear hears music, speech or noise, the tiny vessels in the inner ear open up; when the hand holds an object, blood vessels in the muscles of the hand expand, etc. An organ performs an action tiny vessels open up, speeding up blood flow to the organ. The opposite is also true: when an organ is resting and relaxed, blood vessels immediately close up and less blood flows through its tissues (Fig. 2).

Blood vessels are controlled by nerve endings of the nerve center
The tiny blood vessels open and close depending on the amount of work done. These blood vessels do not passively open or close: they are controlled by the nerve endings of the three great nerve centers. The most important nerve center is the brain which controls all voluntary actions such as holding an object, standing up, lying down, doing push-ups, jogging, running, turning eyes to the right and left, listening to music. Sense organs also perceive light and sound without voluntary control.

On both sides of the spinal cord are two important nerve centers: groups of tiny brains or ganglia. In the chest region, one group of tiny ganglia, **the sympathetic ganglia**, directly control blood flow through tiny blood vessels of regulatory organs: heart, lungs, kidneys, skin, endocrine glands and blood vessels of reproductive organs: uterus, Fallopian tubes, ovaries and glands. Sympathetic ganglia control blood flow indirectly to digestive organs and glands, to sex organs and glands.

The other group of tiny ganglia, **the parasympathetic ganglia**, are in the cranial and sacral regions of the spinal cord: they control blood flow directly to digestive organs and glands, sex organs and glands (Fig. 3, 4, 5), indirectly to regulatory organs and glands, reproductive organs and glands.

What happens to red cells after passing through open blood vessels?
Red blood cells die after passing through open capillaries of an active region;

the stronger and more powerful the action, the more cells die, decreasing overall blood volume. Bits and pieces of disintegrated red cells remain in the circulatory system, later used to rebuild new red cells. Of the five liters of blood constantly flowing in the living body, two liters are red blood cells.

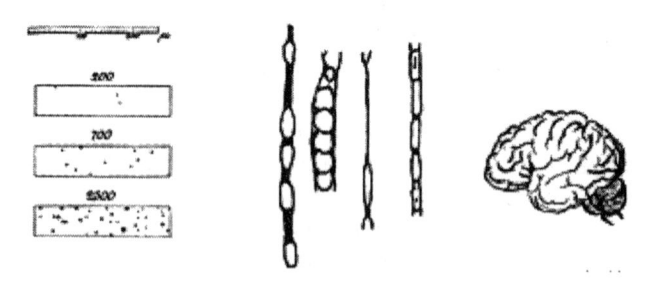

Fig. 1. Preparation from vitally injected muscles from guinea pig. Optical transverse sections (*from Krogh*).

Fig. 2. Muscle capillaries of guinea pig injected during life with India ink, showing different degrees of constriction. (*from Krogh*).

Fig. 3. Left cerebral hemisphere of a human brain (*author's drawing*).

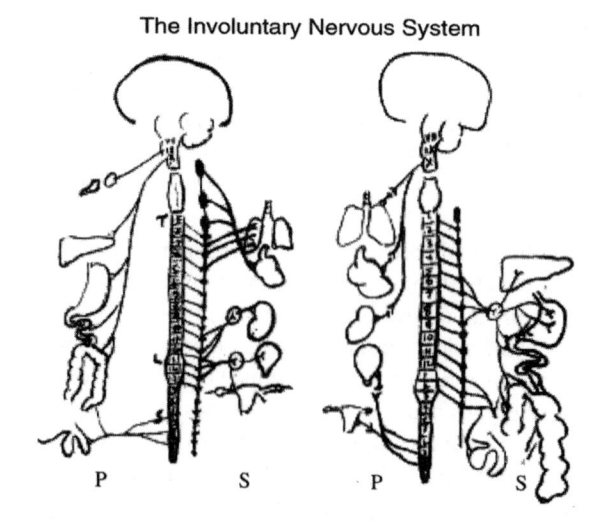

The Involuntary Nervous System

Fig. 4, 5. Notice how parasympathetic fibers control digestive and sex organs directly. Notice how symmpathetic fibers control regulatory organs and uterus directly.

Notice how parasympathetic fibers control regulatory organs and uterus after passing through another ganglion. Note how sympathetic fibers control digestive organs and sex organs after passing through other ganglia. Thus the control is less direct. (Author's drawing after Best and Taylor)

How to Live a Long Life

What happens to blood in a closed circuit of blood vessels?

Similar to Pascal's **Principle of Communicating Vases**, in a closed circuit of blood vessels, active work in one direction automatically depletes blood in other areas. Mild activity exerts a smaller effect on total blood volume, but heavy action depletes blood in all other areas, especially in regulatory organs, the body's motor. In pregnancy, heavy activity depletes the uterus of blood.

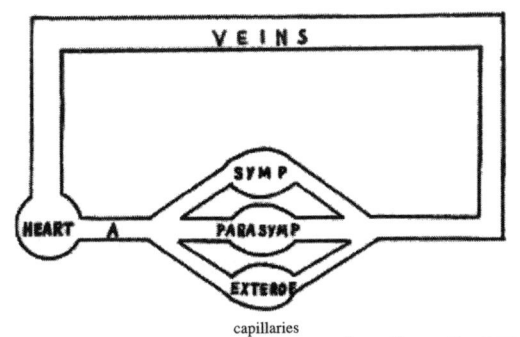

Fig. 6. Systemic circulation. Exterofective = muscles and bones. Parasympathetic = digestive and sex organs. Sympathetic = regulatory and reproductive organs. (*author's drawing*)

Fig. 7. Diagrammatic representations of the three great systems at work:

a) in heavy physical work;

b) after a meal; and

c) during sleep.

(*author's drawing*)

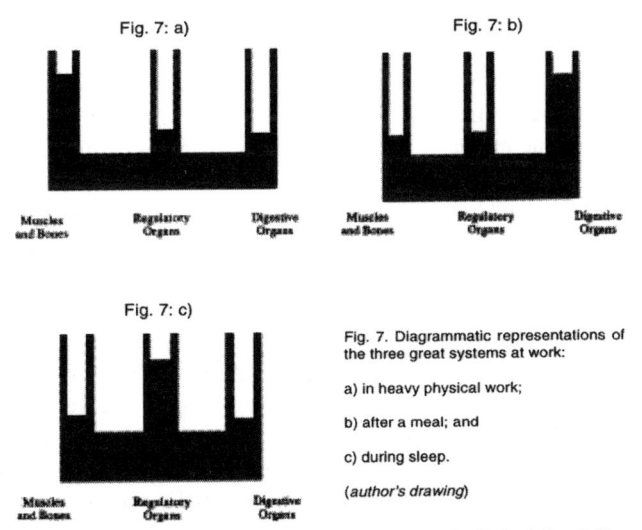

Fig. 7. In a closed circulatory system, blood fluctuates as in Pascal's **Principle of Communicating Vases**. (Author's drawing)

Muscles and bones are the external cover of internal regions. Heavy or continuous physical work depletes internal organs of blood (Fig. 6). The antagonistic organs are similarly affected.

Example: after a heavy meal, heart, lungs, kidneys, skin, and endocrine glands automatically receive less blood supply. In sexual performance, less blood flows to reproductive organs: uterus, Fallopian tubes, ovaries—opposing to sex organs. During pregnancy, avoid sex for the growing embryo would receive less blood (Fig. 7).

Assessing the amount of blood flowing to the many organ-systems

Normally, blood supplies equally all organ-systems. Muscles and bones represent about 50% of man's total body weight. Jogging, running, lifting heavy weights, singing, etc., blood goes to irrigate muscles and bones being used, thus decreasing blood supply to regulatory organs.

The digestive tract is a large system. After a heavy meal almost the entire blood volume concentrates in the stomach and intestines. Do not overeat. We frown on competitions on how fast can one eat how many frankfurters. To hasten digestion and prevent overeating, sit in a comfortable sofa chair and lean back when chewing. Relax when eating: the ancient Romans reclined on a sofa to eat.

The uterus is normally dormant; when pregnant, a woman's uterus becomes a large active organ, and mild activity in other organs must be observed. Normally dormant, sex organs during copulation becomes a large active organ and blood flows to the penis or clitoris for the orgasm.

Eyes and ears are small organs, but when assailed by bright lights, loud music or noise, much blood flows through these small organs. Prisoners have been tortured by shining continuously bright lights on them. Torture forcefully drives blood continuously through the tortured organ; eventually, the regulatory organs are affected, driving the prisoner mad, forcing him to confess guilt even though he is innocent.

Examples of torture: having a goat lick the sole of a foot, drip water on a forehead; In Paris during the 15th century, two young men, the d'Aulnay brothers, were having a liaison with the daughters-in-law of King Philippe le Bel; the brothers were skinned alive in the market place in the presence of thousands of spectators.

Regulatory organs receive the greatest blood supply only at night, during sleep. During the day, blood cells are destroyed by stimuli bombarding remaining organ-systems. To replenish the energy lost, living organisms must sleep at night. In the daytime, whenever possible, relax in a reclined position, lean head back, lift legs up. This position will fill regulatory organs with an optimum blood supply immediately. Your body may be seen at work, internally and externally, at all times of the day (Fig. 8).

How to Live a Long Life 5

Ensure a constant optimum blood flow to the regulatory organs

To preserve regulatory organs, analyze organ size and strength of action and change actions to control blood flow: during singing, dim lights that strike the eyes. Remain silent when traveling. Many singers sing and move their body simultaneously, a danger: many blood cells are destroyed simultaneously. When playing piano, do

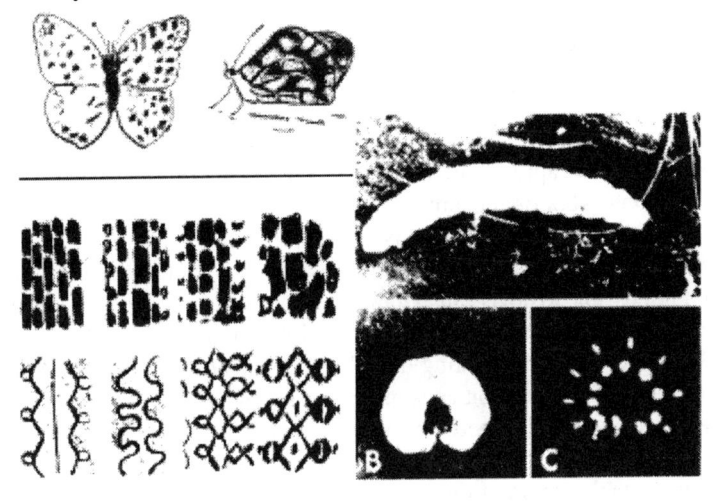

Fig. 8. (*top left*) The pearly butterfly pinned up to show the right upperside and the left underside. (*bottom left*): Pattern variations in Python. A single specimen may have a number of these patterns in different regions of its body. (*after Portmann drawn by author)* and Amanda.)
(*top right*) Female larva of the beetle Phengodes. A) dorsal view. B) lateral view. C) luminous specimen in darkness. (*after E. Newton Harvey, Living Light*).

Fig. 9. Schematic representation of the six systems with five systems at work. Note the depletion of the Regulatory Organs. (*author's drawing*).

not sing: allow the body to breathe freely.

Many jobs do not allow one to sit: guards, policemen, cashiers, etc. When a person is inactive, he must sit—every worker should have a chair. The seated position immediately diverts blood to the regulatory organs.

Make a habit of assessing size of organ and actions performed: if too many organs are involved, stop immediately; when studying, reading a book, working with hands—dim lights, lower music.

Do not overwork large organs with many capillaries for gradually overall appearance will change. Overexerting one large capillary area stirs obesity. Overexerting two large capillary areas stirs thinness. The body will shrink when three or more large capillary areas are overtaxed (Fig. 9). Skin is the only visible regulatory organ. Abnormal manifestations on skin indicates over activity in one of the five active divisions. Self-analysis can solve the problems.

Biology texts explain the living body in nine systems with nothing to unite them, making it impossible to devise an axiom. We observe birds daily; they are extremely sensitive and aware of their bodies. A loud noise—immediately a flock of birds fly away. Birds peck at foods, treating them like poison, and excrete continuously. We marvel at their ability to sit on eggs, male and female taking turns, until fledglings hatch. Birds show us the importance of body heat. We should learn from observing birds.

This immutable axiom of the six systems' function tied by blood flow, enables man to direct blood flow from region to region by decreasing or increasing an action. Control objects penetrating, striking, acting upon; watch wastes collecting in the body and monitor actions that detrimentally affect regulatory organs. Be wary of pain, especially in the head, for the heart is next to be detrimentally affected. Pain in the head is a sign of excess activity in several large organ systems.

If you have difficulty using this axiom in daily living, think about everything done by the body. The action affects the organ itself. Continued stimulus depletes the regulatory organs and glands. Beware of anything impinging upon, penetrating, done by, collecting in the body for the more powerful the action or stimulus, the more wastes collected, the greater the damage to regulatory organs. When all external stimuli, actions, things penetrating, wastes collecting in the body, are removed, regulatory organs immediately receive a greater blood supply.

Claude Bernard predicted that the day will come when man will guide his actions by an immutable theory requiring no further experimental verification. He will then achieve immortality till death suddenly overpowers life.

Chapter 2
Conception without artificial means

To live a long life, normal conception is indispensable. Today many couples seek counseling for conception, others use fertility drugs resulting in multiple births of infants weighing a pound or less each. Newborns of low birth weight have a lesser chance of survival than a normal six or seven pound newborn.

Let us examine the reproductive organs in order to understand them better.

Understanding female reproductive organs

The *sella turcica* is a tiny depression in the brain, where the light sensitive pituitary gland is located. In the pituitary gland are the hormones that control the male and female reproductive organs. Without light, the gland fails to induce maturation of sperm or eggs. Blind hamsters have regressed testes and ovaries because they do not see light; if the pituitary gland is removed or when anesthesia is administered, a similar effect is produced.

Female reproductive organs comprise paired ovaries, Fallopian tubes or oviducts, uterus and their glands. Situated behind the bladder and in front of the rectum, ovaries are small oval bodies about 1 1/2 inch long, 3/4 inch wide and 1/3 inch thick. Each ovary lies in a groove formed by the hypogastric artery and ureter. Ligaments attach ovaries to bladder, rectum, sacrum and walls of pelvis. Ovaries, tubes and uterus are firmly maintained in place by two double-layered broad ligaments extending from the peritoneum (lining of abdominal wall). Blood vessels. lymph vessels and nerves pass through broad ligaments. In the abdominal cavity, female reproductive organs are maintained in a firm position.

A cross-section of the ovary reveals an outer germinal layer, an inner framework of cells, blood vessels and follicles of varying size. The latter are little bags, each containing an egg. Each follicle looks like a chicken egg without a shell. The larger the follicle, the more advanced in maturity.

Fallopian tubes or oviducts are arms of the uterus. About 4 inches long, each tube ends in a funnel-shaped structure with edges prolonged into a number of tapering processes called *fimbria*, some attached to ovaries. Admitting only a bristle, a minute opening from the three-coated Fallopian tubes, leads into the uterus. Through the larger abdominal end of the tube, the mature egg enters the uterus.

Pear-shaped, the uterus is very small and flat, stem pointing downwards. About 3 inches long, 2 inches wide, one inch thick, a neck or cervix leads uterus to vagina. The uterine wall has three coats: outer serous, involuntary muscular and inner mucus. The thick muscular coat, cuts like cartilage. In pregnancy, new fibers develop, increasing in size. Lined by columnar epithelium, the mucous layer's inner surface is smooth, soft and pale red with many tubular glands embedded in its loose tissue.

Richly supplied by blood vessels from the sympathetic nervous system, the uterus is able to receive and sustain a fertilized egg. A slender cavity about 6 inches long, the mucous layer's numerous ridges allow the cervix to expand. Its glandular follicles secrete mucus and the cysts are distended with secretions. The cervix leads into the vagina.

About 2 1/2 inches long, vaginal walls are usually in contact. A cross section of the vagina presents the letter H, with a longer back wall. Shaped like a football, its three-coated wall has an outer muscular, inner mucous and a middle erectile layer. The mucous coat is studded with papillae, most numerous near the opening. At its entrance, the muscular coat's external longitudinal layer has an internal circular layer with a band of striped muscular fibers: the sphincter vagina. In penis captivum, this sphincter suddenly closes imprisoning the organ. During intercourse in the penis, the erectile tissue's wide blood spaces are gorged with blood.

Depending on the bladder's size, the uterus can assume different shapes. On a full bladder, the uterus is erect, lying on the bladder. In menstruation it becomes vascular. At birth, around 100,000 eggs are present in the female. A human egg is 0.016 mm. in diameter, finer than the point of a cambric needle. Three billion human eggs fit into a hen's egg shell. Eggs lie dormant until puberty, at the menses. During this lengthy developmental period a child must be given the best food. Of utmost importance are sufficient light, sunshine, fresh air and moderate exercise.

Female puberty

At puberty, stimulated by pituitary hormones, each month an egg matures. Pushed out of the ovary, the egg is surrounded by a follicle. The follicle breaks open, releasing the tiny egg into the Fallopian tube's funnel-shaped opening leading into the uterus on either side. Travelling outward, backward and downward, the egg leaves the tube by the bristle-sized opening, entering the top part of the uterus. As the egg moves across the Fallopian tube, the discarded follicle develops into a mass of cells with blood vessels: the corpus luteum. If the egg is fertilized, the corpus luteum continues to grow until later months of pregnancy, its hormone exerting a constant influence on the growth and functional integrity of the placenta apposed to uterine wall. If fertilization does not occur, both corpus luteum and egg leave the uterus in menstruation. A woman is particularly sensitive and nervous at this time of the month. Menstruation is similar to spontaneous abortion but less powerful: the egg was not ripped away from the uterine wall. Be sensitive towards a woman during the menses. The menses represent the death of the preceding month's egg. At ovulation, a new egg leaves the ovary. Ovulation is about the 15th day after the first day of the menses, depending on the menstrual cycle of the woman—varying between 25 and 30 days. Four or five days after ovulation, the mature egg moves across the Fallopian tube entering the upper part of the uterus where it may meet a sperm. The mature egg lives only 7 hours and can be fertilized during 24 hours. Spermatozoa stay alive four to five days.

Male reproductive organs

In the male, primordial germ cells arise from specialized cells that cease dividing on the 18th day of fetal life. By the 8th month of uterine life, out-pocketings of the abdominal wall known as genital swellings, lower themselves slowly through two ducts, the inguinal canals, entering scrotal sacs. In their descent, blood vessels, nerves and the ureter are drawn with them, forming the most vital spermatic cord. In their descent, layers of the anterior abdominal wall are brought along, forming coverings of both testicles and spermatic cord. Sometimes testes do not assume their normal position behind the penis but will do so by adolescence.

The scrotal sac is two-layered and has a multi-folded outer layer for testical expansion when replete with sperm; an extremely vascular inner layer, the dartos, allows sperm to leave the testes. A layer of fat separates scrotal sac from testes. The three-layered testes has an outer serous and a thick fibrous inner blood vessel layer. The fibrous layer sends incomplete fibers to the substance of the testis, dividing it into two parts. Slender branches are also given off, dividing the gland into cone-shaped chambers. A transverse section through a testis resembles an orange with 300 wedges, each with 2-4 tubules. Between wedges, blood vessels, nerve and interstitial cells are responsible for attributes of masculinity such as beard, deep voice, firm musculature and development of male accessory sex organs: Cowper's glands, seminal vesicles and prostate gland. Cowper's glands function during the sex act. Seminal vesicles and prostate gland ensure viability of sperm.

Fixed behind each side of the bladder, paired seminal vesicles are branched, saclike pouches about 2 1/2 to 4 inches long, 5 lines in breadth, 2 or 3 lines thick. Each vesicle is a single tube coiled upon itself, the diameter of a quill when uncoiled. It joins the vas deferens of the same side, becoming a straight, 3/4 inch long narrow duct, the ejaculatory duct. From both sides, ejaculatory ducts penetrate the substance of the prostate gland.

Seminal vesicles discharge fructose, the principal carbohydrate substrate for sperm metabolism. Vesicles do not store sperm; their function is glandular. At ejaculation, their secretions form the greater part of the ejaculate.

About 3 cm. high, 4 cm. wide and 2.5 cm. thick, the prostate gland is small, chestnut size and shape. Its substance comprises 30-50 branching tubo-alveolar glands, embedded in smooth muscle tissue. These small glands discharge their secretion into 16-20 tiny ducts converging at the urethra's prostatic portion. The prostate secretes a thin, slightly alkaline milky fluid of a characteristic odor.

Male puberty

At puberty, at 13-15 years of age, stimulated by hormones of the pituitary gland's anterior lobe, germinal cells mature, divide and form sperm. Microscopical in size, each spermatozoon is about 0.1 mm. long, resembling a tadpole with a head, body and tail. In a single ejaculate of 2 cc. a fertile man has around 152 million sperms, 91 million if infertile. Between the ages of 25 and 55, a man produces 240 billion spermatozoa.

Some external factors may affect germ cell formation: X-ray irradiation of local areas and of entire body; birth control pills, hormones, alcohol, induce a deficiency of vitamins A, B, C, E, and detrimentally affect sperm. In rats, peanut oil impaired sperm formation. Obesity and anemia play an important role in infertility. To prevent exposure to high body temperature, testicles hang outside of the body. Direct heat on testes induces sterilization; insulation of scrotum with woolens and tight-fitting suspensoria pressing testes close to the body also cause sterilization. It has been shown that in early stages of sperm development, high temperatures and fever effect a dramatic decline in sperm count. Optimum time for sperm formation is mornings after a good night's sleep. The sexual orgasm is detrimental to viability of sperm or egg. During orgasm, less blood flows through scrotum and uterus: they are tense and contracted. After the explosive orgasm, the uterus remains contracted for about a half an hour. To prevent loss of seminal fluid, women are advised not to change position from side to side or to stand after intercourse. To increase volume of seminal fluid, allow an interval of 4-5 days between ejaculations. The average scrotum weighs about 10-12 grams.

Fertilization of an egg

Mature sperm move to the testicle's outer part. At coitus, muscles surrounding penile canal, contract. An automatic valve prevents bladder from pouring out its contents. At orgasm, forced out of testicular tubules, sperm pass through a series of tubes and joined by fluid from seminal vesicles, end in the coiled epididymus. Straightening out into the vas deferens, the epididymus becomes the urethra and the ejaculate leaves the body through the penile lumen.

Semen is slightly basic, the uterus acidic at a 4-5 pH. When semen penetrates vagina, uterine acidity is neutralized, its action lasts 16 hours. After the 10th hour of penetration all sperm are motionless.

Once deposited in the upper part of the vagina, sperm propel by swimming slowly at 5 mm. per minute, nodding the head from right to left, reaching the egg in 10 hours' time. When a sperm meets an egg, the tail disappears, head and body penetrate the egg. Automatically all other sperm are prevented from further penetration; immediately after fertilization, the egg begins to divide, implanting itself on the uterine wall two or three days after sperm's entrance.

How to Live a Long Life

To ensure fertilization
Because women have different menstrual cycles, to ensure fertilization, have coitus on the 17th, 18th, 19th and 20th day from the first day of the menses. The 19th day from the first day of the menses is the day a woman can most assuredly be fertilized. To prevent conception, have coitus from the first day of the menses until the 16th day, also after the 20th day until the beginning of the next menses or during the menses.

Spontaneous abortion of an embryo
To prevent conception, centuries ago Hippocrates advised a slave to jump vigorously seven times. Running down a stairway a young woman missed the last step; she fell with a thud. She aborted spontaneously the next day; pain and weakness overtook her; a tiny gel-like pouch appeared on her panty. She saw she had aborted an embryo. Induce a spontaneous abortion by jumping several times from an ordinary chair. Jumping rope vigorously is also effective.

Conceive an embryo without fail
To conceive securely, do not copulate excessively; orgasm expels uterine contents and does not help retain the egg. One sexually active woman always experienced spontaneous abortions and was never able to conceive. After a hysterectomy she copulated freely. Our body is made up of so many parts, overexertion in a region detrimentally affects conception. Vigorous activity is dangerous: loud singing, constant talking, large meals, loud music or noise, excess physical exertion, overfilling the rectum with a quart-sized enema, bright lights, injections, strong emotion, etc. One woman spoke very loudly. In her youth, she conceived an infant but about the 5th month of pregnancy, she aborted spontaneously. She underwent all the pains of labor and perceived a tiny infant, perfectly formed, stillborn. She never conceived again.

Besides assuring a continuous optimum supply to regulatory organs, our five liters of blood must perform so many functions, powerful activity in other directions prevents an optimum flow to reproductive organs, thus affecting conception.

CHAPTER 3
Improve prenatal conditions for a developing embryo

To live long, improve living conditions from the first cell division on. Many mothers work full time, often until the ninth month of pregnancy. Some mothers smoke and drink, oblivious to these dangerous products.

A pregnant woman must not expose herself to noise, excitement or powerful emotion; rest, get fresh air/sunshine, take walks and follow a nutritious diet.

The kind of work and tests to avoid during pregnancy

Mothers-to-be must avoid standing at work and must have two hours of fresh air and sunshine daily. She should eat fresh fruits and vegetables, some meat and cheese, light coffee or cocoa, fresh juices and soups. A light diet helps regularity to give the growing embryo more space in the womb. Do not subject a growing embryo to ultrasound. The high-powered waves of sound increase fetal movements and the cord may wrap around the embryo and cause strangulation.

Scientific proof indicates that ultrasound decreases newborn infants' weight. A mother was carrying a baby in her arms; asked if the baby had been subjected to ultrasound, the mother acquiesced. We told her the danger; she said her infant was premature and at birth, the umbilical cord was wrapped around his body, a good reason for premature birth: he could not grow larger, the cord wrapped around him prevented growth.

According to a study published by WHO in 1982, at therapeutic intensities, ultrasound causes platelet aggregation and other hematological alterations. Ultrasound retards bone growth, triggers muscle contractions and alters thyroid function. Exposure of uterus at low therapeutic intensity range increases fetal abnormalities and lowers fetal weight.

A. R. Williams states: ultrasound cannot propagate through a tissue without some of its associated energy being deposited as heat. This heat raises the temperature of the tissue, weakening it. In an adult man ultrasonically damaged cells recover or dead cells are limited in number but reproductive cells are definitely damaged. When temperature rises in tissues in vivo, blood flow increases through the tissue causing erratic growth. No need to apply ultrasound on the embryo. Ultrasound has not prevented Siamese twins or birth defects. A pregnant mother is limited to two ultrasound sessions. Stop!

A pregnant mother is subjected to many tests. At 16-18 weeks of fetal life, amniocentesis is performed: ultrasound is used to locate a pocket of fluid free of fetus and placenta. To withdraw fluid from the amniotic cavity where baby floats, the mother's abdomen is cleansed, the skin numbed. Through the abdominal wall, a needle is pierced into the uterus to withdraw an ounce of fluid with a syringe. Amniocentesis is supposed to detect fetal abnormalities. This is a risky test, it has caused a 3% fetal loss, including injury to the fetus, placenta or umbilical cord, infection, miscarriage or premature labor, with possible bleeding. A preliminary pregnancy test is a vaginal examination: avoid it. Avoid all tests, drugs, anything that deviates from normal living practices. If bleeding occurs, an ectopic pregnancy may have occurred where the embryo is developing in the ovary or Fallopian tube. Terminate this kind of pregnancy by vigorously jumping down from a chair or jumping rope. In industry, ultrasound is used as a pest repellent. The reflection of waves of sound is comparable to radar used to detect airplanes or ships. Should we expose our invaluable embryo to ultrasound waves? Ultrasound is used to detect a child's sex. Why risk a fetus's life? This unknown factor is a mystery. We love the infant regardless of its sex.

Fluctuation of blood to the growing embryo
Joseph Barcroft's important data overlooked until now. He examined the uterine blood flow in a growing rabbit embryo during the entire pregnancy and wrote: as the fetus grows larger in the uterus, blood flow increases steadily until it reaches a maximum after which, regardless of the embryo's size, blood flow does not increase further but fluctuates between maximum flow and slightly below. This indicates that from conception until the maximum size of embryo, blood flow is able to increase up to the maximum or decrease down to a minimum, yet the embryo remains alive. An increase or decrease in blood flow affects the embryo's brain; the brain directs the formation of all body parts. Fluctuations in blood flow arrest or increase the growth of bodily parts, causing malformations.

During the first eight weeks of growth, an embryo is very vulnerable. A woman's body temperature fluctuates with fever and an increase in temperature automatically increases blood flow to the embryo, causing multiple growths. Today, an embryo is aborted if a mother has high fever during the first eight weeks of pregnancy. Blood flow can decrease without temperature drop, causing limited abnormalities. In this ambience, strong vital activity in any direction decreases blood flow to the embryo, causing abnormal formations.

Damaging activities to avoid during pregnancy
A pregnant woman must not exert heavy physical activity or overeat. Many pregnant women have sex. The sexual orgasm is equivalent to maximum effort: one perspires abundantly, the heartbeat increases, blood pressure rises, one pants for breath, culminating in orgasm. This vital activity affects the embryo detrimentally, and every milliliter of reduced blood flow will cause some malformation: mental retardation, skin tumors, tumors in peripheral nerves, blotchy skin pigmentation,

mental defect, calcification of brain cortex, microcephalus, acrocephalus, cleft lip and palate, fused fingers, atrophied limbs, claudication, etc. We cannot list all the malformations of embryos.

Activities to avoid during pregnancy

Medical books advise that it is natural and normal to have sex during pregnancy. According to Joseph Barcroft's findings, powerful vital activities decrease blood flow to the developing embryo, without lowering body temperature. After maximum blood flow to the fetus is reached, if a mother is weak, sex, strong emotion or activity will cause a spontaneous abortion with premature birth. A strong, healthy woman can have sex and not abort until term—with possible minor abnormalities. A young woman about seven months pregnant was subjected to great fear when her mother-in-law scolded her son, screaming at the top of her voice for half an hour. The baby was born normal but died a week later. The best advice for a pregnant woman is to refrain from emotions during the nine months gestation, and avoid sex, drugs, pills, radiation, injections. Get fresh air, sunshine and eat a delicious diet conducive to perfect growth conditions for a developing fetus.

Food is very important. There are cases where members of the same family are born with inherited malformations for generations. This can be traced to eating overcooked foods. See chapter on better cooking.

Embryonic development is also affected by drugs like thalidomide, strong emotion, physical overexertion, blinding lights, deafening noise, deafening music, overcooked foods, powerful penetration of substances in mother's body or powerful activity will detrimentally affect her growing embryo.

Some young women talk very loudly which may cause blindness, deafness, retardation in an embryo, and even cause a spontaneous abortion. Speech is a higher manifestation of life, a feat requiring skeletal system's energy and diverts blood away from all other organs. Science has not yet solved the prevention of birth defects.

Some examples from the medical library

Under extreme nervous tension, a Chinese woman played MahJong till dawn during the nine months gestation. At term, the baby was born severely handicapped. He moved with difficulty, spoke with great effort. Tied to a chair, he became huge and had to be carried by two male servants. An opera singer had two children, one was a deaf-mute, the other, retarded.

In Portugal, at the beginning of the 20th century, a girl had phocomelia. Her limbs were atrophied; she could only sit. Children called her a rat. Another boy in Portugal was born without limbs, he became a schoolteacher and lived to age 35. He punished the children by knocking them with his head. Placed in a padded basket, he couldn't bear clothing on his body. For exercise he would writhe on the floor. He was an interesting conversationalist greatly loved by his mother. The medical library abounds with cases of Siamese twins such as Chan and Eng who worked for Barnum & Bailey, and deformed children, some born without legs, others without hands. One woman had an arm on one side, a leg on the other and was able to give birth to a normal child.

Any defect is nature's message to the adult to arrest the defective region's activity to preserve longevity: a retarded child must not be forced to study; a person with a strong claudication must not walk excessively; the deaf is not supposed to speak or hear, while the blind is not supposed to use his eyes. Strong defects of brain, limbs, voice, are nature's indication of the difficulty of creative activity, walking and speaking which are higher manifestations of life. It is also a warning for normal people not to abuse them.

Saving the lives of Siamese twins

In ancient Greece, to ensure perfect citizens for the state, imperfect children were hurled down a precipice. In the royal courts of France, Spain, dwarfs were kept as pets. Today Siamese twins are separated, endangering their lives. Siamese twins sharing a pair of legs and of kidneys should never be separated. They should be left alone to live out their lives. A single pair of kidneys serving two digestive systems cannot last long. These children should be cared for by their loving parents. Light foods can prolong their lives.

Once in China, my mother took me to a store, and as she was talking with the owner, we heard voices quarreling behind a curtain. Curious, I went over, lifted the curtain and saw two heads discussing violently. Quickly I let the curtain drop and returned to my mother. The Chinese accept things as they are; they realize that Siamese twins do not live long, so let them be. They can be separated if joined by muscle, ligaments, cartilage or bone. If separated, one child should be sacrificed to allow the other to live. Don't leave each child with one leg, hoping both will survive.

Do not induce labor

Sometimes a physician will induce labor if a woman's pregnancy extends beyond nine months. Do not allow induced labor. In Asia, many women have a 10-month pregnancy which is perfectly normal and preserves the fetus's life.

Dwarf uterus

Women with a dwarf uterus abandon hopes of gestation. One Italian woman with a dwarf uterus was advised by her physician to adopt an orange diet—for nine months she ate nothing but oranges. At the end she gave birth to a normal baby girl who is now a pianist.

Chapter 4
A peaceful childbirth leads to longevity

Since time immemorial man has tried to minimize labor pain yet in the year 2002, no method has helped to relieve a laboring woman's pains. Alleviating pains would prolong the lives of both mother and child.

Current means used to reduce labor pains

To reduce pain, some current methods used are mixtures of analgesic drugs, meperidine (Demerol) with a tranquilizer promethazine (Phenergen). These drugs sedate a patient, cause sleepiness and pass through the placenta to the baby, decreasing the unborn infant's breathing. During a Caesarian section, anesthesia is given. General anesthesia slows down the infant's respiration and heartbeat. At birth, the infant is asleep while the mother is *out* for an hour and is unable to see the baby till later.

A mother may be given Epidural blocks: at a numbed spot on the lower back, a needle is introduced in the middle of the spinal cord. By means of a needle, the anesthetic is injected into the spinal cord but not into the canal. With a plastic catheter left in place, at regular intervals or when needed, medication is injected into it. The danger is in lowering the mother's blood pressure while the baby suffers a reduced blood flow with trouble at delivery.

Tests performed on the infant at delivery

To find out how well the fetus will tolerate labor stress, a fetus may be tested for blood pH (acidity). For this test, a dilation of at least 2 cm. is required, and the mother's membranes must be ruptured. It is done as follows: to the baby's scalp an instrument is applied and in the skin a small nick is made. Baby's blood is collected in a small tube to check the pH. This test determines whether labor should be allowed to continue or if a C-section is required.

During labor, a baby's heart rate may be monitored at every contraction: a belt with a receiver is strapped on mother's abdomen, and to detect baby's heartbeat, a principle similar to ultrasound is used. By means of an electrode on baby's scalp, wires connect an internal monitor to a machine recording fetal heart rate. This test is feasible only if a mother's membranes are broken and the dilation 1 cm. The test is supposed to show how well baby tolerates labor contractions. A bad response is a sign of fetal distress.

Preparatory surgical means used on laboring mothers

Forceps delivery may be used, but this method has decreased and instead, a vacuum extractor used, with a similar effect, as follows: a plastic or metal cup is fitted onto baby's head by suction. At birth, the doctor pulls on the vacuum cup as hard as with forceps.

An episiotomy may be performed on the mother: at delivery an incision is made from vagina toward rectum. It is supposed to avoid undue tearing as baby's head passes through the birth canal. The depth of the incision varies: it may be cut through skin only; or through skin and underlying tissue; or through skin, underlying tissue and rectal sphincter; or through all previous tissues and rectal mucous membrane. After delivery, sutures are separately closed with absorbable sutures. This is a dreadful incision never to be performed: it may detrimentally affect both sexual intercourse and bowel movements.

Reduce pain naturally and hasten pelvic expansion at labor

Having given birth several times, we experienced little pain at labor. We instinctively held our legs up in the air or against the wall. The vertical position of legs is one of the most effective means to lessen labor pain, naturally forcing blood towards the abdomen. It is not a dignified position but forget dignity when it means less pain. Pain is due to a lack of blood as contractions increase in strength to separate pelvic bones and the coccyx turns upwards, enlarging the pelvic outlet for the infant's passage.

To increase blood volume, a laboring mother must drink water. Painful contractions destroy red blood cells and lessen total blood volume. Increasing blood volume reduces pain and hastens contractions. Most women must labor in rooms without circulating fresh air. Some women labor during two or three days without expanding enough for birthing, then a Caesarian section is necessary. For quick expansion, a room with circulating fresh air is most important regardless of season.

No hand insertions please!

A pregnant woman is subjected to a pelvic examination every few weeks. Regular pelvic examinations are not necessary. When our daughter was in labor, the midwife inserted her gloved hand every half hour: 6 or 7 times. She suffered trauma and returned home. Having never delivered a child, we were undaunted; we researched at the library and were ready for the delivery.

We delivered our grandson

On a hot August day, we opened the windows wide. After lining the bed with newspapers and towels, our daughter was left alone to expand. It was 2 AM. For scissors and to wash baby's eyes after birth, we prepared two portions of saline water. An hour later, our daughter felt ready to push. We examined her and saw the baby's hair and the perineum was 10 cm. long. We knew the baby was about to come and advised her to push at the next powerful contraction. At the next contraction she grabbed onto to the bed's mattress and pushed with all her might. The baby's head appeared and remained hanging for two minutes. It did not breathe nor move. We said it appeared blue and was perhaps dead. Indignant, our daughter said it couldn't be dead as it had been kicking so hard. We said we can do nothing just now, we must wait. Two minutes later she was assailed by another contraction. Gathering all her strength, she pushed and the baby's shoulders appeared. We pulled and the baby gently came out. A little boy uttered a small cry, like a cat's meow and urinated on our hands. We washed his eyes with salt water and held him close to his mother as we felt the umbilical cord. Now wrapped in a blanket, we held the baby for 20 minutes, always checking the umbilical cord for pulsation. Once the cord stopped pulsating, our daughter confirmed it, the cord was tied in two places and cut in between.

Everything went well. Our daughter's perineum was not torn at all and did not require stitching.

Do not turn an infant at childbirth

Having had occasion to view several deliveries on video, we were appalled by the overall lack of knowledge, despite the billions of deliveries performed all over the world. The usual procedure is to turn the infant at the first push, pulling the baby out by force, tearing the mother's perineum. This is a senseless procedure since the body automatically rids itself of a mass and contractions do happen even if one had to wait a few minutes longer. It is always feared that the infant is dead if it does not breathe immediately. Newborns are slapped repeatedly to induce breathing. No need to fear: at a distance of 5 cm. from the mother's body, the placenta is **still attached to the uterus and the infant continues to receive oxygen through the umbilical cord**. At a distance of 15 cm., the placenta detaches from the uterine wall, the baby receives no more oxygen from the mother and lungs begin to function, **indicated by the first cry as air gushes into baby's lungs**.

If a newborn's head hangs out without breathing, it is at a distance of 5 cm., and the placenta is still attached to the uterus: no breathing is required. At 15 cm. the placenta detaches from the uterus and the baby will breathe on its own naturally without being slapped!

Why pelvic insertions, perineum cutting are senseless procedures

It is futile to examine cervical expansion by inserting a gloved hand. Painful contractions are due to expansion of the pelvic basin as the two innominate bones separate at the symphysis pubis and the coccyx turns back and upward. As a result, the cervix expands from nickel size through 25-cent, 50-cent stages, etc. reflected externally at the vaginal opening: pea-size, 1 cm slit, 2 cm slit, 5 cm., and finally 10 cm. at which point the head becomes visible. Never insert a gloved hand into the laboring mother who is already undergoing so much pain. A gloved hand, though gently inserted at labor is comparable to a rape. Does a birthing mother need more trauma at this crucial time? An external examination of vaginal expansion is sufficient.

It is equally futile to cut the perineum. Circulating fresh air will allow a laboring mother to expand quickly. Contractions increase in strength when oxygen is rapidly delivered by red blood cells to muscles and bones. Without oxygen contractions will be slow in advancing. Every contraction slightly expands the opening of the pelvic basin and uterus, enlarging the outlet.

Before cutting the umbilical cord, wait, for the pulsating cord means that the portion of blood in the placenta belonging to the baby is flowing into his body. When the cord no longer pulsates, it can be safely cut as it serves no further purpose. We hope that an infant will no longer be turned at the first push. When the head appears, wait. Do not slap the baby, think about its distance from the placenta. The infant will now enter the world in a peaceful way.

Damaging effects of circumcision

Removal of the foreskin is akin to the practice of deflowering a maiden by breaking the hymen for fear of blood contamination. The foreskin is as important as one's nose, teeth, eye or limb and has the right to exist. Circumcision uncovers the glans and leads to excessive masturbation. It exposes the penis to all kinds of trauma—zipper injuries, burns, toilet seat syndrome and hair or thread injury. Circumcision diminishes the glans's sensitivity, and the bare tip becomes dry and hard from contact with external substances, causing its skin to turn prematurely old.

Circumcision is a cruel, savage and mutilating practice; it causes bleeding, phimosis (unretractable foreskin) from surgery, concealed penis, distortion of penis, ulcers of the glans and inflammation, stenosis of the urinary meatus, (narrowing of opening), infection in 8% of the babies. Uncircumcised boys never develop inflammation or closure of urinary meatus. No statistics are extant to prove infant mortality from circumcision but hours after circumcision, four cases of infant deaths have occurred. The English Medical Journal also reported cases of deaths. Hebrew ecclesiastics ban or delay a third infant's circumcision in the same family if two previous deaths have occurred from the operation. If circumcision were a life preserver, there should be no deaths from the operation. Surgery becomes a medical problem only after a child is circumcised immediately after birth because the blood coagulation is interfered with. Circumcision has caused more deaths than skin cancer.

Abolish circumcision and prolong men's lives

In the 1950s male infants were automatically circumcised immediately after birth. In the year 2001, mothers must pay the sum of $100-150 for the operation. Circumcision is still performed in the U.S.; in many countries the foreskin is left alone.

According to medical records, circumcision dates as far back as Neolithic times during the Stone age, about 6,000-8,000 years ago. The operation involves cutting the whole or part of the foreskin covering the glans penis. With the exception of the Indo-Germanic, Mongol and Finno-Ugrian peoples, the greater part of the world follow this custom. In ancient Egypt boys were circumcised between ages 6-12 years. Ethiopians, Jews and Muslims practiced it on newborn infants. In 4,000 B.C., it was established as a traditional rite in Egypt where the operation was done before or at puberty. In Arabia, circumcision was performed immediately prior to marriage.

Circumcision is a cruel practice — an age-old practice instituted when people were unable to bathe. When asked why people do not circumcise horses and other cattle, veterinarians replied it would be a horrible and senseless practice. Foreskin is a precious piece of skin — an erogenous tissue, with many greatly sensitive pressure Pacini corpuscles to cover and protect the glans penis. To better satisfy a woman, the foreskin adds bulk to the penis as it rubs the vaginal wall during coitus. Foreskin enables a man to better control ejaculation. Maimoinides (1135-1204) said that a Jewish woman who had intercourse with an uncircumcised man would not want to leave him.

A child's response to pain is acute and a surgeon's knife is traumatic leading to suicidal tendencies. One child was circumcised with long scissors at six years old, he was in such intense pain, his howls echoed throughout the house. Cases of circumcision performed on boys aged 4 and 6 resulted in destructive rages; they developed claustrophobia, played killing games, showed destructive behavior and occasional suicidal tendencies.

Removal of the foreskin was intended to prevent infection. The foreskin is tight over the penile tip for its protection, similar to the hymen protecting the vaginal opening. A tight foreskin is a temporary condition, usually corrected by the first erection. If it can be retracted and cleansed, the foreskin should not be removed. By retracting it once a day for cleansing purposes, by age 70 it would have been retracted 25,500 times, enough to loosen any tissue. Leave the foreskin alone, there is no reason or need to remove it.

Dr. Paolo Mantegazza, an authority on sex, said that the foreskin is an organ of pleasure, augmenting one's pleasure in the embrace of a woman and circumcision is a scourge, a shame, an infamy. In the name of humanity, it should be abolished and the surgeon who practices it without being justified should be considered guilty of malpractice and severely punished.

Circumcision can be equated with foot binding, which crippled half of China's population for 10 centuries. Feet are directly related to the internal organs of reproduction. Foot binding was invented to keep women home bound, unable to walk much or wander far from the house, and warp their internal sexual feelings and response. Out of fear, men imposed the practice of binding feet. Fear that women would be free. For ten centuries women suffered because of men's insecurities of being abandoned by a woman.

Circumcision has been practiced for 8,000 years. Men and boys who were not circumcised proved themselves stronger in every respect than those who underwent the operation. "If circumcision were proposed today for the first time," said J. Lewis, "it would be met with determined opposition whereas its purpose would be considered lunatic, fit for an insane asylum." Men are the law makers; they must demand the abolishment of this cruel practice and women must fight to make sure the foreskin on the penile tip of their infant boys is retained.

Statistics show that women live longer than men. It is difficult enough for a man to carry a mass in the groin—and a most delicate mass! Why weaken the area further? The penile tip is the most delicate part of a man's body. To protect it from injury, nature has provided a foreskin. Man must not go against nature to man's detriment. First try it out on animals then apply it to man. If it is not done on animals it should not be done on men. The foreskin is not a superfluous appendage or a nuisance to the organ's normal function. It is an important piece of skin to be treasured for a lifetime.

Today, 80% of women in Egypt are circumcised. Man's insecurity causes his madness to mistreat women and make laws to keep them cloistered and maimed. In Africa, the clitoris is circumcised—the pea-sized organ helping a woman to experience orgasm. Out of fear, men imposed on women clitoris circumcision. Fear that women would enjoy sex—reserved for men exclusively. At all cost—even death—young women were forced to have their orifice scarred with keloid scars! Without a clitoris a woman can experience the ecstasy of foreplay but rarely orgasm. Our lives are short, and our greatest pleasure and release is orgasm. A woman leads a lifetime of toil; she should enjoy some happiness. A woman's circumcision is equivalent to a man's penis being cut off. This practice must be abolished. All circumcision must be abolished!

Chapter 5
Form a beautiful baby and ensure longevity

Life can be prolonged by improving growth conditions during the first year of life. By the end of the first year, 75% of brain tissue are lain. A child learns to speak, walk, use hands for fine movements; teeth appear, the involuntary function of sleep, the digestion of solid foods are set. Depending on the first year's formation, a person can become autistic, bow-legged, have a cantankerous gait or be affected by seizures as in epilepsy, etc. Many children today are prematurely born or with low birth weight. Infants weighing less than 5 1/2 pounds are considered of low birth weight and placed in neonatal intensive care units (NICU). They lie in isolettes, only with a diaper, the body naked, with an intravenous feeding tube.

Diet of premature infants

If the infant's growth rate matches that of in utero, neonatologists believe that the diet for a premature infant is adequate. As a result, NICUs provide as many calories as possible without placing excess stress on a premature infant's immature organ-systems. Intravenous feeding, also called parenteral feeding, uses a solution of amino acids, glucose in the form of Polycose, a synthetic polymer made by linking a group of glucose molecules into one large molecule; vitamins, minerals, electrolytes and sometimes fats. Given through a peripheral vein, the solution has 25-30 different ingredients and is rarely modified. Babies are monitored to prevent high glucose levels and metabolic complications.

The best source of milk for a premature infant is not known. Some are given milk via a gavage tube inserted through the nose. Glucose water is first given, then diluted formula or breast milk, starting with small portions of 3-5 ml. every two hours. Term babies of low birth weight thrive on term milk but infants of low birth weight thrive best on pre-term milk.

Problems of intravenous feeding. This feeding method gives rise to numerous health problems that affect premature infants: respiratory distress syndrome caused by a lack of an entire group of fatty acids derived substances in the lungs called surfactant, chronic lung disease, broncho-pulmonary displasia, a chronic lung disease of varying duration and severity. Another common problem is apnea, where breathing is arrested for 15-20 seconds or shorter periods. Apnea affects infants who sleep lightly. Many factors affect breathing: tactile stimuli, temperature and mechanical irritation of bronchi's mucous membrane.

Necrotizing enterocolitis may also affect premature infants: a disease of the bowel wall. In the NICU at least one infant suffers from abdominal distension every day.

When the feeding volume is diminished or the formula changed, symptoms disappear. Premature infants may suffer from infection, a major problem in the NICU where 25% of infants develop meningitis. Jaundice is a common problem of the NICU where a baby's skin turns a yellowish orange color due to accumulation of bilirubin, a bile pigment formed by the breakdown of hemoglobin's products. To decompose bilirubin, intense blue light is shone on premature infants. Exposure to phototherapy is a dangerous treatment. To prevent infant jaundice, a pregnant mother should not work excessively. Work destroys red blood cells and excess dead cells produce much hemoglobin, forming much bile, developing jaundice in her newborn infant.

Intravenous feeding is known to produce jaundice. Jaundice usually resolves itself five or six days after birth, but when bile rises to high levels, the liver cannot excrete it fast enough. Some premature infants experience bleeding in the skull, hydrocephalus or water in the brain, or eye problems with a scarred retina—a condition due to administering oxygen. This practice must stop for strabismus or myopia may develop in later life. Intravenous feeding and oxygen administration are dangerous. Pregnant mothers should be careful to avoid having premature babies —a mother has no control over his food intake in NICU.

Empress Josephine brought Napoleon a basket with a little man about 17 inches high, dressed up like a hussar. At the sight of the tiny man, Napoleon was very much disturbed and told his wife to remove him.

People are informed of the danger of ultrasound on embryos. Powerful sound waves increase the embryo's heartbeat. Heart action is tied to brain action, an increased heartbeat causes erratic blood flow to the brain which directs the formation of all body parts and can cause premature birth; in later months ultrasound may cause spontaneous birth. Ultrasound may produce Siamese twins or other abnormalities. More Siamese twins are born now than ever before. Increased blood flow causes the fetus to increase movements with possible strangulation from umbilical cord wrapping around the neck. Ultrasound is used as a pest repellent. Lower organisms are very sensitive to powerful sound waves.

Improve a premature infant's growth

The infant must not be naked in an incubator. The bodies of newborn animals are covered by fur; therefore, infants must be warmly wrapped, clad in shirts, bonnets etc.; the environment around the body must imitate the warm environment of the womb, and they must breathe fresh air. In the summer, knitted silk shirts and pants should cover their bodies; wool clothing is a must for winter weather. They must lie on a warm mattress, preferably wool, to avoid an incubator. Only daylight should strike their eyes. At night, light up the room with several lamps of fabric over parchment shades with 25 Watt yellow bulbs.

Foundling baby cats and dogs are fed with a dropper. If premature infants were fed with a dropper, it would obtain sufficient food. When breast-milk is not available, fresh skim milk is the best, diluted with water. Intravenous feeding is unnecessary. Nothing external should penetrate the body except through the digestive tract: blood from the digestive system is first brought to the liver. Cleansed by liver cells, purified blood is returned via the hepatic vein to the inferior vena cava. Blood flows upward for a short distance, joins blood from the superior vena cava and returns to the left side of the heart; then it is oxygenated by the lungs before being pumped into the arteries. This is nature's means to prevent the liver's cleansed blood from irrigating the body immediately. This indicates to man that **nothing** external should ever penetrate the body unless it is first cleansed by liver cells.

Intravenous feeding introduces foreign matter directly into the bloodstream—a very dangerous practice with disastrous effects on the infant. Premature infants require very little fat and the amount contained in fresh skim milk is sufficient for their needs. It would promote deeper sleep and allow the tiny bodies to rapidly excrete the accumulated bilirubin. After several weeks on skim milk, preterm mother's milk should be given in exactly the same manner: with a dropper. Some freshly squeezed grape juice, diluted with three or four parts of water can also be given. This feeding method will improve a premature infant's formation.

A breast-feeding mother must follow a strict diet with very little carbohydrates. A mother bird regurgitates her food for her fledgling. Once a young girl, curious to know how many fledglings were present, shone a flashlight into a nest of finches. Immediately the mother bird abandoned her fledglings, refusing to feed them. All of them died. Humans do so many dangerous things to our infants. Intravenous feeding, gavage tube feeding, shining a blue light on premature infants, incubating naked infants, etc., besides tampering with the embryo in the womb. Leave a pregnant woman alone. For your precious infant, follow the rule: do not feed an infant anything that you yourself would not eat.

Our daughter breastfed her infant

Having raised our grandson together with our daughter, with excellent results, we would like to share our method with every mother.

Weighing 7 lbs. 11 oz. at birth, our grandson was breastfed from the first day for two years and nine months. The following are highlights of his development with the additional foods given during that period.

At one week, he drank fresh grape juice diluted with three parts of water. Orange juice was tried but removed when he developed pimples on the face.

The ninth day after birth, remnants of the umbilical cord fell off. He was sponge bathed; then he had his first bath.

At one month he drank more dilute juice than breast-milk.

At three months he liked a little mashed banana.

At four months he held his own little juice bottle.
At four and a half months he weighed 18 pounds.
At five months he sat up a few minutes.

Our daughter's diet consisted of some meat, vegetables, very little starchy foods and sugar. If she ate ice cream or chestnuts, her son would develop a rash.

At five months, he ate mashed chicken and eggplant Parmigiana or other freshly cooked, strained foods such as spareribs, string beans, half a teaspoon of blended roast pork, broccoli, water.

At 11 months he said "Mamma" and understood Italian and English. He ate regular milk with meats, vegetables, fruit mixtures and yogurt with milk.

At one year, he was very alert, lifted himself up, without being held, stood for 10 seconds. He waved to people and smiled to everyone.

At 13 months, he took 8 steps by himself.

At one year and three months, he weighed 26 lbs.

At 14 months, he could walk alone without help.

At 14 months, he brought his coat to his mother when he wanted to go out.

At one year and five months, he ate a piece of pear by himself.

At one year and six months, he began to wean himself. The first molar tooth and the 4 upper and 4 lower front teeth appeared.

At one year and seven months, he no longer liked grape juice but wanted orange juice instead.

At one year and eight months he ate with a fork by himself.

At two years and seven months he said many words like I'm happy, I'm tired, I like it. He weighed 46 lbs. People wanted to hold him but he was so heavy, they had to put him down.

At two years nine months our daughter discontinued breastfeeding.

At two years nine months his toilet training began.

At three years four months he was toilet trained.

At three years and 10 months, he was very independent. Very clean, he rarely wetted himself. He knew all the letters of the alphabet and told his mother to write them down to draw over them. He pronounced words correctly in Italian, English, French; he likes music, piano, guitar, colors and history. He slept like an angel.

We developed an infant feeding method

When our daughter was born in Switzerland, we used the Galactina method. The first step prescribed a concoction of cornstarch mixed with whole milk. This was our first experiment. The great scientist Claude Bernard said there is nothing wrong in experimenting to see what would happen provided no danger is involved. Few people would venture to experiment on their own infant. Since the first few days of the experiment were so successful, we decided to continue.

The first change or *experiment* used skim milk. Our baby fared very well, never cried except when hungry or wet. Her sleep was very deep, her body wiry and strong and such a happy baby. After a few weeks on skim milk and cornstarch soup, the next step in the Galactina method prescribed a cocktail of very fine cream of rice soup and whole milk. We made this change but continued with skim milk. Our baby showed such great progress that we decided to continue, and add diluted fresh fruit juices.

The last step in the Galactina method called for a change from cream of rice soup to a mixture of five cereals and whole milk. We made the change but used skim milk for a while, then at five or six months of age, we changed to whole milk and five cereals soup. Our daughter fared very well, but we noted that at a year's age she was small yet strong. She crawled for a year and a half, then suddenly she stood up and walked steadily. Her teeth grew slowly, appearing at seven-eight months of age.

After the first year, we gave her plain whole milk with a little sugar. Of her own free will our baby took milk from the bottle until nine years of age. If poured in a glass, milk was sipped with a spoon or straw. She had no crooked teeth and her occlusion is perfect. Her diet was always carefully under control, her growth, steady yet not rapid. At 12, she was about a head shorter than 12-year old children. Her nature is peaceful, her schoolwork always excellent. In her childhood, she had two or three mild infectious diseases with fever lasting two or three days. On a fresh juice diet the fever subsided quickly. Otherwise our baby was never sick and never received medication. When given a box of cookies she knew when to stop. If not hungry she would go without food the entire day.

When our second child was born, without a moment's hesitation skim milk was substituted for whole milk. We followed through with cream of rice soup but made a major change in the Galactina method: the cream of rice soup was used and the five-cereal soup omitted.

While our baby grew beautifully, we noticed a difference in size between the two babies, the second one was much larger and stronger in every respect, her sleep remained peaceful and deep. She was never sick. When the two children are compared, even today the difference in size is present.

With our last baby, we succeeded in developing the formula that can solve man's problems. Our son was supposed to use one of the many prescribed formulas. Since no special cornstarch for babies in this country existed, we decided to use ordinary cornstarch for cooking purposes; the quality is not inferior to the kind used for babies in Switzerland. Two level tablespoonfuls of cornstarch in a quart of water; boil the mixture, then simmer until it becomes a smooth colloidal mixture. Store in a glass jar in the refrigerator. When a new bottle is prepared, some cornstarch soup is added to the proper amount of skim milk for the age. At three months of age, whole milk was substituted for skim milk, the cornstarch soup remained unchanged. The effect of this formula on our baby's growth was overwhelming; he slept uninterrupted; upon awakening, stretched and tightened his body, like a flower before blooming.

The cornstarch soup was used until well past the first year. This baby has shown us the intuitive powers of the human brain. He ate meat cut up in tiny strips. Until the age of five, he avoided children's swings but leaned on an adult swing and gently swung himself. Instinctively, he plugged his ears to protect them from the deafening noise of subway trains. He wears long-sleeved polo shirts and long pants in any weather. He is very friendly and lovable yet when irritated, his temper flared. He was never sick in his childhood.

Pictures of the children are in our third book.

Convinced that we have discovered a great formula for the formation of babies to benefit mankind, we obtained patents for U.S. and Canada. Though the cornstarch soup is easily prepared at home, it may be bottled or canned for the housewife's convenience. But nothing is better than a freshly home-prepared product.

In **The Brave New World**, Aldous Huxley said that some day babies will be formed perfectly, using a new kind of formula. It is now possible to do so. It will raise the mental and physical level of mankind while bringing about peace and love on the earth. Many mothers' milk cannot compare with this formula because mother's milk contains too much fat.

Once mankind's physical and mental levels are raised, we will solve the problems of misery, poverty, ignorance, illness, prejudice, war, crime and juvenile delinquency. Only a perfect race of mankind will think about improving laws and living conditions for all. There is hope for mankind, but only with a mother's inspired guidance with the right formula.

Extreme care must be given to the rearing of boys; they are weaker, their sex organs are located outside of the body. It is a man's world and men's laws depend on women's execution. A man cannot replace a mother, and children brought up by men are often disturbed or have dark instincts. To be normal, children must live with their mother or with both parents.

Perfect babies smell like perfume, their cry is a musical delight. Today's women breed children who make you sick with their whining, complaining, screaming, a result of improper nutrition. Women can now form healthy beautiful babies they can love and want to stay home to rear them.

Breasts

Breasts are made up of a mass of cells, forming alveoli drained by a branching system of ducts. Much fatty tissue covers the mass of glands, and connective tissue partitions separate masses of mammary tissue. Externally, of a darker pigmented skin, the areola surrounds the nipple of a yet darker pigmented skin whose pore is through which milk leaves the breasts when a baby sucks.

When a mother stops to breastfeed, squeeze the remaining milk from breasts. Stale milk in mammary tissues may cause tumor formation. Check the breasts often to make sure no lump is present. If a lump or pain appears, rub immediately. In three days a lump or painful sign will disappear. When abnormal signs appear, rub for two minutes several times daily to prevent tumors/growths to form or remain; to prevent breast tumors, do not wear brassieres: they bind the body and impede circulation to breasts. Breasts are extremities similar to hands and feet, and blood circulation is difficult to reach these areas.

For successful breastfeeding, a woman must relax and the best position is to lie down, leaning the head back, ensuring a large surge of milk to breasts. To form a very strong child a nutritious diet is essential.

Milk formation: Immediately after birth, the anterior lobe of the pituitary gland automatically liberates into the bloodstream a hormone, *prolactin*, which stimulates the mammary glands to form milk.

Things to watch out for in a newborn infant

To ensure perfect formation of a newborn infant, watch the consistency of his stools. Liquid stools means that the formula is too concentrated, and baby has difficulty digesting it; his growth will not proceed well. An infant's stools must be light brown and pasty which will assure a healthy growth. Change the formula immediately and use the method we have developed, or breastfeed, and add fresh grape juice made as follows:

Fill a blender half full with grapes and blend till very fine. Sieve with a fine plastic sieve and store in a jar. Let it stand till all pulp is at bottom of jar. Dilute half an ounce of juice with water to fill a bottle. Feed as often as desired. Breastfeed baby making sure mother's diet has very little fat and starches. At about three months of age, change to dilute fresh orange juice. An infant formed in this fashion will be perfect.

A baby must have fresh air and sunshine. After the first month at home, dress him warmly in a down overall, cover him well and take him for a walk in the stroller. Let the sun shine on his skin. This is very important otherwise his bones will not grow strong. The first weeks of life are crucial. A newborn infant must sleep deeply 19-20 hours daily. At three months you will see if he is perfect by the round shape of the forehead a tiny mouth, and a perfect nose; his cry must stir every fiber of your being. His body must be beautiful. You will have achieved perfection. Now learn to cook for a perfect body for the rest of 18 formative years. A perfect infant must be beautiful and intelligent, peaceful, kind, and ambidextrous in most common actions, and have unusual physical strength; he functions like a clock in sleep, elimination, appetite, sex, etc.

Eradicate autism and epilepsy by improving the feeding method during the first year of life

In 1932, Dr. Leo Kanner first described autism as a disorder of affective contact. Autistic children cannot develop relationships, speak with difficulty and are unable to communicate. The physical appearance seem normal; change caused distress; otherwise the IQ did not differ from normal children.

All attempts to understand autism have failed; research on autistic children provide us some data. In a controlled group, 80% of autistic children had prenatal complications, low birth weight, bleeding, toxemia, neonatal convulsions, failure to initiate respiration, a need for oxygen, etc., 8% were mild to profound mentally deficient. Cerebral palsy affected half of the group, convulsive disorders affected 75% of them. Among 50 children examined in five years, five died. At 18 months of age, three quarters had lost their autistic behavior. Seven were affected by grand mal seizures. Children who develop autism in later life are weak, have feeding difficulty, refuse food, vomit, experience diarrhea, colic, etc. They have difficulty falling asleep, awaken in terror, or experience long periods of wakefulness.

In the U. S. it has been estimated that about 2,500,000 people have speech disorders. At 12-15 months of age most children begin to say words, and a child is not retarded unless he has passed 24 months without being able to speak. Normally, a child begins to speak at 12-15 months, thus speech is developed during the first year. Therefore, autism and speech problems are due to poor development during the first year. Some infants have difficulty sleeping, and remain awake for long hours because most are given ready-made formulas containing chemicals. These formulae may agree with children born healthy and strong but can be detrimental to infants of low birth weight. Breastfeeding is the solution but many mothers are reluctant, preferring an infant formula. The above-mentioned formula we developed should solve the problem.

Understand epilepsy

Children also develop epilepsy. Epilepsy is described in detail in our 11th book. Characterized by two types of seizures, namely *grand Mal* and *petit Mal*, epilepsy is due to poor automatic function of the sympathetic nervous ganglia, not the brain or parasympathetic ganglia. <u>Proof</u>: seizures occur anywhere, they are not voluntarily controlled. During a seizure, the patient falls to the ground. All voluntary movement ceases: the brain no longer directs blood flow to muscles and bones; foam drools from the mouth; it means that the parasympathetic ganglia are not supplying blood to the digestive organs. The body is in a tight tetanus convulsion, the entire blood flow is suddenly directed to the regulatory organs.

The patient's eyes roll upwards, simulating sleep. After a seizure, the patient is very sleepy and doesn't recall anything about it.

The automatic function of the sympathetic nervous ganglia, or the sleep mechanism, is set during the first year of life when an infant sleeps almost continuously. A discrepancy in the sleep pattern of newborn infants stirs the possibility of eventual epileptic attacks in the adult. Epileptic attacks reflect a poor automatic control of the sleep mechanism by sympathetic nervous ganglia. Sympathetic ganglia direct blood flow to regulatory organs. The earlier an infant loses sleep, the stronger the seizures and the sooner epilepsy will develop. The importance of deep sleep in a newborn infant cannot be stressed enough. Undisturbed sleep is particularly important in the beginning months of life. Many infants remain awake for long hours after birth. Use a more natural infant formula as many infants are not sleeping enough needed for optimum growth.

Help for autistic and epileptic children

A light diet is essential. After a meal, the body must feel light, not logy. The Asian diet is such that after a meal one doesn't feel stuffed. Asian delicacies are the light foods that should be given to autistic and epileptic children. Buy delicacies such as Dim Sun, etc. from Chinese restaurants. Some recipes at the end of this book can also help these afflicted children. Light foods should be always be given. Increase the liquid intake to stir several stool evacuations daily, and the condition should improve.

How to prevent birthmarks

Small birthmarks are inconsequential. Large birthmarks may be due to infrequent bowel elimination during the gestation period. A mass in the abdomen reduces the space intended for the growing fetus and if the child's body touches the uterine linings, a birthmark will form. During gestation, keep regular daily bowel movements to allow space for the growing fetus. Liquids and wet foods help regularity.

Chapter 6
Form a beautiful child during 20 years and ensure a long life

During a child's growth years, 25% of the remaining brain tissues are formed. This parallels the development of long bones, muscles, regulatory organs, sex organs, reproductive organs, etc. During the 20 years' formation, tissues' cellular growth in size is set for a lifetime. A perfect growth prevents illnesses in adulthood. So many factors affect a child's growth that a mother's greater awareness in the growth may be inspired by the following.

When should a child begin to walk
Young parents often hold their toddler in the upright position, forcing him to walk. Never force a baby to walk—his bones are too weak to carry his body weight and he will become bow-legged. We allowed total freedom. Our eldest crawled for a year and a half and walked upright at 19 months. Our second and third walked at a year. Let a baby crawl as long as he wishes.

Babies held in the upright position will cause them to drool. When a baby drools, lay him down. Drooling means that baby's foods are not digesting well. The upright position forces blood to muscles and bones, preventing optimum flow to digestive organs indicating the difficulty of the upright position for humans. Babies often yawn; stop all movement. Yawning means he is consciously bringing blood to his regulatory organs. Let him yawn. Avoid loud speaking in the presence of a small infant. Avoid loud radios, TV, machines. Let birds chirp around a baby.

Should we expose baby to direct sunlight?
Mothers do not put their infants in the sun because of its *detrimental* effects; they turn the carriage to hide the infant from the sun's rays. The sun is life to all living creatures, it is only detrimental if we lie on the beach and allow our skin *to roast* in the sun. We grew an avocado plant in our kitchen where no sunlight penetrates. The plant grew like a stick with big, ugly long and thin leaves. Our daughter grew an avocado plant in her kitchen where it was exposed to two hours of afternoon sunshine daily. It is a healthy, beautiful little plant with broad, oval shaped, deeply colored leaves spread out in a circle.

Like plants, humans require direct sunlight. When our children were small, we went to the park to expose their bodies to the sunshine at least two hours daily; a little bonnet prevented overheating.

Humans need vitamin D for the growth of long bones. Synthetic vitamin D added to milk is not comparable to the vitamin D produced by sunlight. Skin contains cholesterol and when exposed to the sun, vitamin D is naturally formed as sunlight acts upon skin's sterol. Vitamin D promotes the absorption of calcium in the intestines, forming a constant quantity of lime salts in blood, excreting excess calcium through feces. Hydrochloric acid and vitamin D enhance calcium absorption from intestinal food. Calcium absorption is hindered by excess fats and phosphates, oatmeal and certain cereals.

In big cities such as New York, few take advantage of the sun; most apartments receive little or no sunshine. Sun is essential for all vital functions. Children not exposed to the sun during growth years will shun the sun in adulthood. Habits are formed during our youth.

Mothers must try to keep their children clean; some mothers do not cleanse children properly. Children sometimes smell of urine and some even have lice. Some adolescents trail a strong stench. Many people do not know how to cleanse their bodies. Cleansing only needs hot water and soap.

A child's skin should be very clean

Skin is the only externally visible regulatory organ with a large surface; in a newborn, it covers an area of about 2,500 square centimeters, in an adult, 18,000 square centimeters. Skin eliminates poisons from the body and when kidneys fail, perspiration removes body poisons through the skin's surface.

Daily Bath

A bath is preferable to a shower where water beats on the skin's surface with possible damage to the innumerable sense organs important for the sex act. Soap the skin's surface and lightly scratch all over with fingertips. Do it carefully. Do it twice. Soap again. Use a rough natural sponge (not synthetic kitchen/bathroom sponges). Try scrubbing gently with a plastic scouring pad like Pot-Brite or with a small hard body brush. Check for cleanliness by using fingers to rub for dirt. If skin is not squeaky clean and dirt rubs off, soap again—redo procedure five or six times until squeaky clean. This bathing removes all dirt and maintains skin's pores open to breathe. Skin must breathe, if not, one will soon die. Daily bathing is imperative for a lifetime. Hair must also be washed; shampoo twice and scratch, rinse. Don't enter a bathtub full of hot water. Hand test water and enter a half full bathtub and let the water slowly fill tub to keep water very warm. Do not remain longer than half an hour, or until thoroughly cleansed.

Grooming a child's hair

Hair protects. Mankind has hair only in delicate regions of the body: groin, armpits, head. Brain tissue is very delicate. Hair is nature's way of protecting our delicate brain by providing maximum warmth.

For centuries men and women have allowed hair to grow long on the head.

Napoleon didn't have the patience to braid his long hair and created the short hairstyle for later centuries. After his hair was cut, Napoleon became very fat and towards the end of his life he was so fat, his leg muscles rolled over his ankles, as recorded by a young woman who visited him at St. Helena. Since then, the whole world has followed Napoleon's style.

Barbers are quick to cut hair off even though hair is precious. Actor Yul Brynner popularized the bald hair style because he was bald. A shaven head is hardly beautiful, aside from its danger to health.

Should boys and men wear long or short hair?

Keep hair long to the nape of neck as in Renaissance Italy where men were handsome with the pageboy hairstyle. The temperature differs when your hand passes through long hair. A few tenths of a degree higher than room temperature raises breathing rate, hastens digestion and elimination. Young men wear a cap; why wear a cap when hair can preserve your health? Nature provides so well.

In Europe, during the 17th century, men wore long wigs for warmth. Voltaire and Louis XIV lived long lives; perhaps we should wear wigs to protect the brain.

Girls should wear their hair long.

Do not tie little girls' hair in long, tight braids. Leave hair loose and fluffy, regardless whether it is kinky, wavy or straight. A recent article in the Reader's Digest suggests to leave hair alone: do not tie, dye, curl, cut hair too short, even if gray. Hair is important; it increases normal brain metabolism and may prevent brain tumors later in life. Today many have brain tumors. Children are highstrung and nervous when hair is tied up tightly—Stop!

Clothing for health

Synthetic fabrics developed by man are cheap. But people do not realize the danger of clothing made with such fabrics. Synthetic materials do not allow the skin to breathe. Synthetic fabrics are produced by the polymerization of simple compounds derived from coal, air, water, petroleum and limestone. They do not absorb water and collect electrostatic charge such that the fabric clings to the wearer, attracting dust and lint. In cold, dry weather, natural fiber prevents static electricity build-up. Artificial fiber stirs extreme nervousness with a destructive desire. Avoid artificial fibers in clothing, shoes or coverings. Curtains made of synthetic fabric prevent air from penetrating the apartment.

Wear clothes for good health

With the exception of hands and face, do not expose naked parts of the body to air; when exposed, body temperature rapidly falls; water evaporates from bare skin, dehydrating the body. Use leggings, socks or long thigh-high stockings under pants or dresses. Wear loose clothing for health, not binding. Dresses are better than pants and skirts. Belts and neckties constrict important articulations. Brassieres and girdles impede circulation and may contribute to the formation of tumors.

Modern style for boys and men is uninteresting. Men should have attractive, colorful clothing. Designers should examine the ancient Greeks, Chinese, Arabs, etc., who created long robes for men. During the Renaissance, young men adorned themselves elaborately and attractively. Attractive clothes will give boys something to think about. Our clothing habits during our adolescence remains with us for life: a poorly dressed child will be poorly dressed in adulthood.

In 80° F. weather, wear silk. In autumn and winter, wear knitted wool material next to the skin. Wear cotton undergarments. Wool and fur should be worn in winter or when chilly. A cotton hat under a wool hat increases breathing rate. Wear leather or cloth shoes. Avoid clogs or sling back shoes where heels are exposed. Back of shoes sustain body weight. Keep feet warm. Dress warmly in cold weather for long walks in cold air. Insufficiently clad is when one needs to go indoors immediately.

Footgear for growing children

Scientific data indicate that for the same distance covered, twice as much energy is used when walking on a heeled shoe than in flat shoes; at the same time one will eat more and in time, become obese. In the United States more and more people are obese. A city of skyscrapers makes life very difficult. Towering buildings stir speed in action and incessant activity. Buy comfortable shoes for children. They will walk slower, expend less energy and eat less. Obesity is also caused by hormones added to foods.

When buying shoes, feet must spread out so that toes can wiggle. In ancient Rome, only sandals were worn. In the Florence of Lorenzo dei Medici, shoes were completely flat, tips pointing upwards. Shoe designers must create beautiful, flat shoes, with wide soles so that the body automatically rests at each step. It would help solve obesity. Avoid sneakers: they are running shoes, not walking shoes. Notice how fast one walks in them. Buy them for running marathons.

Care of teeth

Children's baby teeth will be replaced by permanent teeth. Avoid filling cavities in baby teeth. Dental students need to work on human teeth, and children's deciduous teeth are an excellent experimental source. Students should practice on dogs or cat's teeth, not on precious children.

A very thin layer of enamel covers the exposed crown of a tooth. To fill a cavity, the tooth must be drilled through the enamel to expose the tooth's dentine. To prevent further decay a metallic amalgam is placed over the hole. A cavity requires no filling for in the pulp chamber's lining, resting odontoblasts (bone cells) become active when decay sets in, **producing another layer of secondary dentine**. This dentine is not as strong as the first dentine, but it is a protective mechanism to counteract losses from advancing decay or wear. In about three days, the sour feeling from the cavity will disappear, indicating that new tissue has been formed.

Because enamel is very thin, avoid using electric brushes or any machine to clean the teeth's surface. Though enamel is hard, with time it will erode. The normal color of teeth is off-white. Avoid exposure of teeth to X-rays. If X-rays are dangerous to body parts, X-rays are dangerous to teeth—teeth are living tissue. Animals keep their teeth during a lifetime whereas man needs so much work done on teeth? We should be able to preserve our teeth for a lifetime. One Italian woman never went to the dentist all her life. At 70, she still has all her teeth; they are not as strong as before but she is still able to use them.

Daily care of teeth. Use a good hard brush (not electric or bent brushes). Brush with a massaging motion between teeth and gums. Use a good toothpaste morning and night. In the evening, massage between teeth with a rubber tip once daily, in and out between teeth. After eating, remove food particles with toothpicks. Avoid flossing for gradually teeth will loosen with pulling the thread out.

To preserve teeth for a lifetime. Teeth are bathed in body fluid of a warm temperature. Notice how we intake hot food. An indication that all foods eaten should be ingested warm which should prevent a tooth's nerve from dying.

What to do when a nerve is dying: A dying tooth has a gnawing pain when hot or cold food is chewed. Do not worry. Tighten up the jaws into a tight GRRR whenever gnawing pain assails a tooth. You will be able to save it for some time longer.

Immediate action to take upon loss of teeth: Teeth may be knocked out by a blow or in a car accident. Do not panic. Pick them up, rinse them in water and immediately replace them in gums before the recess is forever closed. Soon blood vessels and nerves will find their original attachments and teeth will function as before. Never allow knocked-out-teeth to remain exposed to air longer than half an hour: 30 minutes of exposure kills all live tissues.

To remove tartar from roots of teeth

Pyorrhea is treated by a dental surgeon. With the right instrument, adults can safely remove tartar from their children's teeth. One woman was taught to remove tartar with an instrument; she does it now for her husband and daughter. She finds it a great way to save both teeth and purse. Buy a double-headed, half-moon shaped scaler from any dental supply store for about $20. Healthco # U-10-35.

To find out if you have pyorrhea, feel your gums, if it itches, there is tartar—time to remove it. Insert the scaler between gum and tooth and scrape sandy deposit gently. A little blood will appear, which is perfectly normal; use a tissue to dab the blood. After removal of tartar normal circulation will be restored and gums will no longer itch. Do not let itch develop into pain when tartar removal will be more difficult, but still possible. After one treatment, brush teeth gently for a few days — gum tissues are tender. If you fear using an instrument, visit a dental surgeon. A few sessions with a dental surgeon can teach you to do it on your own.

Remove ear wax from the ear canal

A more serious problem is wax accumulation in the ear canal. In western countries, wax is allowed to accumulate until the mass becomes hard and large as a marble or fruit pit. A physician will then flush or vacuum it out. Why do ears eliminate so much wax? We believe that the ear canal is a receptacle for wastes from brain tissues, its innumerable cells, cerebrospinal fluid and ventricles. This must be true for in the embryonic state, ears are out-pocketings of the brain. The neck separates body from head. So many important structures pass through the neck, the latter cannot rapidly dispose of the brain's wastes. Brain cells cannot function normally without a rapid outlet for wastes; the only outlet is through the ears — these wastes should be removed almost every day.

In China, when a man goes to have a shave and/or a haircut, he also gets his ears cleaned with an ear-picker; children are trained to remove wax from ears with an ear-picker, from the time they are able to sit still. With the light shining into the ear, a parent proceeds to remove the accumulated wax. Because it is a surgical process, it is important to train when still a child.

If one has never inserted anything into the ear, one needs training. Of course, it is easier to clean ears with a Q-tip. Ear-drops can also help. They may be purchased from drugstores over the counter. Visit a Chinese doctor, he can show you how to do it carefully; after a few sessions you can do it yourself. In children, the tympanum (eardrum) is closer to the surface, so do not insert the ear-picker too far in. Another alternative is to have the wax removed by an ear-nose-throat doctor who vacuums it out.

After learning to remove ear wax, insert some vaseline, beeswax or coconut oil in the ear, overnight. Some moisturizing cream for extra dry skin is also excellent. The next day, dip the ear-picker in hot water and remove earwax or use a Q-tip. In China, this custom is handed down from generation to generation. We believe it can prevent the formation of a tumor in brain tissue. Recently, a woman removed a piece of earwax as large as an apricot pit from her husband's ear. Despite the removal, he died of a brain tumor at 48. Daily earwax removal allows free circulation of blood in the brain. When ear wax is not removed, circulation is hindered, stirring the formation of abnormal brain tissue.

Ear-pickers cost $2.00 in Chinatown gift shops. They come in bone, wood, metal. Silverstone metal earpicks, 3 inches long, are best. For a rough edge, scrape the spoon tip gently on rough stone. The Chinese use earpicks daily.

Care of the navel
A circular depression at about the middle of the abdomen, the navel marks the point where blood vessels from the umbilical cord, entered the fetus's body. The three blood vessels are two arteries and one vein. The vein carries oxygenated blood from placenta to embryo, some of it passes to the fetus's liver, most flows to inferior vena cava of embryo and empties into the right auricle. During a lifetime, the navel is not completely closed and must be kept very clean. After a bath, use a Q-tip, scrape out the deposited waxy substance. A wood ear-picker is good for a more complete cleansing. If not cleansed, the accumulated dirt will cause itch then pain and end in convulsions.

Serious infectious diseases
Growing children may suffer from infectious conditions. Tonsils and adenoids are removed due to inflammation. Tonsils and adenoids guard the entrance to the larynx and naso-pharynx respectively. Lymphoid glands are sentinels at the entrance to the breathing apparatus. Lymphoid tissue is the home and factory of lymphocytes, the large white blood cells that proliferate and become active in times of infection. Lymphocytes fight off bacteria that have penetrated the body by engulfing and digesting them. If lymphoid tissue is inflamed, modify the diet immediately.

Inflammation of tonsils and adenoids
Adopt a starch-free, fat-free diet immediately. Children usually eat more starchy foods: candy bars, chocolate, ice-cream, potato chips, corn pops, cereals, etc. Children grow up with cereals. Reduce carbohydrates during growth years and infections will subside quickly or never occur.

Some bacterial infections are: mumps, measles, meningitis, rubella, manifest similar external indices: a rash and fever; at the first occurrence, modify a child's diet immediately: the illness will subside in a short time. When our children were small, at the first sign of fever, they were placed on a juice diet and in a few days fever and rash disappeared.

To remove pus from acne pustules
Teenagers troubled by acne with pustules on scalp, face, chest and back. These are due to a disproportion between the capacity of skin's sebacious glands' to secrete and their ducts' transport capacity. Whiteheads and blackheads appear on the face, chest and scalp; they are due to insufficient disposal of excess fat secretion. Pustules are due to fibrous foods. Avoid eating fats, starches, sugars, cereals, breads, rice, beans, whole grains, sausages and cured meats. Mix foods

to prevent eating large quantities of one food. Keloid scars from acne occurs because youngsters are not taught to remove pustules. Never touch a painful pimple; wait until it comes to a head, itches and is soft to the touch, then squeeze until deep red blood appears, and a white root is squeezed out—this method will not leave scars. If a root is not removed, it is still there. If a painful pustule is broken, do not panic. Keep it open. Squeeze it daily until no more pain is felt, then squeeze strongly at the end, until all pus and root are removed and deep blood appears. No keloid will form. Acne affects boys more than girls. Heavy sports cause acne as exercise pours extra carbohydrates into the bloodstream. Abstain from excess physical exertion and the condition will subside.

Do not play around with skin: Youngsters today poke holes in various regions of the body: tongue, ears, face; tattooing skin. One time a young woman with pierced ears soon developed two tumors; they were surgically removed. When ill and circulation slows down, tumors can develop in areas in contact with foreign matter.

Adorning with jewelry. Young people wear jewelry. Metal bracelets move around skin warming them constantly. Bangles cause loss of body heat, bring on colds, and cause masculinity. A young girl wore several bracelets on both arms all the time. She developed a moustache. Warned about the damaging effects of bracelets, she stopped wearing them. Jewelry can be worn but wear bracelets that mold the wrist like a watchband. Wood and leather bangles are better than cold metal, jade or other stones. Rings and necklaces are fine.

Prepare a child for immunization shots

Children must be immunized against infectious diseases; several shots are given gradually. Beware of shots. After an immunization shot a little girl fainted. Precautions should be followed carefully.

1. Shots should be given only in summer mornings after a good night's sleep. After deep sleep, heart, lungs and kidneys, skin, are well irrigated during eight hours of sleep and an injection would not harm a child.
2. Drink some juice and do not eat solid food. It helps maintain regulatory organs in a state of optimum irrigation, maintain blood volume and prevent a sudden depletion of blood after an injection.
3. Inject in a seated position. When seated or reclined, 50% of body weight is relaxed, more blood becomes available to regulatory organs, therefore, safeguarding a child's life.

Blood rushes to the injection site while depleting regulatory organs. A Chinese woman wished to visit her daughter at the hospital but was refused access to the room unless she received a certain injection. She agreed. Upon injection, she died. Another young man of 21 was given an injection after dinner. He immediately turned blue. With massage, he regained normal coloration.

We believe if children were perfectly formed immunization shots should never be required. Shots penetrate the body directly—a dangerous practice. A better alternative would be to administer orally.

Work for a growing child

A child attending school must not work. A child uses his large head eight hours a day; much blood is deviated during these hours, depleting blood from regulatory organs. Working for material gain would deplete regulatory organs further and prevent proper regulation and growth at night. Excess work can stunt growth and even cause a nervous depression.

A young Dominican aged 28 never had his wisdom teeth. Since the age of 18 he had worked as a plasterer, sometimes painter. Especially dangerous is physical work requiring the use of 50% of body weight. At night, sleep can only replace the energy lost from physical work; it cannot allow for growth, which explains why the young man never grew wisdom teeth. After school, children should take music or dance lessons to improve their general performance.

Choose foods for better growth and improve adult formation

Having examined many cookbooks and health books, we noticed that among the immense array, there is no definite scientific guideline for people to select foods. It is important to know what to eat and what to avoid. Some foods are high in carbohydrates, others are heavy in inorganic ingredients protein, calcium, potassium and fat.

Digestion is a process of putrefaction, or rotting. We may state that foods that rot faster when exposed to air are more beneficial than foods that take a long time to rot. Prepared breads, cookies, cakes, are in this category. Fresh meat, pudding, home cooked foods, soups, etc. are superior. Fresh milk is better than Parmelat.

Melting is another useful criterion. An item melting rapidly at room temperature is superior to a product that does not melt quickly i.e., American cheese versus Muenster cheese. When foods turn brown when exposed to air, the faster they will digest and leave the body, preventing over-absorption in small intestine.

Because sphincters are present along every section of the digestive tract, food exits in small bits. Foods cut up finely lessen absorption and prevent obesity. They leave the digestive tract faster than food in large pieces. Though foods are chewed, there is a difference in people's chewing capacity; different people require different numbers of chews for the same meal and the same foods.

Select foods according to the theory of evolution

The theory of evolution can guide us to maintain our own development, man being the highest in the scale. We know that grubs, worms, mushrooms, ferns, algae are lowly organisms, in the animal and vegetable kingdoms. Fruits or fruit-like vegetables are high as opposed to leaves, stems and roots. Thus organisms high in the evolutionary scale are superior to organisms with lower traits. Shoots, stems, leaves, mushrooms, roots are inferior to fruits, fruit-like vegetables, flowers, grains, seeds, nuts. Meats, fowl, fish are superior to grubs or worms. In the same species such as fish, lowly traits are small size, lack of scales, digestive system on the side. Among lower cold-blooded organisms, the lack of bilateral symmetry, vertebral column, are lower traits. A larger organism is superior to tiny organisms.

Choose foods according to determinism

Claude Bernard mentioned repeatedly that determinism must exist in the biological sciences, as in the inorganic science. The same principles govern both sciences and manifestations of properties are tied to environmental conditions of temperature and humidity, best seen in lower animals. "We should be able to arrive at this law ruling living organisms," said Bernard, and what is needed is an idea, a function of the time and place we live in.

We remember how we were inspired to prove determinism in the organic kingdom. We were studying Chopin's Etude in A flat major when we suddenly stopped playing and loudly enounced the following hypothesis: *"Animals feeding on food placed high in the scale of evolution are fast-moving. Animals that feed on food low in the scale of evolution are slow-moving animals."* According to Claude Bernard, one admits the absolute principle by a hypothesis, a workable theory to be modified after submission to nature. *"One must always doubt oneself,"* said Bernard, as well as one's interpretations until one arrives at a law with the greatest number of facts to support its proof.

Audubon's Birds of America finally convinced us to search for determinism among living organisms of a large size, feeding only on one type of food. In our 6th book we have provided the data indicating that large organisms whose food habits comprise lowly organisms are slow-moving animals, large organisms feeding on meat and fish are fast-moving animals.

This law of determinism is especially important for man in case of illness or in old age. The principle of determinism should open up new fields in biology, such as a reclassification of Carl Linnaeus' System where much random placement of living organisms is extant.

Vegetable oils are indigestible

In 1972, Dr. Roy Shepard mentioned in his book **Alive Man**, that vegetable oils produce a kind of waxy ceroid undissolvable by man's body enzymes. Animal fat is more readily dissolved. Two steps are required in the digestion of vegetable oils: first, they must be converted to animal fat, then dissolved by body enzymes, thus more difficult to dispose of. Fats affect voice quality. Both men and women of a previous generation had beautiful singing voices, attributable to the use of lard and butter for cooking purposes. Today, there is no voice like that of Enrico Caruso.

In magazines, on television, notice the limpness of women's hair. This was not the case in a previous generation and may be due to the use of vegetables oils: corn, olive, palm, coconut, etc. For cooking purposes the best fats are: lard, chicken, duck, goose, bacon fat. Do not use lamb or beef fat. They are too concentrated.

Some criteria to observe in cooking

Cooking methods can cause obesity or maintain slenderness. Overcooked foods will cause a child to consume a double portion and never feel he has eaten sufficiently; this causes obesity. Recently the news announced that the odor of a carcass emanated from someone's apartment; it was someone's cooking: a fine example of foul smelling cooking! Some people are incapable of cooking. One woman said she never cooked because she didn't know how. Follow two rules and you will never overcook again: cook slightly beyond the point of smell: the aroma must not reach the hallway or outdoors. Do not allow vegetables to change color. Do not let food cook by itself for a long time; simmer when food is hard. To soften foods, cook it stirring constantly and gradually add a little water. Fire is a killer, and to maintain health and for maximum benefit, use it sparingly in cooking.

Seafood and fish requires very little cooking time. When fish is flaky it is overcooked. Unless frying a whole fish over high heat, cook skinned fish and seafood over low heat until a knife penetrates it easily. Remove from heat right away. Use raw cut up seafood if mixing with other cooked foods. Light browning of mixture is enough to cook the added seafood.

Chapter 7
Preserve the skeletal system to ensure a long life

We do not realize how destructive the modern way of living is: noise of zooming subways, radios, rumbling cars, trucks, buses, etc. We talk, walk, run, etc.—there is no end to the activities.

The way actions are performed affects the function of the regulatory organs. Blood links all parts of the body together. Activity in a region lessens blood flow in another region, particularly the regulatory organs—the body's **engine**. We advise on how to perform daily activities to preserve regulatory organs for longevity.

Walk healthfully

Upon awakening, walking is our first action. Some people walk fast, others take their time. Walk slowly. Watch a turtle walk. Turtles live a long life. Fast walking tears the legs' tiny blood vessels. Slow walking preserves them, maintains metabolism in legs and prolongs life. Skyscraper cities compel constant activity, forcing us to walk fast. To combat this destructive tendency, wear the most comfortable, flat shoes to relax at each step to preserve energy, eat less and live longer.

Sneakers should be worn for running. Sneakers stir fast walking, they rush your steps to the grave. Narrow soles are unhealthy. A sole must be as wide as the picture drawn around the standing foot on paper. The American Indian mocassin is healthful. Today India, Australia, Canada and Brazil make good shoes and boots. Buy a size larger than the usual size; you can relax at each step. This applies especially to shearling-lined boots. Walking uses 50% of body weight; much energy is spent by a rapid gait. According to **Healthy People 2000**, physically active people outlive the inactive. Light to moderate is better than vigorous physical activity. Recently, TV announced that walking is the best physical exercise to help reduce heart problems.

Running and/or jogging

Running is strenuous physical exertion. The heart bounces in the process. In the chest cavity, the sac enveloping the heart is in a very stable position, nature's means to prevent bouncing movements. In nature, animals never run except when pursued or to catch a prey. In running, body weight is lifted against gravity, involving a large part of body weight. At 25 miles per hour, sprinters require brisk reaction time, explosive strength. Abnormalities were heart beats of up to 170-180 beats per minute, breathlessness and high blood pressure. At high temperatures of 23° C. marathon runners had rectal temperatures of 41° C. Athletes have died of heat stroke. Watch out for high rectal temperatures of 40° C. or 104° F. Rising temperature may cause dehydration, diminished sweat secretion and blood flow to skin, with cerebral irritability, hallucinations, coma, irreversible cerebral damage and injured kidneys. If you have to jog, jog for short periods.

Skate, ski, climb and swim

Skating is related to running but more energy is expended. Downhill skiing accumulates large quantities of lactate. At slalom events, for one minute of skiing supra-maximal pulse rates were reported. However, cross-country skiing on flat ground contributes to longevity.

In climbing, there is poor equilibrium as the body leans forward. Vertical force is the greatest effort: always climb slowly. Climbing is good exercise but climb slowly. One woman who lived on a 5th floor walk-up developed breathing difficulty and heart trouble. Some experienced considerable weight gain from running up and down five flights of steps several times daily. To prevent tiredness when climbing, lock up knees at each step; climb slowly.

Swimming requires arm exercise to resist water viscosity, causing a drag. In racing, crawl is the best swimming stroke. Sudden speeding up and slowing down uses more energy. At one knot per hour maximum effort is expended. Never swim or dive alone for fear of drowning.

Calisthenics and bicycling

Gymnastics improve physical condition. In calisthenics, pulse rate rises from 90-100 or more per minute. Persons past middle age should not indulge in vigorous calisthenics; practice Tai Chi or Chinese shadow boxing. Depending on weight, exercising on a bicycle ergometer is postural work. When covering a distance of 33 km. on a bicycle, at 20 km. per hour, a force of 1.8-3.6 kilograms is exerted. Bicycling is an energy-consuming exercise. Cycle for fun at moderate speed. See Table I at the end of this chapter. The table represents the energy expended for different activities.

The table does not indicate the caloric expenditure for creative activity. Perhaps because the person is seated. There is a difference between being comfortably seated and being seated and working with hands and brain. Active hands and brain represent creative activity, requiring the use of the basketball-sized brain and hands. Much blood is expended in creative work: compose music, write a book, knit, sew, crochet, make jewelry, weave rugs, etc. Composer Gioacchino Rossini said he suffered all the illnesses affecting a woman who gave birth many times; he composed 40 operas until age 40, after which he never composed another opera but wrote delightful orchestral music. He reclined in bed to compose. Gaetano Donizetti composed 75 operas. A caricature depicts him writing a comic opera with the right hand, a tragic opera with the left, indicating the rapidity with which he composed. Mozart composed more music than any other composer in this world.

The western world incites one to constant activity. Towering structures are disturbing; three-storied houses in lanes are peaceful. Man can relax and enjoy life instead of working himself to death. The greater a man relaxes, the longer he can live—easily to 150 years.

Why is creative work tiresome

An active organ is in a state of constant contraction. In creative work, brain and hands are active, and muscles and bones are contracted when one stays in a seated position. These organs represent a large body of organs. Contraction uses up red blood cells, depleting regulatory organs and digestive organs—being constantly active. In time insomnia will set in, and indigestion with constipation. Tumors will develop, trouble with heart, kidney, endocrine glands, to end in paralysis, stroke, even death.

To live a long life, reduce creative activities. To minimize detrimental effects of creativity, assume better positions: lean the head back, support feet on a footrest, arms on armrests; recline in bed like Rossini. Work in silence. Often it is difficult or impossible to relax: painters paint in a standing position. Michelangelo painted the ceiling of the Sistine Chapel horizontally. Few painters were handsome. To retain beauty reduce all creative activity.

Dangers of vigorous exercise

Strenuous physical exertion produces much lactic acid, pouring extra carbohydrates into the bloodstream. The impetus for mental work is lost. Blood pressure rises; vigorous exercise precipitates a heart attack. appetite is lost. In strenuous exertion red blood cells are destroyed, inhibiting urine secretion.

A maximum contraction of 70-80% completely prevents blood flow to muscles. Long-lasting contractions affect muscles. Blood thickens, becomes viscous, hastening the clotting process. Viscous blood stiffens muscles. In weight lifting, muscle weight increases but joints lose flexibility. In continuous treadmill-pedalling pulse increases to 140 per minute. In vigorous leg activity, muscles may tear. In rapid breathing, chest and lungs become rigid as work is done against the viscous forces of chest and lungs.

Fatigue is first felt by heart and lungs. Remote parts feel some prostration with pain in arms. Appetite is lost when stomach, intestines and brain are affected. Exhaustion stirs sadness, depression, loss of visual acuity and hearing. Skin receives less blood flow. Exercise dilates blood vessels, precipitating a heart attack. Athletic training enlarges the heart. Normally heart size is 11 milliliter per kilogram body weight. An athlete's heart size may be 14 ml. per kg. body-weight. Increased blood flow causes turbulence and heart murmur. Maximum effort results in breathlessness. A young man's breathing rate increases with effort, reaching 35-45 breaths per minute, 300-400% greater than at rest. From a normal respiratory volume of 4 liters per minute, it reaches 90-120 liters per minute in maximum exercise. In 30 minutes of intense rhythmic effort, blood pressure rises substantially. Vigorous exercise precipitates a heart attack. When blood cannot be expelled from heart, heart ventricles may show irregular writhing contractions, possibly fatal, causing a heart attack. Excess exercise causes violent fever similar to typhoid fever. In marathon running, body temperature may rise to 41° C. with great sensitivity to cold. A marathon runner's face turns ashen. Blood clotting speeds up, precipitating weakened physical states: typhoid fever, colds and tuberculosis. In patients suffering from Addison's disease, diabetes, neurasthenia and bile disease, the least effort caused disastrous manifestations of fatigue. Exercise worsens a pre-existing infection. Vigorous ventilating may activate a quiescent tubercular lesion. The adrenal medulla's secretions are exhausted. The white blood-cell production increases. Liver function and intestinal absorption are depressed, and stomach contents empty at a slower rate. If exercising under unfavorable climactic conditions, sweating could reach two liters per hour.

Take care when exercising: Do not exercise at 104° F. body temperature for fear of overheating. Do not wear synthetic material, it prevents sweat from evaporating, stifling the body, and can cause heat collapse. If an overall sensation of general fatigue and weakness is felt, slow down and stop prolonged activity.

The above indicates that strenuous exercise is not beneficial to the human body, moderate exercise is preferable and five minutes per day is sufficient exertion. Vigorous exercise has no positive effect on general health.

Why exercise with force?

While some people exercise violently, others are sedentary. In North America, the average person eats 50% more food than a primitive tribesman: twice as much protein, four times more fat, large amounts of sugar. Some coronary patients consume 300-400 lbs. of sugar per year and are addicted to coffee and tea. From a low intake of 5 lbs of sugar per year in 1770, modern western man has increased it to 25 lbs per year in 1870, reaching a climax of 120 lbs. per person yearly in 1970.

All prepared foods contain polyunsaturated fat. We have mentioned the danger of this type of fat. Remove it from the diet. Reduce the use of sugar, cream, all fats. People indulge in starches as scientific texts indicate that muscular energy is due to the burning of glycogen/carbohydrates, yet blood contains less than a tenth of a percent of carbohydrates and glycogen can be formed from proteins, starches or fats. Snacks contain more starches. Is the craving for physical exertion an instinctive need to rid the body of excessive starches, sugars and fats? Blood normally contains 7% protein, 0.1% carbohydrates, 1% minerals and 92% water. Excess starch and sugar cause aging, stir bad temper, violence with murderous instincts. The daily excess intake of carbohydrates and proteins is detrimental to the body, causing erratic behavior.

Every body action represents work: pumping air into chest, pumping blood around body, carrying materials across cell membranes against a concentration gradient, breaking down of tissue protein and synthesis. Energy is required to grow new tissue in adults and growing children.

A man normally has a caloric intake of 3,200 kcal., women 2,300 kcal. In competitive cycling, an athlete requires the consumption of 6,000-12,000 kcal per day. With less exertion fewer calories are needed. The ordinary city dweller is inactive. His daily activities boil down to a short walk or climbing a few stairs, shopping, housework. Except during sex or emotional excitement pulse rate rarely reaches 110 per minute. Whether athletic or sedentary, to obtain the required amount of proteins, a well-balanced diet is required.

Dilute foods containing little carbohydrates and protein will preserve a constant state of health and prevent the craving for bursts of energy in violent sports. Observe animals: they seldom show signs of aging and never perform strenuous feats unless stirred by self-defense or hunger. Aside from exercise, a body assumes different positions.

Preserve energy when seated

In the seated position, stroke volume is 80 ml. per beat, considerably less when reclined. In the seated position, energy is preserved because a portion of the musculature is relaxed. Chairs must have a backrest, high enough to lean the head when desired. Chairs with armrests relax arms. Be comfortably seated otherwise the desired rest is not achieved. A chair is only good when one feels at ease when seated. Raising the feet on a footrest preserves yet more energy. When the head leans, notice how stomach muscles immediately relax. At work, counteract fatigue by leaning back occasionally.

The detrimental effects of constant standing

In a quadruped, stress is concentrated on front legs. Man, in the upright position, stress is concentrated on feet that support the entire body. In the standing position, circulation to head and neck is at a low pressure. Negative pressure in neck veins causes vessels to collapse. When standing, blood is pooled in legs, reducing stroke volume through the heart. When the brain receives less blood, changing posture suddenly becomes difficult and one may faint. Do not be alarmed. Purse your lips and tighten up the entire body, breathe deeply and strength will be regained.

When standing, 9% more energy is used than when lying down. Blood shifts to lower limbs when position is changed from horizontal to vertical. When working in a standing position, lock the knees and less energy will be expended. Good posture minimizes static work. Bad postures are indicated by a protruding abdomen, round shoulders, poke chin, head thrust forward. On a hot day, with prolonged standing, limbs swell, and it is easier to faint; equilibrium is unstable in a standing position.

Feet are the body's mechanical support bases. At 120 lbs., feet provide full support when standing on a solid base of good shoes, wider than the foot with soles one centimeter thick. As a weight-sustaining structure, heels require full contact with the ground. The heel's principal support is the first metatarsal bone. Body weight must fall on the first metatarsal of both feet. High heels concentrate body weight on metatarsals 2 and 3. Pressure on metatarsal 2 causes burning or sharp local pain with formation of skin calluses.

Each foot supports half of body weight. At 120 lbs., each foot supports 60 lbs., each heel, 30 lbs., 10 lbs. on metatarsal 1, 5 lbs. by each of other metatarsals. High heels shorten calf muscles, throw the body off balance, causing sway back, tilting the uterus, and developing a paunch. The upright position is a sign of evolution. Treasure your higher development and walk with flat shoes. Man's upright position was made possible by perfect blood properties. Not everyone has perfect homeostasis or is entirely bipedal. The upright position is a very trying position, not to be abused.

How to carry weights

Carry weight close to the body. Rest an armful of groceries on the hip, it will be less weighty. Lift weights slowly and deliberately. Young men age 16-18 should not lift weights heavier than 20 lbs., girls, 15 lbs. Weightlifting for physical fitness raises pressure and adversely affects the heart. In weight lifting, the breath is sometimes held—a dangerous practice for a weak heart. Injuries affect about 1.5% of weightlifters. Some accidents occur affecting the back, shoulder and fingers also hernia and sudden death.

Physical fitness

If vital parameters show a smaller displacement from resting values, one is deemed physically fit. This shows physical endurance. A good overall formation withstands wear and tear. Some vital parameters are slow pulse rate at rest and at sub-maximum effort, rapid recovery of pulse after exercise, greater vital capacity, increase in heart volume as cardiac muscle mass increases in size and a greater number of blood capillaries in muscles.

To retain physical fitness some exercise is needed. At home or at work, machines take over many duties, forcing inactivity causing man to lead a sedentary life. Families own one or two cars but rarely ride a bicycle or walk. Man's daily activities last 1-60 minutes and only a small amount of calorie expenditure is necessary. To increase heart and breathing rates, exercise with adequate intensity: use a dry mop and dust the apartment, avoid using the loud vacuum cleaner. Alternate sweeping, dry-mopping, wet-mopping and dusting every other day; walk a mile a daily. These activities increase heart rate, deepen breathing and are sufficient exercise.

Teenagers should not practice excess violent sports which may cause disproportionate growth. One hour of continued effort stirs excess secretion of pituitary gland's anterior lobe with peak output at growth. Competitive sports exert psychological and social pressures on young people. Avoid them. A better exercise is social dancing. Join a dance club. Meet people, dance and exercise at the same time! It has been recorded that by a peculiar movement of muscles called body shivering, the female python can raise her body temperature. Bali dancers are beautiful: the movements are short, body muscle tightening. Imitate Balinese dance movements to increase body temperature—tightening is similar to shivering.

Plan daily exercise. Women: use a 5-lb. weight, bend the body down to the toes, twist yourself to the right, to the left, make counterclockwise movements with one arm, then with the other. With a weight in the hand walk backward. Do a few hard boxing punches in the air. Physical activity is excellent to increase depth of breathing without expending energy.

Gymnastics teachers often punish students with a dangerous practice of 20 push-ups at a time. Muscles and bones are 50% of man's body weight; push-ups forcibly drive blood through muscles, depleting regulatory organs of an optimum blood supply. School children use their basketball-sized head eight hours daily. By driving blood through muscles and bones during study hours can cause a heart attack. Some young people have died after strenuous exercise.

A sleeping limb

When a position is held for a length of time, a tingling sensation is felt, preventing the use of the limb. Do as you feel: do not walk, stand, move or use the limb. Remain still and wait till numbness disappears, reestablishing circulation. Forcing the use of a sleeping limb may cause its permanent impotence.

Table 1
The expenditure of energy in calories per hour

Rest and light work .... **cal/hr**
Sleeping 70
Lying quietly 80
Standing at ease, Conversation 110
Personal toilet 110
Singing 120
Manual labor
Farming chores 230
Road repair 300
Stacking lumber 350
Masonry 380
Chop wood 405
Pick and shovel 400
Planting, hoeing, raking 280
Hazing, plowing 400
House-painting 210
Carpenter 230
Moderate work/Sports
Strolling, Driving a car, Play violin 140
Acting on stage, Housekeeping 150
Kitchen Work 200
Wash clothes 190
Pitching horseshoes 240
Baseball 280
Rowing for pleasure 300
Calisthenics 300
Bicycling 300
Dancing moderate 250
Vigorous 340
Hiking 350
Continuous swimming 500
Mountain climbing 500
Long distance running 900
Sprinting 1,400

(Source: Morton & Fuller, **Human Locomotion and Body Form**, Williams & Wilkins, 1952, p. 187.)

CHAPTER 8
The use of vocal activities to ensure a long life

Man performs visible muscular activity, and muscular action audible to the world. How the latter are performed may shorten or lengthen life.

In New York City people have a tendency to speak continuously: radio announcers, TV shows. Speech is a higher manifestation of life: only humans can speak—it should not be abused. If lower animals emit sounds constantly, they would soon die: a constantly barking dog cannot live long. Lower animals lack certain essential parts of speech production. Without sinuses snakes hiss; giraffes have vocal cords but no sinuses; sheep have sinuses but no vocal cords. Animals can only communicate with their own kind. Man is the only species able to speak and sing.

Aristotle said that the heart has its share of work in tone production and vocal cords, brain and heart are interconnected. Speech in man is due to optimum blood flow to brain. People who suffer a stroke are often speechless. To produce sound from the throat, optimum blood volume is indispensable. The 10th and 11th cranial nerves convey sensibility to larynx and trachea, vocal cords and heart respectively. Man speaks because his brain wills blood flow to muscles activating vocal cords. A lack of blood flow to the brain prevents the power to speak. Voice is a very delicate mechanism.

Our voice box

A valve guards the entrance to the trachea; the larynx is the voice box. During breathing, air, after leaving the nasal passage, passes through the trachea whose upper end expands into the larynx. Three pairs of large and three pairs of smaller pieces of cartilage bound together by ligaments form the larynx. At the top, the ligaments attach the larynx to the hyoid bone, the skull's lowest part. The larynx is in a sturdy, immovable position.

In the center of the larynx, lined by folds of mucous membrane, a slit allows air to pass through. Of fibrous elastic tissue, the edges of the chink are the vocal cords attached, in front, to the laryngeal wall, behind, to a pair of small cartilages activated by laryngeal muscles. In its mucous membrane, many mucus-producing glands and hairs drive foreign substances away from larynx. The larynx or voice box is the main speech apparatus, functioning with the diaphragm's help. The diaphragm is responsible for 60% of the air breathed in. Aside from larynx and diaphragm, the head is the seat of sound. It is the most perfect, ideal machine ever conceived for tone production, and sounds are produced by passing breath through the head. Sound is not music and there is a difference between music and noise. Other important structures for voice production are the cheekbone's nasal and maxillary sinuses, acting as resonators. Continued speaking ability is ensured by good health, optimum blood volume and deep sleep.

The larynx when speaking
When silent and breathing regularly 18-20 breaths per minute, vocal cords lie against the voice box's wall and the laryngeal slit is wide open. As soon as a word is uttered, activated by muscles, the two tiny pieces of cartilage tied to vocal cords are swung together. Sound is produced when vocal cords vibrate as air passes from lungs through trachea into larynx.

When different vowels are pronounced in speech, the mouth cavity changes shape as mouth and tongue continuously move. When expired air is interrupted in various parts of the vocal pathway, consonants form. In loud speech, vocal cords vibrate with greater breath pressure, made possible by combined efforts of nervous system on breathing muscles and voice apparatus. In continuous speech it is impossible to breathe. When speaking or singing, one breathes through the mouth. To breathe through the nose, one must always stop speaking first. This rule is applicable to any action done with the mouth: whistling, blowing a musical instrument, humming, swallowing. Breathing is impossible when the mouth is active, so beware. During speech regulatory organs are depleted of an optimum oxygen supply.

Speech is the great distinguishing characteristic of humanity. No other sound is as beautiful as a singing voice or a well-modulated delightful, mellow speaking voice: it has great persuasive charm. It multiplies neurons in the brain, develops mental faculties, communication, perception, everything a mind can conceive of and it projects feeling, body and soul. Voice is the measure of a person's mental capacity, alertness or incapacity, and physical well-being or illness. It can warn, persuade, attract, repel, excite or flatter, beg or command. A resonant speaking voice is a voice of gold, promising a good life. A beautiful speaking voice is conducive to longevity, wealth and good fortune. A poor speaking voice belongs to a poor person. Surely a muddled brain would produce an unintelligible pronunciation and voice.

Effect of the spoken language on longevity
Depending on the spoken language, one can remain youthful or age quickly. A young woman during gestation, spoke French to her husband, German to her mother-in-law. She was exhausted; her baby was prematurely born and didn't survive, an indication that language and speech can be exhausting.

People using pictorial languages, Korean, Japanese, Chinese, and Arabic, being monosyllabic, require much lip movement. Of the languages spoken today, English may be the easiest. French is beautiful, most sounds use the tip of the tongue. Its refinement is transferred through generations and French babies are born with a special look found in no other peoples of the world.

Countries with pictorial choppy monosyllabic languages should adopt a romance language. Pictorial languages should be reserved for scholars to maintain a country's tradition and culture. In the beginning of Christendom, Egyptians adopted the alphabetical languages. In most African countries today, children are taught French, English, German and their native tongue. Guttural and spitting sounds similar to expectoration stir meanness and cruelty.

Detect illness by the voice's sound

A brilliant voice indicates excellent health while a dull voice, emitted with effort is a sign of illness. A metallic speaking-voice indicates poorly regulated physical and chemical properties of blood, with possible impending illness. Loss of voice indicates poor blood flow to the brain, a need of complete rest.

Work using voice forcefully is a danger to life

Extensive vocal activity such as acting—also exposed to extreme danger and fear, is a threat to life. In the Pink Panther, sudden fright continuously assailed actor Peter Sellers. Sellers died a sudden death. Acting in TV series is often dangerous. Both Elizabeth Montgomery and Michael Landon died young. Limit your acting work, retire when you are tired, and allow other young people to take your place. Life is not forever, give yourself time to enjoy the fruits of your labor. Children are given the opportunity to make ads on TV, to speak in shows, to act. This can be dangerous, together with schoolwork, it can hinder growth. When obliged to act, do not speak rapidly. Some musicians choose wind instruments, with a career in an orchestra. The same principle underlies the playing of wind or wood instruments: when breathing to produce sound, one cannot also breathe for the regulatory organs: all blood being concentrated to produce sound on the instrument.

Besides speaking, voice is used to sing. The singing voice carries unspeakable love, passion or peace to the soul. It can rouse from extreme sadness to happiness. Singing cures melancholy and terminal states. After Princess Pignatelli's husband died, she was in a state of stupor; when her condition did not improve, her family asked the famous castrato Farinelli to sing in the garden. When the princess heard his beautiful voice, she cried for three days and was cured of her condition. When very ill, harmonious music with a calming effect, is more restorative than jazz and discords.

Singing

Singing is tone correctly placed and undisturbed by physical effort and muscular contraction. Sound is produced when breath passes through vocal cords. Vowel sounds can be sung with exact pitch and precise and definite value in length. It is impossible to sing on a consonant. Before passing out through the nose, air must travel some distance in the nose to reach nasal sinuses behind turbinate bones.

To sing and control breath, skill and training are required. Women and children's shorter vocal cords enable a high pitch. Men's longer vocal cords produce a deeper voice. In singing, only about five or six breaths per minute are inhaled. Voice is the result of muscular and air activities. In loud singing, vocal cords vibrate with energy and the diaphragm exerts greater pressure. Lungs work passively but lung volume changes are brought about by changes in chest cavity's capacity, made possible by the combined action of diaphragm and muscles between ribs. Excessive singing is similar to physical exercise and causes lassitude, depression, lessened appetite and sluggish vital functions. Several principal singers should sing at each operatic performance. Why not four different Violettas, one for each act in Verdi's La Traviata, in one evening?

If you want longevity, do not embrace the singing profession. Control yourself and refrain from speaking or using the mouth. Once one has learned to remove earwax one will be able to remain silent the entire day.

Laughter and its effects

Sense organs feel the pleasurable stimulus but laughing depends on brain activity. Conducive to health, a happy and joyous mood releases nervous tension, however, overpowering happiness can be destructive. Once a young girl died on her wedding day, overcome with joy, her heart burst. Great excitement accelerates heart rate, constricts small blood vessels, increasing arterial blood pressure.

Strong emotion causes changes in blood pressure, heart rate, induces sweating and concentrates some hormones. In great excitement, heart, lungs, brain, skeletal muscles are over-abundantly supplied by blood taken from lesser organs. Adrenalin pours into the bloodstream, blood clots faster, which explains the young woman's death on her wedding day. Sudden explosive bouts of laughter can cure illnesses. Affected by an abscess in his throat, a cardinal burst out in irresistible laughter on seeing his pet monkey don his miter; the abscess broke, pus poured out and the cardinal regained his health. Sudden laughter stops sneezing. Hiccups can bring down high fever. In France, sanatoriums present comic plays to alleviate sufferings of the mentally ill. Late night TV shows induce laughter. Man is the only animal able to laugh, beginning from the 20th week of life.

The danger of crying

The first inspiration causes a baby's first cry. Later, various situations induce crying. Similar to laughing, crying is an uncontrollable, involuntary physical eruption almost always caused by sadness. One of the sense organs causes crying: eyes or ears. Once stricken by sadness, the brain and later the entire body will be affected. Beginning with a wail, tears stream from the eyes, corners of mouth turn downwards, the brow furrows, the body is gripped by incessant sobbing, sighing, whimpering: the whole world seems dark and gloomy. An overpowering sadness causes oppression and lassitude. A person dissolves in tears as consciousness is drowned by emotions. Every inspiration is a sob. Weeping is warm with emotion and bound by feelings. The loss of a loved one causes great sadness, bringing on weeping: we capitulate before grief, yearning and despair. Deep feelings well up tears, stir intense grief and crying without respite. Intense sadness brings on terminal states or temporary loss of the mind as in shock.

Fear, grief, and strong emotion first strike the sense organs. The message is brought to the brain and as long as emotion lasts, blood will be driven through the brain, depleting other regions of the body. Regulatory and digestive functions come to a standstill. Deep emotion and weakening are coupled together and shock develops into flaccidity of muscle as lips begin to tremble, setting in a feeling of estrangement and isolation. Great sorrow causes intense weeping. In such a state, resistance to disease lessens, blood cell types change, growth rate changes, specific diseases such as asthma, stomach ulcer, worsen. Glandular secretion of pituitary gland increases and excessive adrenalin production hastens blood clotting. For longevity, live a calm, quiet life and avoid excitement.

Do not weep excessively at the loss of a loved one for soon your turn will arrive. Creative work such as music or art can counteract the loss and turn sadness into gain. It is better not to live too closely to family members for sooner or later someone will die. Living farther away will cause less sadness and save your life. One young woman cried her heart out after her mother passed. She became terminally ill and was placed on disability. Actress Romy Schneider cried so much after the death of her son impaled on a pike that she soon died. Had she been properly advised not to weep, she would not have deprived her other child, of a mother.

Humming, whistling

Humming is similar to singing. Its effect on breathing is similar for when humming, breathing stops. Whistling: the louder the whistle, the greater the energy expended, a proof that silence is gold.

The thymus: gland of muscles and bones

Until recently, the function of the thymus gland has been a mystery. The gland is closely associated with the muscular system. Every organ-system has its own particular gland. The thymus is the particular gland of the skeletal muscular system. Thymectomy on experimental animals indicated atrophy of lymphatic system, poor resistance to infections and before death, signs of endocrine glands' exhaustion.

Thymectomy on animals gave rise to asthenia (deficient vitality, loss of strength), disabled gait, anorexia (loss of appetite), diarrhea with coarse and dirty fur. Thymectomized frogs, mice, tadpoles and guinea pigs develop a wasting syndrome, weak, fragile bones and atrophied skeletal muscles. Lymph nodes shrink, lesions in heart muscle are indicated, etc. Thymectomy should never be performed on humans.

In most living organisms species the thymus is the first lymphoid organ to develop; as fetal age advances more lymph cells are progressively formed. Total body X-irradiation inhibits immune competence in thymectomized rats. This is applicable to humans and defective prenatal development is related to cases of myasthenia gravis and ataxia. Paralysis of muscles with abnormality of histological elements or tumor growths in thymus are manifested in myasthenia gravis. Patients with cerebellar ataxia have tiny thymuses. Under stress, blood will produce an increased amount of corticosteroids, causing thymus to involute—an occurrence in almost every serious illness. The ingestion of steroids causes lymphatic tissue to involute. Many living organisms form steroids from lipid materials of cells, natural substances connected with many processes of life. Sex hormones, adrenal cortical hormones contain steroids. Cholesterol is a precursor in the biosynthesis of steroids. Avoid fats of any kind as all fats form cholesterol.

The thymus is the master gland of the neuromuscular system.

Location and structure of thymus

Extending from the 4th costal cartilage upward, as high as the lower edge of the thyroid gland, the thymus gland lies behind upper part of breastbone. Partly situated in the superior mediastinum, partly in the neck and covered by the sternum, it sits on the pericardium.

Of two lobes of differing sizes, sometimes united, forming a single mass, the thymus attains its full size by the end of the second year of life and at birth, weighs about 12 grams or 1/2 oz., reaching maximum size of about 37 grams or 1 1/3 ounce at puberty. It begins to decrease in size at puberty, weighing only 6 grams or 1/2 ounce at about 60-70 years of age.

In infection, poisoning or when fasting, the thymus gland involutes faster. Patients with myasthenia gravis or ataxia show abnormal histological elements in the thymus.

About 2 inches long, 1 1/2 inch wide, 3 lines thick, the thymus is pinkish gray in color, soft and lobulated on its surface. A thin layer of connective tissue penetrates the gland's interior, forming walls which branch and fuse, dividing the gland into numerous interconnecting lobules of .05-2 mm. in diameter.

Structured like a lymphatic organ, microscopically it has a large number of lymph follicles, each with an outer cortex and an inner medulla. Both regions have cells of two types: lymphocytes embedded in a meshwork of slender branching cells, more numerous in cortex where branching cells are coarser. Also present are concentrically arranged Hassall's bodies surrounding a mass of granular cells.

Chapter 9
The three important nerve centers

Muscles and bones do not function alone. Controlled by the brain, blood flow to muscles and bones is guided by the nervous system. Blood does not automatically flow to tissues.

Living organisms must have a heart of some kind before a brain of any kind can be developed. The gradual formation of a tube-like heart in earthworms to a two-chambered heart in fishes, through the three-chambered heart in frogs, to reach the four-chambered mammalian heart with perfect separation of arterial from venous blood, reached the final complex brain development.

The three separate divisions of nerve centers gave rise to speech, abstract thought, upright posture, internal fertilization and formation of an infant, sexual powers to be aroused at will, internal skeleton, etc. The above indicates we must have a better understanding of the brain, sympathetic, parasympathetic ganglia and of human behavior.

The brain's external appearance and between arachnoid and pia

The brain resembles the kernel of a giant walnut. A lengthwise fissure divides it into two equal halves. Both hemispheres are the seat of man's highest functions: memory, intelligence, moral sense, sight, hearing, smell, taste, body sensations. For protection, a thick membrane, the dura mater, wraps around the brain. Adhering to the skull, this membrane's internal surface is smooth. To protect different parts of the brain, the dura sends four processes into the skull's cavity. Under the dura, the arachnoid membrane dips deeply into fissure between hemispheres. The third innermost membrane, the pia mater dips deeply into every fissure of the cerebral cortex.

Between arachnoid and pia lies cerebrospinal fluid under a water pressure of 90 mm. in the lying position, zero when standing. When coughing, sneezing, blowing the nose, straining at stools, lifting weight, cerebrospinal fluid rises. Cerebrospinal fluid fills the four ventricles, enlarged spaces in brain tissues. Fluid provides buoyancy to both brain and spinal cord.

The brain: its internal appearance and fissures on the brain's surface

In the brain's substance nerve cell bodies form the outer layer of gray matter; nerve cell fibers make up the inner layer of white matter. Fibers ascend or descend from cells into the spinal cord. Fibers may also arise from cells within hemispheres, connecting both sides of brain.

The brain's gray matter covers an area of 2,200 square centimeters or 2 1/2 square feet. Besides nerve fibers, supporting cells and blood vessels, the cerebral cortex contains cell bodies of around 14 billion nerve cells.

From the brain's hemispheres, fibers lead to the midbrain, pons, medulla obblongata and cerebellum, extending into the spinal cord. In the brain, descending fibers cross over at a certain point so that one side of the brain controls all voluntary movement of other side of body and vice-versa.

The surface of the giant hemispheres has many fissures. The fissure of Rolando is the most important, transversely dividing the brain into equal halves. The area surrounding this fissure represents motor and sensory areas for voluntary movements, mapped out into more than 200 areas. To best visualize this control, picture yourself a cut through the fissure of Rolando down one hemisphere, much like a slice of cake. From upper border through lateral surface, the brain controls toes, ankle, knee, hip, trunk, shoulder, elbow, wrist, hand and face. The motor region lies in front of Rolando's fissure, behind lies the sensory region.

Very large cortical surfaces control complicated movements of hands, smaller areas control limited movements of feet. Particularly thick is the area's gray matter, around 3.5-4.5 mm., containing the giant pyramidal cells of Betz whose cell bodies may reach a height of 60-120 microns. These cells transmit impulses for all voluntary movements from cortex to spinal cord's lower motor nerve cells. One hemisphere is larger than the other; left-handed people have a larger right hemisphere and vice-versa. Areas in front of the fissure of Rolando, on its side and behind it exert a controlling influence on the motor.

The temporal region interprets sound, the occipital region, sight. etc. Damage to ascending or descending nerve fibers or to cell bodies causes extensive damage to conducting pathways with erratic movements. Beneath the pons, nerve fibers cross and begin to assume the spinal cord's outer position.

<u>Brain growth</u>: By the first year of life, 75% of brain tissue are lain and by five years of age, 90% of brain and head are formed. Brain size continues to increase from 2 to 10 years of age, until full growth at age 20.

Nervous structures leading to the spinal cord

Immediately above the midbrain, the optic thalamus is buried in each cerebral hemisphere. It is a large mass of gray matter. Both optic thalami are separated by the third ventricle. The corpus striatum separates outer side of thalamus from internal capsule. It is a bottleneck pass through which all fibers must pass to reach lower levels of the nervous system.

The internal capsule comprises ascending and descending nerve fibers. Numerous fibers connect thalami, internal capsule, cerebral cortex, cerebellum and spinal cord. Impulses of pain, temperature, touch, muscle sense, enter the Thalamus. It is an organ of crude consciousness.

Appearing as two separate gray masses, the corpus striatum is a large gray mass bent on itself. Its numerous fiber connections with other parts of the nervous system exert a steadying influence on skeletal muscle tone.

At the brain's base, behind the optic chiasma, the hypothalamus contains several groups of nerve cells. These centers control sympathetic and parasympathetic function. Entering the hypophysis' neural lobe, a bundle of nerve fibers, the hypothalamic hypophyseal tract controls liberation of pituitary hormone.

Immediately under the optic thalamus lies the midbrain, a short, narrow, pillar-like portion of the brain. A narrow canal runs through it: the cerebral aqueduct, communicating midbrain with third ventricle, above, with the fourth ventricle, below.

In front of the cerebral aqueduct, the greater part of the midbrain comprises two cerebral peduncles transmitting tracts from cortex, frontal and temporal regions of brain's respective sides. These fibers form the tegmentum, fusing at the back. Three gray masses lie on each side of the midline: the red nucleus and nuclei of oculomotor and trochlear nerves. At red nucleus fibers cross, forming the decussation of Forel.

The brainstem comprises the medulla obblongata, pons and midbrain. The brainstem largely controls postural motor functions, thus equilibrium, normal upright position in the field of gravity without conscious intervention. Behind cerebral hemispheres and brainstem lies the cerebellum with two lateral masses, the cerebellar hemispheres, and a central elongated worm-like structure, the vermis. In its cortex several layers of cells form flat leaves one against the other. The cerebellum comprises masses of gray matter. Three compact bundles of nerve fibers, the cerebellar peduncles, connect cerebellum with remaining parts of the nervous system. The cerebellum controls voluntary movements. Above medulla obblongata, the pons communicates cerebellum and cerebral hemispheres and prolongs into the spinal cord.

Brain ventricles

In the substance of the brain lie ventricles, cavities containing fluid, lined with a thin membrane, the ependyma. There are four ventricles: right and left lateral ventricles in cerebral hemispheres, the third ventricle in the thalamencephalon, the fourth ventricle in the hindbrain.

A small opening, the foramen of Munro connects lateral ventricles and 3rd ventricle. A narrow channel, the Aqueduct of Sylvius, connects third to 4th ventricle. The foramina of Luschka and Magendie communicate 4th ventricle with central canal of spinal cord and subarachnoid space. In ventricles and subarachnoid space, cerebrospinal fluid serves as a mechanical support for brain and spinal cord.

The brain: its blood supply. At the brain's base, communicating with each other by the circle of Willis, two paired arteries supply the brain: two internal carotids and two vertebral arteries. A system of dural sinuses returns blood to jugular veins. Nerve fibers descend through the midbrain, pons, medulla obblongata, cerebellum, entering the spinal cord. About 45 cm. (18 inches) long, the cord extends from the first vertebra, the atlas, to the first lumbar vertebra. Because the backbone continues to grow after the cord has reached its full length, the spinal cord does not occupy the full length of the vertebral canal of about 70 cm.

The spinal cord's enveloping membranes

Similar to the brain, three membranes envelop the spinal cord: the dura mater, arachnoid and pia mater. Attached to the foramen magnum of the occipital bone, to the axis (2nd vertebra) and to the third cervical vertebra, fibrous slips running down the column fix the dura to the vertebral column's posterior common ligament, thus ensuring the cord a firm position in the spinal column. The dura extends as far as the 2nd and 3rd pieces of the sternum, ensheathes the filum terminale and descends to the back of the coccyx, blending with the periosteum. Under the dura, a delicate tubular membrane, the arachnoid invests the entire surface of the cord. Slender filaments connect arachnoid with pia mater. The subdural space separates arachnoid from dura mater. Continuous with that of the brain, the pia is more vascular, with bundles of connective tissue fibers. The subarachnoid space separates arachnoid and pia. On each side of spinal cord, between each pair of vertebrae, emerges a pair of spinal nerves. There are 33 pairs of spinal nerves, covered by three membranes. Long roots at the spinal cord's tip form a horse's tail, filling up the lower third of the vertebral canal: it is the filum terminale.

Cerebrospinal fluid

Cerebrospinal fluid bathes both brain and membranes of spinal cord. It is a clear, colorless fluid with a specific gravity of 1.004-1.007, containing a little protein and glucose, larger quantities of potassium and salt, traces of sulfate, phosphate, calcium and uric acid. A few lymphocytes circulate in it. The fluid is produced by folds of cells lining the four brain ventricles. It maintains a constant intra-cranial pressure, acting as a cushion for the central nervous system, removing waste products of metabolism from nerve cells of brain and spinal cord.

The spinal cord, its internal configuration

In contrast to the brain, nerve cells in spinal cord are condensed in the center. Nerve fibers ascend or descend from the brain at the periphery. Nerve cells form the letter H or a spread-out butterfly, easily seen on any cross-section of the cord. This arrangement is present throughout the entire spinal cord. At the cord's cervical and lumbo-sacral regions, two enlarged areas may be seen.

These enlarged H's correspond to larger connections with brain, to better control hands and feet. The upper part of the H receives stimuli from sense organs. Cells from lower part of the H bring messages from the brain or connecting cells leaving the cord. They enable glandular secretion, muscle contraction or expansion of blood capillaries. Surrounding the gray matter H, the white matter represents fiber tracts running up and down the spinal cord. The myelin sheath surrounding nerve fibers imparts a glistening white appearance. When the cord is damaged, below it, all sensation diminishes.

Nervous tissue, general information

Nervous tissue involves cells and fibers. Nerve cells comprise gray matter of brain, spinal cord, ganglia and sense organs. White matter is composed of fibers of nerve cells, also called extensions: axons and dendrites. Cells and fibers are embedded in a ground substance or neuroglia with radially arranged fibers and cells. A myelin sheath or neurilemma surrounds axon fibers of nerve cells. It is also called primitive sheath or nucleated sheath of Schwann. Messages are always transmitted from axon to dendrite. First felt by the axon, the message is transmitted to dendrites; a synapse is made with the axon of another nerve cell, and so on until it reaches the brain. Motor nerve cells bring the message back, down the spinal cord, to end on a pre-capillary sphincter: blood vessels expand, increasing blood flow to the area.

Cranial nerves control structures in the head. They arise from a region in the cerebrospinal center and leave through foramina at the cranium's base. There are a total of 12 cranial nerves: olfactory, optic, motor oculi, trochlear, trifacial, abducent, facial, auditory, glossopharyngeal, pneumogastric or vagus, spinal acessory and hypoglossal nerves.

The cranial nerves

The olfactory nerve arises from an oval mass above the ethmoid bone's cribriform plate. Composed of unmyelinated fibers with 20 nerves, an inner group spreads out over the upper third of the nasal septum, the outer group is distributed over the surface of the superior turbinate and ethmoid bones.

The optic nerve is the sense of sight's special nerve. Solely distributed to the eyeball, it divides into two bands, external and internal. At the optic commissure optic fibers cross.

The motor oculi nerve supplies all muscles of the orbit except the superior oblique and external rectus. Originating from the inner surface of the crus cerebri, the motor oculi raises eyelids, dilates pupil, moves eyes in one direction and accommodates to distance.

The fourth or trochlear nerve supplies the superior oblique muscle. It rolls the eye downward and outward.

The largest cranial nerve is the fifth or trifacial nerve. Of five divisions, it is the sensory nerve of the head and face, the motor nerve of masticatory muscles.

The sixth or abducent nerve supplies the eye's external rectus muscle and prevents squinting.

The seventh or facial nerve is the motor nerve of all facial muscles of expression, taste sensation, salivary secretion and hearing.

The eighth or auditory nerve is the special nerve of hearing with fibers exclusively distributed to the internal ear.

The ninth or glosso-pharyngeal nerve innervates tongue and pharynx.

The tenth pneumogastric nerve, also called vagus nerve, is very extensively distributed with both motor and sensory fibers. It supplies speech and breathing organs: the pharynx, esophagus, stomach and heart.

The eleventh or spinal accessory nerve supplies the soft palate. It has two divisions: an accessory nerve to the vagus and a spinal portion.

The twelfth or hypoglossal nerve is the motor nerve of the tongue.

Notice how four cranial nerves innervate eyes.

Direction of spinal nerves after leaving the cord. Leaving the cord on both sides the 31 pairs of spinal nerves enable muscles and bones to move and perform their various activities. Of a mixed character, spinal nerves contain fibers receiving messages from a sense organ and fibers bringing the message back to a gland, blood vessel or skeletal muscle, increasing blood flow to the organ.

Upon leaving the cord, spinal nerves divide into two: a posterior division supplies back of body, an anterior division supplies front of body. Before dividing, each spinal nerve gives off a small recurrent branch to the sympathetic division, supplying dura mater, bones and ligaments. Smaller than the anterior division, the posterior division supplies muscles and skin behind the spine. The anterior division supplies regions in front of spine, including limbs. Hairless regions contain a greater number of sense receptors. Each spinal nerve has a ganglion. There are a total of 31 oval-shaped, reddish colored ganglia on each side of the cord.

Immediately beyond the ganglion, the two roots join. Their fibers intermingle, and the trunk formed represents the spinal nerve, receiving fibers from sense organs, and fibers bringing the message to muscle spindles, skin's sense organs and blood vessels. When a stimulus is set up in a sense organ: ear, eye or touch corpuscle, the message is brought to a nerve cell body within a ganglion, then conveyed to the brain by groups of nerve cells. The message is brought back by motor fibers and either permits a gland to secrete, a muscle to contract or a pre-capillary sphincter to open up a capillary area.

Spinal nerves' ganglia are not to be confused with ganglia of the autonomic nervous system forming a chain much lower than those of spinal nerves. A fine branch connects sympathetic and parasympathetic ganglia with spinal ganglia, thus tying all parts of the body with the nervous system.

Voluntary action, its nervous control

The 12 pairs of cranial nerves and 31 pairs of spinal nerves control all voluntary movement. Emerging on the ventral side of the brainstem, cranial nerves supply every muscle and internal organ in the head, with movement: eyes, ears, nose, mouth, teeth, chewing muscles, etc. Some nerves are sensory, transmitting only impulses to the brain. Others provide only movement, still others are mixed nerves. The 10th cranial nerve or vagus, a famous nerve, supplies muscles of bronchi, heart, esophagus and a third of large intestine.

The 31 pairs of spinal nerves supply various segments of the body. Each segment is a band encircling the body from mid back to mid front. Body segments are supplied by two, three sometimes four spinal nerves. They control the body as follows:

Cervical spinal nerves 1-5 control neck muscles and diaphragm for head movements.

Cervical spinal nerves 6-8 control trunk movements and abdominal muscles.

Thoracic spinal nerves 1-11 control trunk movements and abdominal muscles.

Lumbar spinal nerves 1-5 control movements of lower extremities, inner thigh, genitals, extension of legs, flexion of toes, ankle jerk.

Sacral spinal nerves 1-5 control erection, bladder evacuation, pinching of penis, contraction of external rectal sphincter, coccyx.

Terminals of spinal nerves branch out and join, forming important plexuses where fibers regroup: the cervical, brachial and lumbo-sacral plexuses. At plexuses, the spinal cord's gray matter is larger, indicating a greater number of nerve cells required for movements of head, hands and feet.

Ventral roots of first four cervical nerves join, forming the cervical plexus.

Cervical nerves 5-8, first thoracic nerve with a contribution from cervical nerve 4 join, forming the brachial plexus.

Lumbar nerve 1, sacral nerve 2, a large portion of sacral nerve 3 and a contribution from thoracic nerve 12 join, forming the lumbo-sacral plexus.

Cranial and spinal nerves bring messages to the brain. Sense organs are receptors of messages from all over the body: eyes, ears, nose, taste buds, touch skin corpuscles, muscle spindles, sense organs in respiratory and digestive tracts.

Reflex action

The simplest reflex arc involves two nerve cells: the knee jerk is a good example. When the knee is jerked, a stimulus is set up and transmitted to a nerve cell in a spinal nerve ganglion. Fibers relay the message to a nerve cell in gray matter of spinal cord's dorsal region, reaches a cell in ventral region and the message is returned by motor fibers, causing a muscle contraction. Most reflexes are relayed by a chain of nerve cells to a brain center. From brain's motor area, it returns to stimulate a muscle contraction, glandular secretion, or relaxes a capillary sphincter, increasing blood flow through vessels. The larger the stimulated area, the more connections are made. An impulse travels at a speed of 100 meters per second or 325 ft. The distance between two nerve cells at a synapse is 200 angstroms.

The number of brain cells
The brain's 25 billion nerve cells and 25 million peripheral nerve cells connect the central nervous system. Synapses are more numerous than nerve cells. Surrounding nerve cells, glial cells comprise half the central nervous system's cell volume. Glial cells called Schwann cells enclose peripheral axons. A distance of 15-20 milli-microns separates nerve and glial cells where substances are exchanged. Interstitial space represents 12-14% of total brain volume.

Processing information
To process information, a membrane potential must be present across the lipoid protein membrane bounding all nerve cells. For muscle and nerve cells, this membrane potential must be negative, from -55 to -100 milli-volts; for smooth muscle cells, -30 milli-volts. This resting potential is due to an uneven distribution of various ions in extra and intracellular spaces. The greatest difference lies in the number of potassium and sodium ions within and without cells. Most important are 100,000 potassium ions within and 2,000 potassium ions outside a cell. Similarly required are 108,000 sodium ions outside a cell and 10,000 sodium ions inside a cell. Only under such conditions can information continuously be transmitted throughout the nervous system. (intra-cellular ions are in the form of large protein ions).

A necessary condition of nerve cells: oxygen in the atmosphere
Sufficient oxygen must be present in the atmosphere. In oxygen lack, changes in ion distribution occur and water enters nerve cells, preventing normal information processing. Any stimulus acts as an electrical discharge, a membrane depolarizes with a consequent exchange of ions across nerve cell membranes. Man's central nervous system consumes around 20% (50 ml. per minute) of the total resting oxygen uptake. If blood supply is interrupted for 10 seconds, pronounced cerebral function disruption occurs with possible unconsciousness. The brain is permanently damaged if deprived of oxygen for five minutes. On the undersurface of the brain, two pairs of arteries supply oxygen. Branching out like a tree over the hemispheres, arteries continue downward on the undersurface of the spinal cord, branching out along its length. Even at rest nerves use up oxygen and produce carbon dioxide. When nerves are stimulated, both factors increase considerably.

Speed of nerve impulses
Nerve impulses travel at a speed of 90-100 meters per second, as rapid as the

speed of a bullet, the faster if fewer cells are involved. After an impulse, nerve is unable to conduct for about 0.01-0.02 seconds. The rapid conduction of voluntary impulses is due to the myelin sheath enclosing nerve fibers. Imagine a delicate filament of protoplasm enclosed in a layer of fatty material. The myelin sheath insulates impulses, preventing passage to other nerve fibers. Synapses between nerve cells limit the passage of impulses, preventing widespread excitation to induce tetanus or convulsive contraction of all voluntary muscles.

In widely separated regions, every motor nerve cell is similarly connected with sensory fibers. Thus when slapped, the arm jerks away, trunk and shoulder move, head and eyes turn, an exclamation is uttered, indicating that many muscles take part in the action. Many nerve cells from bottom of H supply bodily muscles while a stimulus excites many skin receptor endings. Stimuli in reflex arcs always stir a movement or maintain posture.

How nerve fibers obtain a myelin sheath: At birth, nerve fibers are incompletely myelinated but are completely myelinated by the time a child walks. Association fibers in the brain myelinate still later. Covering the myelin sheath, Schwann's sheath dips deeply into the nodes, imparting a nerve fiber's segmented appearance. To regenerate nerve fiber an empty Schwann's sheath is an absolute requirement. Nerve fibers supplying all internal organs are not myelinated, impulses here are conducted at the rate of two meters per second, which accounts for the slow movements of internal organs.

The conduction of nerve impulses: Nerves with large diameters conduct impulses faster than otherwise. Nerve fibers divide into some 100 branches, each supplying a muscle fiber. When the arm moves, impulses travel to the cortex at the rate of 5-50 or more impulses per second. Weaker movements cause fewer impulses. Mammalian nerve has a maximum frequency of 1,000 impulses per second. Large fibers conduct sharp pain, slender nerve fibers conduct dull pain of an enduring type. Every nerve fiber conveys a message peculiar to its type of fiber. Fibers transmit impulses but the brain perceives the different types of sensations, whether visual, auditory, pleasurable to the touch, painful, libidinous or burning.

For proper conduction, nerve requires oxygen and circulating air must be always available. Leave windows open all year round. Take daily walks. In an airtight atmosphere, nerve fatigues and actions slow down considerably.

The sympathetic ganglia. In the spinal cord's chest and lumbar regions, sympathetic ganglia form two long chains on both sides. These ganglia's position is much lower than that of spinal ganglia. Sympathetic ganglia are aggregates of nerve cells with fibers to all internal organs: heart, lungs kidneys, endocrine glands, digestive tract, bladder, rectum, reproductive organs, sex organs, etc.

Originating directly from ganglion cells, sympathetic fibers to regulatory organs, digestive organs and other internal organs are not myelinated. Fibers to the digestive tract must pass through another group of ganglia, the celiac superior mesenteric and inferior mesenteric ganglia, before the message is relayed to digestive organs and glands. Thus the action of sympathetic ganglia on regulatory organs and reproductive organs is immediate. Their action on digestive organs and sex organs is more remote. This proves that when much blood flows to regulatory organs, as during sleep at night, less blood is available to digestive organs and to sex organs. When sleeping on a full stomach, blood is continuously used to digest food, preventing deep sleep and other regulatory functions.

The parasympathetic ganglia. In the cranial and sacral regions of the spinal cord, parasympathetic ganglia form two groups on both sides. They comprise the cranial-sacral outflow whose fibers provide a greater blood flow to digestive organs and sex organs, a lesser blood flow to regulatory organs and reproductive organs. When digesting a meal, both regulatory organs and reproductive organs receive a lesser blood supply despite their irrigation by parasympathetic ganglia (see Chapter 1).

Ganglia of the autonomic nervous system comprise the following:
1. The gangliated cord: three pairs of cervical ganglia, twelve pairs of dorsal ganglia, four pairs of lumbar ganglia, four pairs of sacral ganglia.
2. In front of the spine, three great gangliated plexuses in the thoracic, abdominal and pelvic cavities, namely the cardiac, solar and hypogastric plexuses.
3. Some other microscopic ganglia found in the heart, stomach, and uterus.

The three divisions innervate blood vessels of thoracic and abdominal viscera. Sympathetic fibers communicate ganglia with one another, supplying internal viscera and coats of blood vessels.

How to assess human behavior

As a bilaterally symmetrical human, man moves in a definite direction. The large brain is a central coordinating mechanism for the three great sense organs of sight, smell and hearing, the three supra-segmental portions of the nervous system directing man's actions in life.

Internally and externally, sense receptors from all over the body bring impulses through cranial and spinal nerves, to the spine, the meeting place of nerve paths from all over. Received by nerve cells and transmitted to the brain, stimuli from impulses come in touch with cells carrying the message away, modifying muscular or glandular activity. The various reflex arcs bind one part of the body with another and action in one region either stirs movement or refrains action. The various sense organs prevent confusion of reactions, limiting stimuli to particular reactions. This selective excitability is self-protective in nature.

At birth, the nervous system is not fully developed and responses are poorly organized. With learning and mnemonic (memory) reactions, experience relations are made with objects and the latter are avoided or sought according to whether harmful or beneficial in nature. Pavlov felt that conditioned reflexes form the basis of training and are biologically of great significance.

The acquisition of skill in life allows discriminative reactions by memory, reducing unnecessary movements, improving speed and accuracy. For survival in society, training is most important yet instinctive behavior has a single objective: to preserve the conditions of life in a constant internal environment. All vital mechanisms, no matter how varied, disrupt the constancy of blood's physical and chemical properties. Man instinctively protects himself by plugging ears when noise is excessive, by jerking the hand away from burning fire, by remaining silent after much exertion, by retiring to a quiet spot after a day's work, etc.

Normal values of blood allow performance of daily activities. After a day's work, this constancy is slightly offset. Daily sleep restores normal values. Joseph Barcroft showed that changes in the normal limits of blood's values affect the brain. The more perfect the brain, the narrower are the limits of blood's properties. According to J. Barcroft, the proper amount of oxygen inspired during growth determines the perfection of the brain's higher functions. Brain size is not particularly indicative of intelligence, but breathing in the proper amount of oxygen is a more definite sign of mental capacities. Thus a nose with the least strain indicates a most peaceful nature, a sign of great intelligence and physical strength. Brain size determines mental and physical stamina.

The brain integrates the animal in its life of external relation. Breathing movements are regulated by the hind-brain, containing centers to maintain posture, to stand erect. The cerebellum provides the feeling of gravity. It controls accuracy of movements. smoothness of voluntary actions. Cerebral hemispheres are especially concerned with associative memory.

By age 20, man's brain is fully developed, whereby the importance of an excellent infant formula during the first year of life where 75% of brain tissue are lain. During the following 19 years, 25% of remaining brain tissues are formed. To ensure perfect physical and mental development, a growing child must be given the best food for 20 years of growth.

Dying explained

For normal function, air is the important necessity. How then do we explain fainting and death despite the presence of air? Factors other than air can cause erratic behavior, fainting or death. Humans are affected by something done on the body, penetrating the body or collecting within the body. Excessive activities cause erratic behavior, fainting or death. F. Scott Fitzgerald's wife Zelda became mentally unbalanced and was institutionalized as a result of her intense training to become a ballet dancer.

A heavy blow induces fainting, one dies from a fall, a death in the family causes intense sadness with possible fainting, even dying. One dies when impaled upon a pike, excess impacted wax in ears or navel causes pain, then convulsions and dying, excess fecal accumulation causes consulvions, sexual activity in a weakened state causes death, etc. Activities use up oxygen and when excessive prevent normal blood supply to regulatory organs and brain, with ensuing death. Death occurs when a blood vessel bursts, pouring blood into the system. From a punctured digestive tract, wastes pour into the body cavity causing blood poisoning with eventual death. One dies from an improperly cared for infection. Anything impinging on the body, entering the body, striking the body, performed by the body, collecting within the body, when excessive, can cause death. Aging and dying are much feared.

Approaching death. The inability to relax is a sign of approaching death. External signs are constant muscular activity: continuous speech, jaw movement, convulsive muscular activity, constant activity, tartar on teeth, etc. These conditions are usually caused by a mass collecting in the body: earwax, feces, excess food, a tumor, dirt in other body orifices. When finally all living activities exceed regulatory capacities and involuntary action dominates over normal function, death will ensue by increasingly greater convulsive attacks.

The death agony. Convulsive attacks such as epileptic seizures precede the death agony. The epileptic is not a dying person, and seizures most often lapse into deep sleep. In death agony, blood volume is much reduced and increasingly painful contractions assail the individual until blood vessels collapse and death ensues. Convulsive attacks indicate a lack of control of sympathetic ganglia, the nerve center directing blood flow to regulatory and reproductive organs. When sympathetic ganglia no longer direct blood to regulatory organs, convulsive seizures become so powerful that death ensues.

Accumulated wastes in body will result in the death agony: fecal masses, impacted earwax, a full bladder, nose bugger, dirty skin, dirty navel, tartar on roots of teeth. Be wary of involuntary contractions or twitching—precursors to convulsions. Remove itch and pain from ears, nose, navel, teeth, skin and delay dying.

Sudden death

A living body functions in six communicating systems.

The sympathetic ganglia directly control blood flow to two passive systems:

reproductive (uterus, ovaries, testicles), and regulatory (heart, lungs, kidneys, skin, endocrine glands) organs.

When weak or terminally ill, strong action in the four active systems (muscles and bones, sense organs, digestive organs, sex organs) not under direct sympathetic nervous control, can trigger sudden death. Injections, intravenous feeding; powerful emotion, anger, fear, a blow, being robbed or attacked, screaming, blinding light, deafening noise, sex, a large meal, creative work, singing, incessant talk, physical exertion, travel, etc. When weak or terminally ill, a quiet life is recommended.

Dying is painful because a large blood vessel bursts. Dying cannot be felt during sleep. Prevent the death agony by removing body wastes.

Sudden pain indicates overworking one of the four active systems: heavy food, excess talk, a public life, excess physical exertion, mental exertion, sexual excesses, excess light or noise, impacted earwax, fecal masses. Determine the excess activity and remove it: erratic behavior inability to cope, impatience. If the problem is not resolved, death agony will ensue. Avoid all blood tests, injections, intravenous feeding, surgery, etc.; pain accelerates death.

Extreme terminal state

An extreme nervous tension is characterized by haggard eyes, a very pinched lower jaw and shuffling gait. Do daily chores, walk a mile a day, slowly in the sun and perspire. Do not sit and wait for the end. Keep busy and remain silent.

Cook mixtures of foods till soft. Chew every mouthful till the consistency of baby food before swallowing, and avoid large meals. Eat custard-like foods. The reason is: when blood vessels are very clogged, little blood flows to regulatory organs. Large quantities of foreign substances draw blood immediately to the site, triggering death or the death agony.

Emerge from a terminal state by partial fasting on orangeade, grapeade and salted tea. Approach liquid dieting slowly to prevent fecal impaction. Remain on this diet until hunger pangs return. Stool evacuation may be a problem and low squatting on a potty and pulling on a bar solve the problem (see chapter on cooking).

Remove poisons rapidly

Perspire heavily during hot summer days with 90° F. temperatures and reduce fasting time. Wear silk and wool-lined boots. When soaked in perspiration, bathe. Eat light: cooked fruits, aspics, custards, light coffee or cocoa, soups etc. Stay in the sun daily for an hour, and two to four hours in fresh air. Take long walks, continue to perspire.

Do not stay a great length of time in an air-conditioned room because cold penetrates the body. Drink a cold beverage to lower body temperature. Open windows wide and adjust to the heat.

Poisons must be removed

Fasting removes poisons clogging blood vessels. When fasting urine darkens in color. When blood vessels are cleansed enough, normal blood volume will be restored to regulatory organs. Sleep will deepen, involuntary convulsions will disappear, and blood will flow to active organ capillaries.

Life is the motion of blood to capillaries to sustain the increased metabolism required by vital activity. This is the vital force of the vitalistic concept. We can now explain why some people are born without motion or with motionless parts: useless hand, eyelid, legs, total body. These sad cases are due to non-functional nerve endings in motionless parts. Sufficient blood flows to tissues to maintain a motionless life but capillaries cannot expand due to non-functional nerve endings of capillary regions. Nerve endings are an absolute requirement for all manifestations of life.

Chapter 10
Control external stimuli and live long

We have analyzed active actions done by the living body. Passive actions detrimentally affecting the organism shall now be analyzed. We see and hear despite ourselves: sight and hearing are passive actions. However they become active when lights and sounds are extremely powerful. Sense organs direct us away from dangerous situations, providing awareness of the external world to adapt it to our own use.

The eyes
Eyes are most precious sense organs giving us freedom of action. Global out-pocketings of the brain, their protected position and overlapped visual fields ensure an extensive range of sight, endowing humans with three-dimensional vision, a great improvement from animals' monocular vision. Enclosed in a bony case, the eyeball sits in the fat-padded cavity of the orbit.

How eyes are protected
Eyebrows, eyelids, lashes, tears and blinking protect eyes. Two arched eminences of skin thickened with short hairs surmounting the upper circumference of the orbit, eyebrows control the amount of light striking eyes. In contact with the front of eyes are eyelids, movable folds protect eyes from dirt, dust and injury. At the inner margin of each lid, a small conical eminence pierces the inner margin of each lid: the lachrymal or tear gland's pore.

To better protect eyes, two or three rows of short, thickly curved hairs fringe both upper and lower eyelids: eyelashes. Within upper eyelids lies the tendon lifting and lowering lids. Close to the free margin of the lids, several rows of glands appear like parallel strings of pearls. 30 glands adorn upper lid, fewer on lower lid. Their secretion prevents lids from adhering together.

Above the orbit's outer angle sits the almond-shaped lachrymal gland. In the concave orbit lie the convex eyeball and the superior external rectus muscle. At the eye's inner edge, draining into the nasal cavity, 6-12 ducts run obliquely from lachrymal gland and empty into the tiny lachrymal duct. To prevent dryness or inflammation, tears wash and lubricate eyeball.

Similar to leaves of a book, eyelids comprise seven layers (skin, fatty layer, involuntary muscle fibers and two thin plates of connective tissue, Meibomian glands and conjunctiva). When eyes blink, like a swab, eyelids spread the film of tears over the eyes' cornea, excess tears are pumped out, preventing dryness of cornea.

The eye: its external formation

Segments of two spheres form the eyeball: a small one in front, a larger one behind. Except for a tiny, pin-hole sized pupil in the front, the eyeball is entirely closed to the outside world. The eyeball measures 23 mm. long, slightly more horizontally. A thin membrane completely envelops the eye. This capsule of Tenon is pierced by the optic nerve at the back, ciliary vessels and nerves, in front; its thick lower part forms a hammock-like suspensory ligament attached to cheek and lachrymal bones. To the outermost coat of the eyeball, about half an inch behind the corneal circumference, six muscles allow eyes to move around. Under the capsule of Tenon, three layers enclose the eyeball completely: the outermost sclera, the middle choroid, and the inner retinal layers. Within these layers is the lens, the various humors of the two chambers and lastly the liquid vitreous body. The lens is suspended in the liquid-filled eyeball. In front of the pupil lies a contractile curtain, the iris, varying in color. It controls the amount of light penetrating the eye.

The eyeball's three layers - The lens

The outermost sclera comprises nine layers of connective tissue, united by bridges. Of a brown color on the inside, it has no blood vessels but many grooves to lodge ciliary nerves and blood vessels. A large hole in the center back of the sieve allows retinal artery to pass.

The middle choroid layer firmly adheres to the sclera. Also called uveal tract by dint of its purple pigmentation, it maintains the eyeball in total darkness. The choroid layer's numerous blood vessels and wide blood spaces provide nutrition for lens and retina. The choroid lines 5/6th of the globe, accompanying retina to the edge of the lens where it modifies into the ciliary body, an asymmetrical ring, a contraption of ciliary muscle, nerve and pleated blood vessels, surrounding the lens. Aside from elastic and connective tissue, the choroid has five layers of cells with blood vessels of different sizes within its three middle layers.

The last tunic of the eye is the innermost retina, an extremely sensitive membrane a fraction of a millimeter thick. Soft, purplish-red in color, the retina lines the interior of the eyeball up to the lens. The retina's ten layers of nervous elements lie close to the liquid vitreous body. Farthest from the vitreous body lie a layer of rods and cones, nature's means to prevent overexposure. There are around 7 million cones and 75-170 thousand rods.

The lens of the eye: suspended in the vitreous humour and immediately behind the pupil is the lens, a tiny onion-shaped body. Of concentric lamellated layers, it has a jagged, dentated edge surrounded by pleated blood vessels of the ciliary body.

When light strikes the eye

When light enters the pupil of the eye, it passes through all retinal layers to reach rods and cones. Retinal ganglion cells transmit nerve impulses to the brain. At low intensities of light, rods are stimulated. At high intensities, cones are stimulated. The retina presents a blind spot where the optic nerve leaves the eyeball. It also has a point of clearest vision called macula, yellow spot or fovea centralis with numerous blood vessels. Here vision is most acute.

When an object is perceived

When an object is perceived, rays of light are refracted by aqueous humor, lens and vitreous body. Ultrafiltration of plasma from the ciliary body's tiny capillaries produces aqueous humor continuously. In front of the lens, humor fills anterior and posterior chambers of the eyeball. Very little aqueous humor is produced, only about four or five grains, of which a $1/5^{th}$ is chiefly salt. This humor maintains normal intra-ocular pressure of 20-25 mm. Intra-ocular pressure falls prior to death.

For close or far vision, the lens changes its refracting power. Beyond 20 ft. to infinity, rays of light need not be refracted, all light rays striking eyes are parallel, easily refracted to form an image on the retina's yellow spot. An object closer or less than 20 feet's distance forces greater convexity of the lens, a means to focus rays of light sharply on the yellow spot. To do so, the ciliary muscle relaxes, fibers of the suspensory ligament tense up, pulling the equator of the lens, flattening it up. At the same instant, pleated blood vessels of the ciliary body unfold themseives without fail, to better irrigate the flattened lens. The vitreous body is the last refracting medium. It is a gelatinous, colorless, transparent and semi-solid mass, filling $4/5^{th}$ of the entire globe from retina to lens.

How an object is seen

Upon perceiving an object, the retina's sensory cells carry the message to the brain's vision center where motor neurons bring the message back to the retina's 9th layer stimulating the tiny blood capillaries. In dim light, a few red blood cells flow through open blood vessels. In increased intensity of light, blood cells will rush through tiny vessels. In blinding light, large clumps of red cells force their way through tiny vessels whose walls may burst into a million bits, with resulting blindness.

In adequate light, blood gently flows through blood vessels at the yellow spot where an inverted image is formed. Vision is dependent on the presence of many structures. Sometimes upon perceiving excessive light, pain is felt. Pain is a warning, indicating that the lighting is excessive and must be lowered. Because the pleated blood vessels surrounding the lens must unfold themselves for close work, lights used must be dim: it would prevent bursting of capillaries when lens adjusts, and preserve capillaries at the yellow spot. Excessively bright lights may cause fainting, even death—excess light draws blood to eyes and away from regulatory organs, thus affecting the brain. In antiquity, blinding lights were used on prisoners who eventually fainted or died.

Vision: the ill effects of faulty nutrition
Poor nutrition affects everyone with deleterious effects on vision. Avoid heavy fried foods, the use of cream, sour cream, in recipes. Oil hardens arteries. Exposure to bright lights for close work will burst eye capillaries. In close vision, 80% of the incident light is reflected back to the eyes. Beware of reflected light from glass, paper, plastic, metal or other shiny surface. Retinal capillaries are extremely delicate and easily torn into shreds. Pictures of an eye affected by glaucoma show pulsating blood vessels with many capillaries torn into shreds at the yellow spot.

The best lighting to maintain youthful eyesight and ensure longevity
For close work, use one or two 25 Watt yellow bulb with a fabric over parchment shade. In a large room, several 25 Watt lamps are better than one 100 Watt lamp. It prevents deformations such as far-sightedness/myopia. Equally dangerous is too dim a light as eyes may suffer strain with dull pain. To combat strain or tired eyes, close the eyes and tighten repeatedly. Do not open eyes until tears lubricate them completely. When moving from a dark room to a bright place, consciously tighten the eyes. The sight of sudden blinding light causes fainting, even death. In 1510, Lodovico Sforza, duke of Milan, was released from his ten-year imprisonment at the castle of Loches in France. After ten years in a dark dungeon, daylight struck the poor man like a thunderbolt. He died on the spot as soon as his eyes saw the sunlight.

At times a very large, bright spot may be perceived with closed eyes. This can occur after looking at a bright object or having been in the sun for long periods. Do not panic. Sit down and close eyes until the blinding light disappears, about five minutes' time. Open eyes when the light disappears. Always heed an anomaly immediately otherwise blindness may result.

Take immediate action
When bathing, washing hair, making love, one may knock an eye out of the socket. History recalls the case of a Frenchman who lost an eye while making love with his mistress. Do not panic. If ever an eye is lost, pick it up immediately, dip it in saline water and replace it in the socket. Blood vessels and nerves will soon find their original attachments and sight will be restored. Do so immediately or else leave it in salt water until you reach a physician.

When exposed to the air for half an hour, a vital organ becomes totally useless: dead. Never let that happen. The same applies to a knocked-out tooth.

To prevent eyes from ever being knocked out of the socket: when bathing, washing face or hair, close your eyes tight. Keep them tightened as long as hands are busy washing the face.

When working with hard materials: when prying open plastic objects, working with leather or wood, wear goggles or close eyes. Braille, inventor of the Braille method for the blind, was playing with his father's leather tools when a piece of leather flipped up into his eye, it became infected and spread to the other eye, thus, he lost his eyesight in both eyes.

Maintain perfect eyesight for a long life

Do not wear glasses. They impinge on the nose, leaving a deep mark, worsening eyesight, and every few years, a stronger prescription is required. It prevents normal breathing, reducing the volume of inspired air. If glasses are a necessity, hang them around the neck and use only when required. Light plastic glasses do not leave a mark on the nose.

Never look at the sun. Look into the distance. Beyond a 20-foot distance, the lens does not alter its shape. When eyes feel tired, close and tighten repeatedly, move eyeballs around until tears bathe eyes.

Do not look at red color. It tires eyes and exerts a deleterious effect on the mind. The writer Victor Hugo's wife used red curtains in her home; it may have had an effect on their daughter Adele who became mentally ill.

Do not look excessively at rapid moving objects or pictures. For good eyesight, a dark TV screen is better. Cable TV may cause pain in the eyes. To prevent pain, place a special screen on the set.

Avoid using high wattage light bulbs. Several 25 Watt bulbs in a large room will prevent the need for glasses or contact lenses for life. Contact lenses are closely apposed to the cornea.

Ancient Assyrians had huge, egg-sized eyes. It is not good to have very large eyes. Sight being automatic, when constantly stimulated, blood irrigates them continuously. With large eyes, constant stimulation would drive blood away from regulatory organs and rapidly cause death. A recent article in the Reader's Digest told the story of a little girl with very large eyes. She did not live long. Careful preparation of foods during growth years prevents the formation of large eyes.

Noise - Medication

The most abused of organs are the ears. Ears are constantly exposed to sound. Decibels of sound are molecules of an elastic medium moving back and forth as a pressure wave. Sound has energy and noise is sound with unrelated frequencies. Through the external ear, waves of sound reach the hearing system, travel along the external auditory canal, and strike the eardrum whose waves excite the middle ear to stimulate the inner ear.

Several medications can cause permanent deafness: Aspirin and aspirin-based products, Valium and other tranquilizers, sleeping pills, etc.

The external ear & the three divisions of the ear

In the embryo, ears develop as out-pocketings of the brain. Shaped like a question mark, the outer ear is a single piece of yellow fibro-cartilage. Similar to a seashell, the external ear has a twirl or concha. Facing the exit, a movable cartilaginous tragus closes the opening. Above it lies an antitragus. The earlobe has no cartilage. Elastic and pliable, the auricle's skin has hairs and numerous sebacious glands. Two extrinsic muscles and two intrinsic ligaments attach the ear to the head; three extrinsic muscles and six intrinsic muscles hold it in place. From auricle to tympanic membrane, the S-shaped auditory canal leads to the middle ear. About 1 1/2 inch long, the outer third of the canal is cartilaginous, the remaining two thirds, is bone. A fibrous membrane lies in its upper and back walls. Underneath the auditory canal lie numerous wax glands lined by a very thin layer of skin. Externally flanked by skin, internally by mucous membrane, the tympanum is a firm fibrous tissue. Between tympanum and inner ear lies the middle ear.

Wedged in at the base of the skull, between ethmoid and occipital bones, the middle ear lodges in the pyramid-shaped petrous bone. The middle ear is filled with air from the Eustachian tube running from floor of middle ear to larynx. Except when swallowing, the Eustachian tube is always open.

Lodged in the middle ear are three movable bones in a chain: the malleus, incus and stapes. Like a hammer, the malleus' head articulates with the incus, a bicuspid-shaped bone whose longer process articulates with the stapes' head, resembling a stirrup. The tympanic membrane is connected with the malleus' handle. The stapes' footplate is fixed onto the margin of the inner ear's oval window. The three tiny bones are tied together by two muscles and their ligaments. Within the middle ear, muscles and nerves form vascular folds, imparting a honeycomb appearance. Mucous membrane covers the tiny ossicles, and six arteries supply the tympanum.

Beginning at the round window, the inner ear is channelled in the substance of the petrous bone. The inner ear or bony labyrinth comprises three semicircular canals, each at right angles to the other two, united to the cochlea by a tiny ovoid shaped vestibule. A fifth of an inch long, the membranous labyrinth lies in the bony labyrinth.

The transmission of sound particularly involves the cochlea. About 5 mm. high from base to apex, the cochlea resembles the shell of a tiny snail. Three parallel canals totaling 30 mm. in length, are coiled 2 and 3/4 times around a central bone or modiolus. These canals are the scala media, scala tympani and scala vestibuli. At the cochlear tip, perilymph communicates scala tympani and vestibuli. The scala media with endolymph is sandwiched between the previous scalae. In the living state, two membranous partitions divide the snail-like cochlea completely from top to bottom of the modiolus' projecting shelf. Two membranes join all three scalae:

Reissner's membrane separates scala vestibuli and media, basilar membrane separates scala media from tympani. On the inner part of the basilar membrane a tiny swelling: the organ of Corti, winds its way throughout the scala media's length.

The organ of Corti resembles a piano keyboard with layers of thousands of cells. Similar to the eye's retinal layer, the basilar membrane's sound sensitive cells are the inner and outer hair cells with fine hairlets.

How sound is heard

The tiny snail-like cochlea lies on its side, base directed towards the cranial cavity, apex pointing outward and forward. Directed to the auricle, waves of sound are transmitted to the eardrum with a force ten times greater than at the oval window. At each sound wave, the malleus' handle moves to and fro, making a 0.43 mm. excursion, driving inwards a certain distance. Acting like a plunger at the inner ear's oval window, the stapes' series of inward and outward movements set up corresponding motion of fluid in cochlear scala vestibuli.

The oval window moves inward, the round window pushes outward toward the middle ear, equilibrating pressure. By alternating swinging movements, from base to tip of the cochlea, the waves generated displace the scala media, bending basilar membrane's hair cells. Mechanical deformations convert into neuronal excitation, stirring nerve filaments around hair cells' bases.

Excitations pass to central fibers in organ of Corti's spiral ganglion, they are transferred to the medulla obblongata, then to nerve cells of cochlear nuclei. Secondary nerve cells ascend to mid-brain and nervous nuclei in temporal lobe's auditory center. By the same route motor fibers return the message to cochlear blood vessels, increasing blood flow to spiral lamina wound 2 and 3/4 times around the bony modiolus.

What happens when one hears sounds

High-pitched sounds affect organ of Corti's short hair cells at cochlear base. Low-pitched sounds affect long hair cells at the cochlear apex. Loud noise sets up wild vibrations in the middle ear's three little bones. Simultaneously blood cells rush in clumps through inner ear's tiny blood vessels, forcing their way through. Loud noise of great intensity may cause deafness as capillary walls burst into a million bits. A half hour's exposure to 120 decibels of noise may cause loss of hearing. Sudden explosive sounds may rupture the eardrum or the tiny blood vessels, with permanent hearing loss. Especially affected by loud noise are those with hardened arteries and arteriosclerosis.

Sudden loud noise can cause fainting, even death. When hearing the sudden outbursts of a trumpet at a doctoral ceremony, one young man had an epileptic attack; he died two hours later. Strident sirens should be lowered. Ambulances, fire trucks should emit intermittent middle-range beeping sounds. Humans can hear a pin drop in a crowd. Limiting the speed of cars to 20 miles per hour would preserve both the driver's ears and reduce noise pollution. Though unaware, most drivers are partially deaf from years of driving.

Music: its beneficial effect on health

For centuries, music has been used as an antispasmodic: the mesmerizing tub helped cases of depression. People forgot their sufferings when hearing suave, veiled harmony from combined sounds of hidden flutes and oboes. Music cures depression and brings people out of stupor.

Music has cured insanity, catalepsy, epilepsy, the plague, sciatica, deafness and syncope. The instrument used was individually selected. Low tones affected lower parts of the body and vice versa.

Play a musical instrument or listen to classical music. The different modes of western music contain the nature of passions: Phrygian mode excites anger, Mixolydian induces sadness, and Dorian sounds produce stability and temperance. Iranians believe their music stirs the soul deeply for its tranquillity, has the tones of nature, similar to water flowing over stones and pebbles or wind among trees. Iranians feel that western operatic music destroys the feeling of deep, strong and tense emotion whereas Iranian music of quarter-tones is similar to a Gregorian chant. Music is a highly personal choice, whether Gregorian chants, opera, popular music or jazz. Learn to appreciate silence: our tiny sense organs of sight and hearing are the most precious yet most abused organs. They are the first organs to show signs of aging.

How to preserve hearing

Besides removing earwax daily, plug ears when trains pass. Never listen to loud deafening music. Avoid fried foods and excess starches. Plug your ears when driving. Living quarters should be far from trains, highways or at crossroads of several lanes of cars. Noise not only destroys hearing, it is damaging to regulatory organs. In antiquity, high-pitched sounds were used to torture prisoners.

Excess noise may cause loss of equilibrium, even falling. Living organisms must have a definite posture, which is provided by the sense organs of equilibrium; it is important to know something about these sense organs of equilibrium. Together with sense organs of sight, hearing, touch, the organ of equilibrium provides the ability to maintain upright position.

The sense organs of equilibrium: their exact location: Tiny organs of equilibrium are lodged in the inner ear. They are the semicircular canals, utricle and saccule: in the inner ear's petrous bone, the three parts are continuous, one after the other. Foremost are semicircular canals, utricle in the center, then saccule, and behind them, the cochlea. Separated by perilymph, these membranous organs are inside a same shaped bony case.

The sense organs of equilibrium: About 1/3 the size of the bony case surrounding them, semicircular canals are 1/20th of an inch in diameter. At right angles to each other, two canals are vertical and one horizontal. With a diameter twice the size of the canal itself, a swelling or ampulla is present at the bottom of each canal. On each ampulla, bristle-like hair cells called crista, form an elevation, surrounded by a gelatinous material, the cupula. Crista or hair cells are the sense organs of each semicircular canal.

From semicircular canals, five orifices lead to the utricle, one common to two canals. Between semicircular canals and cochlea lies the vestibule, containing two membranous sacs: the utricle, measuring 1/8th of an inch in its longest diameter; of a globular form, the saccule, a smaller sac. The utricle is connected behind with semicircular canals. The saccule lies near the cochlear scala vestibuli's opening. Thicker than elsewhere are anterior walls and floor of both sacs. Each sac contains a sense organ: the macula, a plaque of hair cells covered by a layer of gelatinous substance to which otoliths are glued.

Otoliths are masses of tiny crystalline grains of carbonate of lime, cemented together by fibrous tissue. Each sac has two otoliths.

Walls of utricle and saccule are three-layered: an outer blood vessel layer, a middle papilliform layer, an inner layer of supporting cells and hair cells. Endolymph fills semicircular canals, utricle and saccule. Between membranous parts and bony walls of petrous bone numerous fibrous bands are stretched across the space, holding canals, utricle and saccule in place.

Macular organs: their purpose

Macular organs informs about the head's position in space. In the erect position, the macular organ is horizontal and the otolith membrane applies no shear force to the underlying sensory epithelium. Tilting the head tips the utricle's macula at an angle. The heavy otolith membrane slides a short distance over the sensory epithelium, cilia bend, stimulating receptors. Vestibular nerves' sensory fibers bring the message to the brain's vestibular nucleus and connections are made with other parts of the central nervous system. Motor fibers return the message to motor nerve cells in spinal column, innervating muscle capillaries. A flow of blood fills capillaries of muscles and eyes and muscular contraction maintains balance.

Maintain optimum spatial position without feeling dizzy

Liquid fills the inner ear: 1) perilymph contains sodium, 2) endolymph has potassium. The eyes and ears are tiny structures pervaded by liquid. A sufficient amount of fluid is necessary every day to keep these liquids constant. The diet should have sufficient amount of salt (sodium) and protein such as meat (potassium). In winter, keep legs and feet warm; feet are poorly protected; living organisms stand on the ground, and cold rises from the feet upwards. Wear wool stockings and fur-lined boots. Cold affects extremities first. With age dizziness can be felt dress warmly and never allow hands and feet to get cold. When we touched the icy cold hand of an older man we knew that death was imminent: two weeks later, he died.

A daily diet of clear broth, light coffee or cocoa, dilute fresh juices, cannot be overemphasized. Voltaire drank several cups of coffee daily and lived to age 84 (1694-1778).

Excess carbohydrates cause dizziness and sleepiness. When dizzy, reduce carbohydrates: cereals, rice, flour products, cookies, cakes, sweets, tropical fruits. When weak, prepare foods very carefully. The young and healthy can eat most foods. With advancing age, the lengthier the preparation of foods, the better.

Taste guards the entrance of dangerous products, poisons, chemicals, excess food. Let us examine the sense of Taste.

The location of taste buds

Attached to the hyoid bone at the back, the tongue is free at the tip, surface, side and part of undersurface. Interposed with much fat and supplied by vessels and nerves, the tongue is made up of muscular fibers in various directions. The tongue has three layers: outer epithelial layer, inner mucous layer and innermost sub-mucous fibrous layer; along the midline a fibrous septum divides the tongue into two symmetrical halves whose surface is studded with tiny projections of mucous membrane.

The presence of 8-12 large papillae gives a rough texture to the tongue's back third. Near the tongue's base, circumvallate papillae form an inverted V, with a row of papillae on each side. Shaped like a truncated cone, each papilla's smaller end is attached to the tongue, the broader part projecting on the surface. The presence of small filiform, fungiform and simple papillae gives a velvety texture to the tongue's anterior two thirds. Filiform papillae's cells are long, thin and thread-like. At tongue's side and apex are numerous mushroom-shaped fungiform papillae. On the tongue's entire surface there are simple papillae, microscopic elevations of the corium, with a papillary loop covered by a layer of epithelium.

The exact position of taste buds: Taste buds are buried in the epidermis of larger filiform, fungiform and circumvallate papillae. Circumvallate papillae have over 200 taste buds, but filiform and barrel-shaped taste buds contain only a few. With long cells, a large nucleus and a hair cell, taste buds sit on their broad base and are interspersed with supporting cells grouped into 40-60 elements. At the gustatory pore converge the cells' innumerable hair-like filaments.

How food elicits taste sensation; taste protects: When food enters the mouth, sensory nerve fibers at the bottom of taste buds, bring the message by cranial nerves

7, 9 or 10, to the medulla obblongata's solitary nucleus. Motor nerves convey the message back to blood vessels of taste buds, eliciting a flow of blood to the capillary network, resulting in a taste sensation. With a lifespan of 10 days, taste buds are replaced by new cells. To elicit taste sensation, a substance must be dissolved. Dilute foods elicit a small flow of blood to capillaries, concentrated foods induce a large blood flow. In fever, sudden blood flow to the capillaries of taste-buds may be intense, causing pain. To prevent pain in fever, eat very dilute foods or pick at foods.

It is dangerous not to perceive taste. Taste sensation warns us of biologically significant objects: food, water, poisons, preserving from ingestion of fatal or toxic substances.

Immediate action after swallowing poisonous substances: If inadvertently a mouthful of cleaning fluid or other poison is swallowed, drink a cup of cold milk. Then induce vomiting. In the upright position bend over the toilet bowl and put a tongue depressor or a finger in the back of the tongue or scrape with a toothbrush to induce regurgitation.

Different taste sensations perceived: When the tongue is moved around taste sensation is sharper. Humans perceive four fundamental taste sensations: **sweet, sour, bitter** and **salty**, sometimes the alkaline and metallic tastes can also be sensed. Combinations of one or other fundamental taste sensations are also experienced. The tip and forepart of tongue perceive sweet and salty foods; taste buds on the side are sensitive to sourness. The back of tongue and epiglottis sense bitterness. The central portion of tongue arouses no taste sensation. Food edibility and digestion are affected by taste sensation. Sweetness is detected in a dilution of one part in 200, saltiness, one in 400, sourness, one in 130,000, bitterness, one in 2 million.

Taste perception and disease: Disease can damage taste perception. At age 45 taste buds begin to atrophy, diminishing steadily beyond age 70. The ingestion of drugs, caffeine, smoking, reduce acuity of taste sensations. Taste sensation is less sharp when the nose is held or if affected with a cold. Very hot or very cold foods may temporarily arrest taste sensation. Food or drink near or slightly below body temperature elicits optimum taste sensation. To preserve taste sensation, avoid dry, creamy, fatty and concentrated foods. To rid accumulated wastes and preserve taste sensation for a lifetime adopt a fruit diet or fast occasionally.

Ten thousand times more acute than man's sense of taste is the sense of smell found in the nose. Dangerous odors can combine with red blood cells' hemoglobin, prevent their oxygen-carrying capacity and deplete air from body tissues, causing rapid death.

The sense of smell: its exact location

A bony septum, the bridge, divides the nose into two equal halves. From the bony wall three parallel spurs of bone project outward, incompletely dividing each septum into four passages. Bony shelves, these conchae or turbinate bones are covered by mucous membrane. The three lower passages conduct air, communicating nostrils with the pharynx (part of digestive tract between mouth and esophagus). Olfactory receptors are mostly found in a blind pocket on the topmost shelf, embedded in a small patch of epithelium about 2.5 cm. square. The middle concha has other patches of olfactory epithelium; 10 square centimeters of membrane-like tissue with a sense of smell are present on the entire nasal surface. Externally, the sense organs of smell are roughly located close to the brain, between the eyes.

Sense organs of smell: their cellular structure

Two kinds of cells characterize the olfactory epithelium's mucous membrane. Long, yellowish supporting cells without cilia and slender, spindle-shaped olfactory cells with a large, round nucleus. Throughout the entire thickness of the olfactory epithelium extend blood vessels and branched tubular Bowman's glands. To reach the surface, thick cylindrical dendrites of olfactory cells individually penetrate small gaps between supporting cells. The 6-12 hairs of each cell form a continuous covering on the mucous membrane's surface. Hairs are kept moist by secretions of Bowman's glands.

In the mucous membrane, axons of ten million olfactory cells combine in groups, forming a number of slender bundles called fila olfactoria. Passing through perforations on the skull's floor, they penetrate the olfactory bulb where nerve fibers end in basket-like clusters called glomeruli. A glomerulus receives impulses from about 26,000 receptor cells sent through 24 mitral cells and 68 tufted cells. On their way to the olfactory center at the brain's base, most mitral cell axons pass into the lateral olfactory tract. The majority of tufted cells cross over to the olfactory bulb of the opposite side.

How smell is perceived

When an odor stimulates olfactory cells, the message is sent to the brain's olfactory bulb. Returned by motor nerve cells along the same route, the message ends on the sphincter muscle of tiny blood capillaries supplying olfactory mucous membrane, eliciting a flow of blood and the odor is perceived.

Humans are very sensitive to odors. They either give rise to a feeling of enjoyment or of aversion that can alter the affective state. Temperature and humidity affect an odor's strength but smell receptors adapt rapidly and cease to respond to a particular stimulus. Man distinguishes thousands of odors, generally classified into a few groups: ethereal (fruity), fragrant (flowers), resinous, spicy, putrid (foul), burnt. In Japan's 1978 Symposium of food and Chemical Sense, the following primary odors were established: **sweaty, spermous, fishy, malty, urinous** and **musky**.

As indicated by their structural formula, odors are amines, aldehydes or ketones, aliphatic compounds. Odors are of a polyhydric nature, compounds formed by oxidation of alcohols, easily reduced to alcohols in an airtight atmosphere. Several alcohols combine to form ether. When inhaled, brain cells can rapidly become unconscious. When ether, chloroform or ammonia is inhaled, a hysterical attack results. One young girl died when she slept in a roomful of lilies. A young officer slept his last slumber in an alcove decorated with twigs of laurel rose.

Odors, their danger. When sick or weak do not sleep in a roomful of flowers. Some people are addicted to the smell of certain substances. German poet Schiller kept a drawer full of rotten apples at his writing desk—he enjoyed the smell. Complex ethers in roses, violets, jasmin or lilac, exert a powerful effect on both vascular and nervous systems.

Asphyxia may occur when increased carbon dioxide fills the atmosphere by chemical decomposition. Perfumes and aromas cause nausea, regurgitation, vertigo, convulsions and dysentery. In a closed room, strong body odor causes nausea. Certain food smells can cause nausea and diarrhea. Cardiac failure can be attributed to certain scents. Though body odor is usually associated with hirsute persons, certain people have natural body scents. History recalls that Alexander the Great's tunics were soaked in his own body scent while Walt Whitman's body had a naturally perfumed scent. Natural body scent can be attributed to an excellent formation during growth years.

Not everyone is endowed with a good sense of smell. There was a cook who could not smell a bad egg! Others are insensitive to coal gas. In general, darker-skinned peoples have a keener sense of smell. Some are born insensitive to smell, others are totally genetically deprived of the sense of smell, the equivalent of being blind or deaf. A loss of the sense of smell affects taste sensation and everyone has experienced it during a bad cold. At one of our best hallowed colleges, some young men put feces on the lunch plate of a classmate who had an atrophied sense of smell; the young man ate it, all the while wondering and asking what it was!

Today many household items are made of synthetic fabric. One woman purchased a Japanese shoji screen. It emitted such a strong smell she couldn't fall asleep. She dumped it. Plastics can cause allergies.

Breath odor may indicate certain diseases: Some diseases are detectable by breath odor. A sweet-smelling breath characterizes the later stages of diabetes and the plague. There is a mawkish odor in typhus, the smell of smallpox is horrible. Rheumatism smells acrid and a smell of mice is detectable in favus, a skin disease. Between lovers, sweetness of breath is very important. Women have used perfume, flowers and jasmine to attract their husbands. Aroma therapy is effective, and there is less desire to eat when the central nervous system has been satisfied by a smell. Others have fasted for days by smelling jars of different foods. Those who prepare and cook large quantities of food for others, eat

sparingly because they smell the food during the preparation.
Advancing age and the sense of smell. With advancing age, the acuity of the sense of smell deteriorates. Dilute foods, partial fasting can help maintain an acute olfactory sense for a lifetime.

Our skin is a very sensitive cloak. Sense organs of touch are in the skin's dermis. Scattered over the entire skin's surface are over half a million touch spots, they enable us to feel qualities of hardness, softness, roughness, smoothness, etc. When skin is gently brushed with a wisp of cotton wool or pressed with a stiff hair, the sensation of touch is felt.

The various sense organs of touch

Meissner's corpuscles and Krause's end bulbs transmit touch sensations. Numerous on skin's undersurface, they are most abundant on the tip of tongue, fingers and mucous surfaces of lips, nipples, vagina and penis—in every square millimeter of skin; corpuscles are in clusters of two or three.

On the windward side of hairs, close to the epidermis, in dermal papillae, lie Meissner's corpuscles. Shaped like an onion cut in half, they appear layered, covered by a thin capsule of connective tissue. About 100 milli-microns long, in sensitive areas of skin; sometimes as many as ten touch spots can be found.

Krause's end bulbs are minute cylindrical or oval bodies with a capsule containing a soft, semi-fluid core. Both Meissner's corpuscles and Krause's end bulbs are present in the eye's conjunctiva, the mucous membrane of lips and tongue, the epineurium of nerve trunks and finger joints. Directly connected with parasympathetic nervous ganglia controlling blood flow to sex organs, they are mostly associated with erotic sensation.

Entwined around roots of hairs are special hair follicle receptors—Pacini corpuscles. Varying from 0.2-1 mm. in diameter, they respond to pressure, touch and vibration. Embedded in the dermis' deep fatty tissue, they are numerous in fingers, clitoris and penis. The palm of the hand has over 300 clusters of Pacini corpuscles. Shaped like an onion cut in half, its nerve endings are enclosed in layers of connective tissue and Schwann cells.

Greatly sensitive touch receptors are the slowly adapting Merkel's discs. Barely visible to the eye, forked like the letter Y, with two discs balancing on the apices, Merkel's discs are about 0.2-0.4 mm. diameter. More complex in hairy skin, abundant on the neck and abdomen, they project in the dermis and lie in dome-shaped corpuscles like a papilla. In hairy skin, Merkel's discs comprise several twigs with discs at each end.

In the dermis' lower layers lie Ruffini's corpuscles, oval-shaped with a bar within and an expanded tip. They respond to deformation.

Fifty percent of dermal nerve endings are free nerve endings. Directly in connection with internal organs they are unmyelinated postganglionic nerve fibers, blood vessel constrictors and dilators. Many skin receptors transmit, without a nerve cell, messages by axon reflexes, passing from one receptor nerve down another branch, onto a blood vessel, dilating or constricting it, thus affecting blood flow.

Also in the dermis are found myelinated free nerve endings. They are cold or warm spots, temperature receptors. More numerous are cold spots, about 16-19 cold points in each square centimeter of the face. On the hand, 1-5 cold spots per square centimeter, to 0.4 warm spots. In the hand, cold spots are at a depth of 0.18 mm., warm receptors at a depth of 0.3 mm. They participate in the regulation of body temperature. Each square millimeter of skin has around 50 receptors. Each receptor receives only one kind of sensation but in mechanical stimulation, several receptors are simultaneously stimulated to different degrees while the sensation cannot be ascribed to a particular receptor.

When closely stimulated, some areas of skin can distinguish two points to immediately note the size, texture and shape of objects. From tip of tongue and other mucous surfaces through fingertips, underside of skin, back of body, heel of foot, there is a decreasing ability to discriminate two points.

How touch sensation is transmitted: When skin is stimulated, the sensation is transmitted to the brain. Motor nerve cells bring the message to nerve endings at entrance of a muscle capillary network and blood flows to the area. Light touch elicits a small blood flow, resulting in itch. As more sense organs are stimulated, pain is felt, indicating that with continued stimulus, tiny blood vessels will soon burst as so many blood cells are flowing through them.

Blood flow through skin: Every minute a liter of blood flows through skin but when all sense organs of skin are stimulated, blood flow can rise to 10 liters. When trapped in a burning high rise, small wonder people prefer jumping to death than be burned alive. Skin's sense organs warn us of impending danger, for excess stimuli draw blood to the skin, depleting blood flow through regulatory organs, with impending death. Warm spots preserve the body from cold or burn.

Cold warns us to dress more warmly for abnormal cell division can occur. Every 45 days the entire epidermis regenerates, cell division or mitosis lasts 60-90 minutes. Cold hands or feet indicate inadequate blood flow through the region. Itch may indicate the need for warmer clothing or better cleansing. Itch always precedes pain. When pain is felt, abnormal cell division is taking place. Avoid rough, tight fabrics for underwear; soft knitted cotton should touch bare skin. Wear wool over soft cotton or silk garments all year round. At 80° F. wear woven silk; knitted silk and wool fabric is good for all seasons.

Importance during growth, sense organ stimulation

A child deprived of maternal love becomes a misfit in society while a child loved by parents will be an outstanding adult. Ashley Montagu believed that for the human infant, breast-feeding is a fundamental requirement. These children become superior adults. In all measured physical traits, infants fed with artificial products ranked lowest.

Stimulation of skin's sense organs is extremely important. There are national and cultural differences in tactility. England's upper classes maintain absolute non-touchability. Latin-speaking peoples, Russians and some other peoples give full expression of affection through touch whereas Jewish and Asian people express deep affection and care for their children. The case of Helen Keller is proof that when all other sense organs fail, skin's sense organs provide awareness of the world around us.

Beneficial effect of touch, massage. The privilege of touching with hands was ascribed to the kings of France. Touched by King Saint Louis, scrofula patients observed a seven-day fast, drank water and were cured of their illness.

Stimulation of skin's sense organs invigorates health. It has been known throughout the ages that massage stimulates Pacinian corpuscles—directly connected with sympathetic and parasympathetic ganglia; these ganglia control blood flow to internal organs. In Bosnia, the practice is to rub vigorously with pressure to restore displaced organs back to their proper places. Another practice is slow massage from brow over back of head, neck, shoulders, arms, trunks, legs and heels cures arthritis, rheumatism, muscular and neuralgic pain. Hippocrates believed a physician should be experienced in rubbing. Rub upwards, advised Hippocrates. Hard rubbing binds, soft rubbing loosens. Some massage techniques are stroking, kneading, friction, tapping, hacking, clapping, beating, pounding. Pinching and digging deeply into muscle are other beneficial strokes. Wave-like massage stimulates intestinal movements, gentle tapping, hacking, pummeling activate regulatory organs.

Sense organs of touch in later life. Safeguard all sense organs. With advancing age, touch sensitivity decreases. The tiny encapsulated sense organs decrease in sensitivity, pricking pain lessens but tolerance for superficial pain rises: may be due to fatigue or getting used to a diminished numbers of capillaries, lessening the capacity to respond to a stimulus.

Allow gentle stimuli for sense organs: dim lighting, subdued music/noise, mild food/scents. Avoid sauna baths, icy/hot showers where water beats on skin, concentrated juices, large pieces of meat, heavy fried or concentrated foods, intense massage. Mild stimuli won't damage sense organs. To prevent inhalation of noxious fumes or odors, do not hold breath but breathe through the mouth. Holding breath can cause fainting. Once in a while, remove the hard bugger in nostrils: it will ease breathing. Do it in private, however.

Chapter 11
Control fatigue, emotion, pain and live a long life

Different types of fatigue
In the Middle Ages the average lifespan was 20 years. Today it is 70 years. People have been known to have lived 160 years, Methuselah lived 800 years. Improved living conditions should allow a longer life, but modern living stresses result in cardiac vascular diseases. In the U.S., each year 7,000 hospitals admit 30 million patients; more than 40 thousand children are born with a defective heart.

These conditions are due to the fast pace of living; plants and animals show that we must relax. Work hours are reduced to a 40-hour workweek—still excessive. The seat of fatigue is in the brain that directs us to work. When blood is driven through an active organ, mental or physical energy is expended. The larger the size of the organ performing work, the greater the number of blood cells destroyed, depleting regulatory organs of an optimum blood supply. When fatigued, all organs are affected, with the following ill effects: loss of appetite, slow digestion, constipation, intestinal disturbances with eventual random tumor formation.

<u>Examples of passive fatigue</u>: jolting of cars or trains, plane rides, the sight of huge, towering structures, rapid moving pictures and objects, loud noise or music, insistent sirens of ambulances, fire-trucks, honking of cars, etc. Emotions are as tiring: grief, worry, crying, affecting the brain, provoking muscular exhaustion, slowing down body functions. Work conditions cause fatigue: sitting without a backrest or standing; the danger is in static stationary stance when the same muscles are constantly contracted, standing or sitting without a backrest, expends a continuous muscular effort.

Some people are intrinsically weak, feeling intense fatigue with the slightest exertion. After a marathon race, one boy stayed away from school for two years. Another man's pulse was 92 when lying down, 144 when standing. He was discharged from the army. Some of us are naturally weak and expending energy is a trying feat. Concentrated physical activity is even more tiresome. Much blood is consumed in creative work: sewing, writing, composing music, knitting, crocheting, painting, etc. The amount of fatigue can be assessed by the size of the active organ. The larger the organ in active use, the greater the force and speed of action, the greater the fatigue experienced.

Activities dangerous to health are: cold showers, massage, sauna baths, indoor exercise without air, heavy outdoor sports. Excess physical exertion produces abundant carbonic acid, removable from blood only by breathing freely. The following activities are tiresome: excessive social affairs, nights at the theatre, dining out. The worst type of fatigue are long hours of fast, intense work in an airtight atmosphere. It increases body temperature and fatigue causes one to tremble with cold. Those who experienced extreme fatigue have been affected by insomnia, dizziness, woe even despair. Rest and relax. Five minutes rest in an armchair does wonders.

All activity destroys red blood cells. In our industrial age, working hours should be reduced to 6 hours a day. Surveys have shown that production increased with reduced working hours. Less working hours allow more hours for play and time to develop a hobby in preparation for retirement. In turn, it lessens aggressiveness and eradicates violence. Our age of violence is stirred by the increased crowding of cities and competition for material possessions.

Factors causing fatigue. Several factors may cause fatigue. Blood flow is impaired if body's glycogen stores are exhausted. Due to their higher myoglobin content dark red muscles are more resistant to fatigue.

The more tired a muscle, the more phosphate is released. In lack of oxygen, phosphate accumulates, but blood vessels can be stimulated to relax and cause hyperaemia (blood congestion). In heavy physical exertion, the most immediate cause of fatigue is the shifting of blood volume to muscles. In strenuous work, splanchnic region organs, kidneys, lungs, endocrine glands, heart, receive a reduced blood supply. The less oxygen breathed in, the faster fatigue develops. Oxygen is required to remove lactic acid produced during contraction. In overworked muscles, avoid jerky movements and vigorous contraction. Rest between contractions; insufficient relaxation causes fatigue; during heavy exertion pause 10 minutes per hour. A tired person has increased sensitivity; he is morally sensitive and is physically and morally depressed. Work performed strenuously without movement is more tiring than if done with movement, where weight and effort are shifted.

Combating fatigue: Eat light: soups and light mixtures of foods; avoid pastries, cookies, cakes, heavy starches, soda, overcooked foods. Remain silent and work in silence. In a noisy atmosphere use earplugs. It saves energy and allows hard work without detrimental effects. Many workplaces play detrimental music on the radio all day long. Silence at work expends less energy, promotes continued health, youthfulness and thereby, stirs longevity. We are often subjected to powerful emotions. Many volumes have been written about primitive experiences man shares with lower animals: hunger, fear, anger and rage. Understanding has advanced, yet doubt exists concerning the exact way powerful emotions affect us.

Powerful emotions affect the organism. Powerful emotions always rouse us through one of the principal sense organs: the eyes, ears, skin. What stimulates a sense organ can act as a powerful emotional trigger: a shape, a contact, an odor, a noise stir fear, anger or rage.

A sense organ is the direct terminal of a brain center: brain, sympathetic or parasympathetic ganglia. A powerful stimulus striking a sense organ involves conscious effort of the entire brain and ganglia. Due to the head's basketball-size, powerful emotion uses up energy: blood; therefore, energy=blood. The brain being highly vascularized, while the emotion lasts, blood will forcibly be driven through the head. Since a human body contains around 5 liters of blood, in powerful emotion, at least two liters of blood may be driven through brain vessels. When strenuous effort strikes an area, remaining parts of the body are depleted of an optimum blood supply. Immediately visible are surface manifestations: pallor, cold sweat, arrested saliva flow, rapid heartbeat, dilation of pupils, hurried respiration and muscle twitching.

Dangerous effects of powerful emotion. Scientific data indicate that during powerful emotion the sexual instinct is repressed. Pregnant women have had spontaneous abortions. Digestion is immediately arrested. Blood clots faster and urine increased in sugar content. Sudden intense emotion galvanizes body functions and cases of sudden blindness, deafness and convulsions, overnight gray hair have occurred. Strong emotion may stir asphyxia and in a weak patient, delay recovery, so much blood being driven to the brain, preventing an adequate flow to regulatory organs. In these instances sudden goiters have developed, and metabolic rate increased by 25% to 11.7% above normal.

Beneficial effects of music. Sudden emotion subjects the organism to imminent danger, but slight emotion acts as a spur to creative activity, increased alertness and effort. Music causes this beneficial emotion. When obliged to display energy, bodily changes automatically provided greater effectiveness. Martial music stirs troops into battle. The ancient Romans sounded trumpets. Germans were spurred into action by drums, flutes, cymbals and clarions. Music raised pulse rate from 74 to 124 per minute. In battle, music stirred the mind into activity, providing strength to fight or fortitude to continue with a fierce exertion.

Anxiety and fear affect the organism. Medical science has often belittled the importance of anxiety and fear. In diagnosing a condition anxiety and fear must be regarded as emotional elements in disease and brought out. One must always inquire whether there has been emotionally disturbing factors: sudden deaths, loss of money, being robbed, etc. In illness, no question is too embarrassing to ask and the cause of a condition can rapidly be pinpointed.

Robbed of her purse, one woman had great pain in both kidneys and was unable to walk for several days. Realizing the damage, she rested, drank juices and fasted. In time her body began to function normally again. Strong emotional excitement depletes all organ-systems of an optimum blood supply. Relax. Recline in an armchair and lean back. Light food eases digestion, providing more energy to other body parts, particularly regulatory organs. Until the condition improves, avoid physical exertion and creativity.

Healthful feeling to fear death. Fear death: it stirs the desire for self-improvement and sometimes complete recovery from an otherwise incurable condition has occurred. One terminally ill woman had been on a strict diet ever since her illness was detected. Whenever her condition worsened, she adopted a liquid diet. She believed she will live quite a long time in spite of her condition.

Jealousy and envy affect the organism. Jealousy and envy may cause dizzy spells, headaches. A dearly loved child will never be jealous. Laughter and happiness lessen sorrow and anger. Take advantage of comic situations on TV. Laughter eases tension in the family and with oneself. Living alone can be beneficial: it compels one to remain silent all day. Some people frighten you for fun—a dangerous prank. One young woman died of cancer before age 20. Her young husband used her as a toy, often throwing her over his shoulder. Brought up in the marine, he had similar training and continued the practice with his wife. It frightened her to death. Prior to her demise her unborn infant was removed from her womb.

Some men frighten their wives for no reason. Stop! Should we frighten those we love? Hopefully no one will frighten a loved one or anyone else, for fun.

Besides fatigue and emotion, pain shortens life with a deleterious effect on the organism. According to Sir Thomas Lewis, every attempt to define pain has served no purpose and the mechanism of pain remains a mystery. Solving the effects of pain would soothe some conditions for pain exerts a damaging effect on heart, lungs, kidneys, endocrine glands and skin.

Pain can be understood as capillary distension. Pain can be defined as follows. When the hand is gently stroked with a feather, itch is felt. Press it further with a pencil and pain is felt. In the first instance a few red cells flow through blood vessels of the stimulated area and itch is felt. By pressing further with a pencil, increasing the stimulus, so many red cells rush through blood vessels of the area where itch turns into pain. Further pricking with the pencil tip causes acute pain as blood cells force their way through tiny vessels. One will scream with pain. If allowed to continue, pain will destroy walls of tiny vessels of the stimulated area. Before this happens however, we will run away from painful situations to preserve blood vessels from further damage. Since the living body can be subjected to an enormous array of stimuli, pain can be felt in four main ways:

1. **When the body performs an action.**
2. **When something is done to the body.**
3. **When an object penetrates the body.**
4. **When something leaves the body.**

Painful stimuli can be divided into *local pain* for small areas, and *systemic pain* for large regions, immediately affecting regulatory organs. Pain-transmitting fibers are nerve endings attached to blood vessels, and pain fibers are present where capillaries are found. Only stimulation of nerve endings on pre-capillary sphincters expand or close tiny capillaries. Painful sensations perceived are either bright, pricking, or burning pain on body surface. Deep pain is an aching pain, a nauseous pain.

1. Pain when the body performs an action: A heavy package held in hands will eventually cause pain—blood vessels fill up with blood when a package is held, the heavier the package, the more blood cells flow through capillaries. When the package becomes weighty, one can bear it no longer as blood cells cannot flow sufficiently fast through tiny vessels, forcing one to drop the package. If one continues to hold the package, the tiny blood vessels may break into a million bits and the hand may become impotent. Only insensitivity will stir one to continue holding the package. Due to the limited number of blood vessels, there is a limit to bodily activities. Excess action will detrimentally affect the organ involved and later, the regulatory organs due to blood deviation and depletion. Especially detrimental is hitting a ball with a heavy bat or racket. He who plays tennis or baseball does not do himself service. Soon they realize the blood capillaries will be destroyed, reducing sensitivity for fine work. A better game would be Badminton or Ping-Pong.

2. Pain from something done to the body. When skin is lightly touched with a feather, itch is felt. When heat, cold or pressure increases the stimulus, pain occurs. Pain here is again due to capillary distension. To maintain the increased metabolism in the stimulated area, more blood cells are required. Due to the limited number of blood vessels of the region, blood cells cannot flow sufficiently fast and pain intensifies. Instinctively man recoils from intense pain for regulatory organs will be the next affected organs. This explains why one screams with pain when it is intense.

In 1887, Dr. Clinton Dent stated that when weak or sickly, slight sounds or degrees of light are unbearable. Pain warns us of possible protein inactivation with irreversible damage to body cells. In intense pain a region or organ can become impotent, capillary distension is so great that vessel walls may burst.

Bright light, loud noise, loud music, heavy noxious smells, bitter or strong-tasting food, fire, also affect the body. Shield yourself from detrimental stimuli. In ancient times, torture inflicted on prisoners involved either pain on the skin (burning with red hot iron), blinding lights, deafening noise, quartering, skinning. The prisoner may faint, become blind, deaf or die.

    a. **Coping with a sudden deep bruise:** A sudden bruise is the most common type of pain. Care for it immediately otherwise it will become black and blue or, in poor circulation, develop a tumor. Rub the bruise. Rub gently until the bruise turns pink. Rub again five minutes later until normal color resumes. It is usually advised to place ice on a deep bruise—not a healthy practice. Ice lowers body temperature. A better alternative would be to run pleasantly hot water on a bruise until it turns pink.

b. **A sudden burn:** A sharp burn from spattering oil can stir skin growth. A young woman was frying food when oil spattered onto her face. She experienced a burn but did not attend to it. Shortly after, a little growth above her eyelid became noticeable. After five months only did she pick at it and remove it. When suddenly burned on the face, arm or hand, rub immediately to activate circulation and prevent abnormal growth formation. Burns on large areas of the body require complete rest. Leave the burn alone, eat light and healing will be more rapid.

c. **Coping with a cut:** If a cut is small, cover it with a band-aid. Leave it alone a few days then remove it when retiring at night. When the cut is deep, doctors prefer to sew up a wound, cut or gash. Sewing up wounds leaves a long scar. Cover it with a large piece of gauze and adhesive. It will soon heal by itself. While washing dishes one day, a young man cut his hand. Though wrapped up it didn't stop bleeding and the school doctor proceeded to sew it up while a team of nurses watched the operation. Today this young man has a long scar on his hand. Never allow a wound to be sewn up but let it heal naturally.

d. **Coping with a burn on mucous membrane:** A burn on the mucous membrane will most probably induce a tumor growth. This could happen at the anus. Do not be alarmed if blood appears in stools or if a tumor develops. Normal people have had blood in stools from straining during elimination. Tumor tissue is not dead tissue and can expand. A light diet is recommended for the rest of life. Better cooking techniques can improve the diet and in turn, improve the condition. After surgery on a rectal tumor, the anal sphincter is frequently sewn up, requiring a colostomy where only small amounts of stools leave the body. One woman had surgery on a rectal tumor. After a few months she realized too late that she should not have had the operation: she died shortly after. Another woman has a tumor in the rectum for 20 years and is still alive. King Louis XIV was the first king who had a surgical operation of a growth on the rectum; he survived.

Fear is instilled in the patient when some abnormality occurs: rectal tumor, breast tumor, brain tumor, etc. Surgical excision of tumors provide little survival chance, a few months, at most five years. Since death is inevitable perhaps it would be better to leave it alone and instead, control the diet. Rubbing can cure a breast tumor. Rub daily, four or five times, five minutes at a time and you will soon feel the tumor diminish and disappear with time.

A brain tumor is due to non-removal of wax in the ear. Learn to use an ear-picker or have a surgeon vacuum the wax periodically. Meanwhile, rub the head. Adopt a starch-free, fiber-free diet and soon it will subside and disappear. There are many cases of brain tumors in the U.S. No need to despair. A dilute diet with frequent stool evacuation will rapidly improve the condition. An internal tumor is always wet. It is easy to deal with internal growths. Rubbing increases circulation while a light diet will help a growth to disappear.

Two organs should never be subjected to the knife: the heart and the brain; and do not tamper with vital organs like kidneys and endocrine glands.

Tumors in the digestive tract are usually surgically removed by cutting off a large segment of the digestive tract. Resection of the stomach causes multiple nutritional deficiencies. About 95% of patients suffering from stomach cancer die from it. In resection of the duodenum, pancreatic and bile secretions are introduced at different sites of the tract. Resection of the distal ileum decreases absorption of vitamin B12 and bile salts, causing secondary anemia. Large resections of the small intestines give rise to gastric hyper-secretion with diarrhea and loss of nutrients. Surgery is dangerous. Resection of the esophagus is followed by diarrhea and excess fat in stools; 15-30 minutes after a meal, the patient experiences gastric distress known as the dumping syndrome where stomach contents rapidly empty into the small intestine causing weakness and sweating. This is a warning to not subject the body to surgery, alter the diet instead.

   e. **Coping with back pain:** We have mentioned that living organisms are attached to the ground. In bed, we are tied to our mattress, which is not warm. No wonder people have back pains. Most mattresses are made of coils of metal padded with horsehair, yet we will cover ourselves with wool blankets, eiderdown quilts, etc. Place a 100% cotton comforter above the mattress. In winter, wrap a shawl around the waist at night or place a down pillow under the back. Many vital organs are at waist level. Many clothes expose at the waist. Wear a long dress or robe — superior to pants or skirts. Avoid bare wood, metal, cement or marble furniture. These materials draw heat away from the body, which can cause colds/influenza/bronchitis. Use cushions on sofas/chairs. Unless in the sun, don't let a body, even clad, from contacting these materials. Never buy iron, cement or marble furniture for your home. Body heat is rapidly lost and illness will strike.
   f. **Pain when hit on the head:** Rub the head immediately and eat a light diet. In the 8th century a beautiful 19-year old girl was hit on the head by a ball. She died in a week. When hit on the head, rub the head immediately until pain disappears and rest. A semi-liquid diet should help the pain to subside.

3. Pain experienced when something penetrates the body. When a foreign object penetrates the body, intense pain is felt from laceration of the region and excessive demands upon the regulatory organs. To prevent infection, remove a foreign body

How to Live a Long Life

immediately otherwise internal organs may be detrimentally affected.

A splinter is an example of local pain. Remove it immediately but do not panic if it cannot exit easily. In a few days, skin cells will push the foreign object to the surface and the splinter will drop out miraculously.

a. Pain from blood-poisoning

Blood poisoning may develop if a cut or wound is improperly treated. When the poison reaches the upper part of the body pain is felt. Physicians may proceed to amputate a limb which may not be necessary. Adopt a liquid diet immediately. Circulation will improve and poisons will leave the system. Diet is most important. A light diet enables white blood cells to proliferate and engulf the foreign matter. Soak the affected limb in peroxide water. Penicillin injections can help. Understand the condition and help yourself immediately.

A 30-year old woman had pain from blood-poison due to an improperly covered wound on her foot. Told to soak her foot in peroxide water, a nurse gave her penicillin injections. In a short time, the poison concentrated itself at her foot but could not leave her body, the wound being closed. Spraying liquid CO_2, on the wound, the hospital physician made an incision on her foot and removed the pus. Her leg was saved. In blood-poison we must try everything possible before opting for amputation.

Acute infection is more dangerous than A.I.D.S., syphilis or gonorrhea. If infection is improperly treated the limb must be amputated. Try to prevent the infection from reaching the heart. If the limb must be amputated, adopt a juice diet for a few days to see if the infection disappears. In an acid diet, bacteria or viruses will not grow. White blood cells will proliferate and rapidly kill these foreign microorganisms. The limb will be saved.

When a wound is red, swollen and painful, acute infection is present. Use a topical disinfectant, paste and liquid, over sterile gauze and wrap the wound. Never let an infected wound touch unsterile material or dry up. If body hair is around a wound, shave it off so that the gauze and tape will securely cover wound. Never let the wound dry up. As long as the wound is open, white blood cells will move to the area and kill the bacteria. This is indicated by pus. Pus is dead white blood cells with ingested bacteria. It is a good sign. If a scab forms and the infection is still present, go to the doctor. The scab indicates that the wound is healing over the infection and when the scab drops off, blood poisoning will occur. It is all right if a scab forms and the wound is still open, white blood cells will move to the area and engulf the bacteria again. Only when the red swelling has disappeared and abundant pus is present, is the infection out of danger. It is so important not to expose the infection to air but to keep it wet with disinfectant, covered and secured with gauze.

Do as directed by the physician who prescribes antibiotics in pill form and indicates how many times topical disinfectant must be changed. A liquid disinfectant and a paste-like disinfectant can be used together. Eat a light diet and soon pus will appear at site of wound. The above must be followed to the letter because: White blood cells do not have a brain. They will only move to an open wound. A dry wound will soon close up the cut and white blood cells will no longer work their way to the infection's site. Bacteria will move upwards in the body, prevent walking or other movement, the pain being powerful. Once the pain reaches the heart, one will die. Before that happens, a physician usually amputates the limb. When a 30-year old woman's pain had reached her hip, she went to the hospital; she was told to soak her foot and penicillin injections finally saved her from amputation.

This is a warning to everyone affected with an acute infection to care for the wound. A child must be made aware of its danger and an adolescent must care for it himself. His wound must be covered until it heals completely and the infection disappears. When it is open, it should not touch water. When bathing, prevent wetness with a plastic cover secured with two elastic bands. Only when a hard scab forms, drops off, and the redness or swelling has disappeared will the wound have healed completely.

b. Coping with appendicitis

When appendicitis is detected, immediate operation is suggested. If the infected appendix is caught on time the body can heal it. Varying one to nine inches in length, the blind appendix juts out from a sac-like pouch, the *caecum* and marks the beginning of the large intestine. It has a firm position in the abdomen. The appendix seems to serve no purpose but contains many lymphocytes, meaning that it may have a connection with the body's immune system. Sometimes hard feces, undigested material or tomato seeds, may fall into its cavity, causing inflammation.

The first symptom of inflammation is pain over the entire abdomen, localizing on the right side about six hours later, with nausea and vomiting feeling. At the first sign of pain avoid all solid foods and shun a cathartic. When the appendix is unable to empty its contents, edema, swelling and distension occur. A cathartic would increase pressure in the appendix, leading to bursting. Two glasses of hot water with one level tablespoonful of Kosher salt would cause a stool evacuation.

When blood vessels close up, the appendix swells excessively, leading to gangrene with bacteria proliferating in the blind sac-like pouch of the appendix. When the appendix ruptures, the pus pocket spills from intestine into the peritoneal cavity. Peritonitis develops with a very serious and often fatal condition.

Do not fear appendicitis or peritonitis for the living body has its own protective mechanisms. Often a sheet of fatty tissue, the omentum, wraps itself around the inflamed appendix. At the site of the inflammation, an exudate develops, acting like paste or glue with clot-forming properties of fibrin. Helped by the omentum, this exudate seals the appendix off from the surrounding peritoneal cavity to prevent spreading of intestinal contents into it. Instead of a generalized peritonitis, a ruptured appendix may be a simple abscess. When finally pain subsides, the appendicitis will have disappeared.

The appendix has peristaltic movements and with a light diet, it can expel its contents. Fasting and application of heat to the inflamed area will allow the abscess to subside. Hold a hot water bag over your abdomen. During the inflamed period, a juice or liquid diet with aspic or gelatine dishes, light custard, eases bowel movements and hastens healing.

An appendectomy is a small operation; but no part of the body should be removed. The appendix has lymphocytes to maintain the immune system in function. Avoid eating tomato seeds, grape seeds or any other small hard seeds. Eggplant seeds are soft and tiny—not harmful.

4. Pain when something desires to leave the body
a. A painful tooth. A painful tooth is a good example of something desiring to leave the body. A person usually runs to the dentist who extracts the tooth and upon extraction, shows you a beautiful tooth. It could have been saved. Here's how.

In slow digestion, stomach acid rises to the mouth, settling around roots of teeth, gnawing at the bony structure, developing tartar. When tartar accumulates, insufficient blood supplying gum capillaries causes pain. Intense pain makes a person run to the dentist for immediate extraction. Painful contractions warn you to remove the tartar, not the tooth.

During a very strong painful contraction, insert the scaler, lean over the bathroom sink and scrape. Some blood will drip in the sink. When the contraction disappears, stop scraping. Like at childbirth, wait for the next painful contraction. Use the scaler again and scrape. If painful contractions stop, do not use it again, and the tooth will be saved. It will be slightly weaker but it will be there, and you can use it as if nothing ever happened. This is an ingenious way to save a tooth.

b. Immediate action when several teeth are painful. Never let this happen for painful contractions destroy red blood cells rapidly and death can quickly ensue. When there is tartar in several teeth, only you can scrape it out. Scrape quickly for painful contractions are excruciating. This is a good example of a systemic pain in a large area—several teeth.

Two cases are known to us where women experienced such pain during the dental surgeon's treatment that both decided to have all their teeth extracted.

c. A fecal impact. Though uncommon, some people have suffered from this condition.

A young woman once attempted a lengthy fast but ate solid foods too quickly and suffered a fecal impact. She was unable to have a stool evacuation for a month. She realized she should not add more bulk to her diet, and for a month she ate only juices and clear soups. She then helped herself by using a surgical glove to remove the impacted feces, and gradually resumed a normal diet.

Coping with an excruciating headache

Besides the above four main types of pain, reflected pain can assail us and a headache is a good example of a systemic pain in a large region such as the large size of the head. Attend to it immediately. A headache is the reflection of over-activity in other large areas of the body: the rectum, muscles and bones, digestive overwork, excess stimuli bombarding sense organs. Stop the activity, quiet the body: the headache will subside. A stool evacuation is another cure.

Napoleon's sister, Pauline Borghese, often suffered from headaches. She spent most of her days reclined on a sofa. Pauline Borghese was her mother's sixth child; she lived 45 years. A weak constitution, an active social life, receiving guests, chatter, laugh, noise, can cause headaches.

A cure for headache is to drink fluids. Light coffee, broth, juices, increase blood volume and can prevent headaches. Another cure for headache is to tighten up the entire head to a tight tremolo, like a grrr... breathe deeply and let go. Like yawning, it is a creative way to cure a small headache, with instant results. Repeat it slowly, until the headache disappears. A nap is another solution: sleep is the simplest cure. Excess clothing can cause a headache.

Coping with pain from abnormal regeneration of cells

This pain assails cancer patients. To lessen needle-like pain from abnormal regeneration of cells, patients are given pain-killing drugs. There are natural ways to alleviate this pain.

Cells die and are regenerated constantly with no pain. Ingesting nutrients beyond the normal composition of blood causes abnormal regeneration of body cells. The most harmful is carbohydrates whose accumulation forms ether with high body temperature. In chemistry, carbohydrates turn into sugar, then alcohol, and finally, ether. In an environment of ether, abnormal cell regeneration occurs with needle-like pain.

Proteins are broken down into amino acids, then peptides, finally, peptones. In an environment of ether and peptones, normal regeneration cannot occur.

In cancer, feed yourself isotonically to normal values of blood or body composition and you should be able to lead a fairly normal life even though afflicted. When preparing foods, think about the normal values of blood: 7% protein, 92% water, 1 percent minerals, 0.1% carbohydrate. Or of the body: 75% water, 5% minerals and carbohydrates, 20% protein. The same may apply to growth pains. Feed children the same diet, and many illnesses can be averted.

How to be rid of a cramp

Sometimes a spasmodic contraction, a cramp, assails us involuntarily, causing intense pain. Physiology texts say that cramps are due to inadequate calcium ions in blood. We believe all cramps are due to overexertion. When several muscles contract at once blood cannot flow fast enough to several places at once resulting in terrific pain due to a lack of blood.

When experiencing a cramp do not cringe, do the opposite, relax. For an abdominal cramp, bend the body backwards. For a severe leg cramp, jump up immediately and stand on the leg. The cramp will dissipate. Don't let pain continue for a long time: muscle protein may be inactivated and muscles may become impotent.

The present theory of pain is in accordance with all previous theories of pain

The present theory of pain and capillary distension is in agreement with the following theories on pain:

Von Frey's theory of specificity designates free nerve endings as pain receptors. They are found where capillaries occur.

Goldsheider proposed the stimulation of sensory receptors of skin to provoke nerve impulses resulting in pain.

Wedell and Sinclair maintain that pain is produced by intense stimulation of non-specific receptors.

Melzack and Wall's gate control theory contends that a neural mechanism in dorsal horns of spinal cord acts as a gate, increasing or decreasing the flow of impulses from peripheral fibers to the central nervous system.

Chapter 12
Sleep deeply, prevent aging and prolong life

Due to a lack of understanding of the mechanism of sleep millions of people suffer from insomnia. Sleep problems can be solved only when its mechanism is understood.

The sleep mechanism, an ancient physician's impression
The ancient Greek physician Alcmeon had a very scientific-sounding explanation for the mechanism of sleep. He believed that when falling asleep, blood flows out from organs and pools in veins. Blood flows back to its proper place upon awakening. Alcmeon was correct in his visualization of the sleep mechanism but at that remote time in history, scarcely would he have been able to prove his point.

The mechanism of sleep revealed through research
During sleep blood fills the entire regulatory organs: heart, lungs, kidneys, skin and endocrine glands. Five liters of blood circulate in our blood vascular system of which two liters are red blood cells. These cells allow performance of daily activities: digestion, sex, exercising, speaking, singing, etc. As red cells pass through tiny capillaries, delivering oxygen to sustain the increased metabolism demanded by vital activities, blood cells die. The more powerful the action, the more cells die. Usually, we do not think of the effects of our actions on total blood volume, but when we relax, in the seated or horizontal position, we will soon fall asleep, Sleep occurs when muscles and bones relax. If your body were transparent, your blood can be seen concentrated in the heart, lungs, skin and endocrine glands to perform the process of regulation. This is visible in the transparent bodies of lower species: the butterfly, the snake, etc. (see Fig. 8)

Muscles and bones represent almost 50% of our total body weight. Blood is diverted to the muscles and bones when they are at work; when they relax, blood goes to irrigate inner parts of the body, especially the regulatory organs. Therefore, sleep occurs by a reflex action of the blood flow, where the relaxation of muscles and bones allows blood to fill the regulatory organs. On the other hand, when we work with our muscles and bones, blood is diverted to them again for work. Work in any of the other five systems will divert the blood flow away from the regulatory organs to supply any of the other systems.

Why does blood fill up the regulatory organs during sleep?
Blood fills up regulatory organs to regulate body fluids for growth and repair. Blood's physical and chemical properties are normally maintained at a fairly

constant level. During our work day, slight variations occur daily but within narrow limits. During a lifetime, our daily sleep regulates blood properties to maintain constancy of values.

On a publicity drive for the March of dimes, disc jockey Peter Tripp stayed awake for 200 hours. By the seventh day he became so confused that he saw swarms of worms around him. He had the impression that everyone was conspiring against him and mistook the physician for the undertaker! One full day's sleep restored him to normal. This shows the importance of sleep. Joseph Barcroft showed that when blood properties are altered, the brain is seriously affected. Sleep regulates homeostatic properties of the blood to maintain them within narrow limits and preserve normal brain function. Take man's body temperature. The normal daily variation is between 36.3° and 37.3° C.; 24° C. is not lethal but lower than compatible with life and activity. At 42-43° C. there is danger some nerve cells' proteins become coagulated.

All physical and chemical properties can be examined: sugar, protein, fat, water, sodium chloride, calcium, oxygen, internal secretions, osmotic pressure, temperature, acidity or pH. Walter Cannon's **The Wisdom of the Body**, analyzes every property of the blood with effects of variations.

Causes of insomnia

From the sleep mechanism, we can deduce that insomnia is the inability to fill blood vessels of all regulatory organs and glands due to blood's insufficient red cells, to begin the process of regulation.

Red blood cells die as they pass through tiny blood vessels of an active organ, to deliver oxygen to tissue cells. When too many red cells are destroyed, an insufficient quantity fills the regulatory organs which will prevent sleep at night. Excess activity during waking hours can cause insomnia. Let us analyze some activities performed daily.

Physical work requires the action of skeletal muscles which are almost 50% of total body weight. Blood is destroyed in heavy physical work. Singing and speaking when excessive, become dangerous. Creative activity, sewing, knitting: these activities drive blood to hands and brain, destroying many red cells and may lead to sleeplessness. Daytime, our eyes and ears are constantly active. Fortunately their small size prevents disruption of regulatory organs' automatic function. Excessive stimuli bombarding eyes and ears can destroy many red cells: be careful with the computer screen, TV, 100 Watt lamps, loud music, heavy machinery's grinding noise, subway trains, airplanes, zooming cars/buses, etc. Excessive stimuli bombarding sense organs destroy many red cells and may lead to insomnia.

Mental work requires concentration. Using the basketball-sized brain is detrimental to a weak person. Many composers lived short lives: Mozart, Chopin,

Field, Gershwin, etc. Music composition requires total concentration. If your head is large, refrain from excessive mental work, especially creative work. There is less danger if the head is smaller. If you must create music/art, assume better body position: lean the head back, lie in bed as did Rossini, use dim lights and turn the radio low. Silence is important.

Sexual activity destroys much blood. In the male a cupful of blood may be destroyed at orgasm. Women lose less blood. If you suffer from insomnia refrain from sex. Sexual activity during pregnancy disturbs the embryo's growth and mother's sleep.

It is better to not have many children. In pregnancy the digestive system is in a cramped position, disturbing digestion and sleep.

Comprising several large organs, our digestive system is 30 feet long—mouth, esophagus, stomach, small and large intestines. After a big meal the entire blood volume concentrates in the digestive tract. Excessive food disrupts the sleep mechanism. Limit yourself at meals and eat dinner before 6 PM drink light beverages until bedtime. Some foods prevent sleep. Tea and coffee contain caffeine. Refrain from stimulating drinks. At night, if you have difficulty falling asleep, analyze your daily activities and determine what excess activity was performed. If your sleep is not restful one day, do not engage in many activities the next day, and you will sleep well the next night.

Ensure a good night's sleep

A body must have a heart before a brain can be developed; these two organs are closely interrelated. To cause the blood to flow to the brain and other regulatory organs, one must quiet the body through relaxation; listen to a droning voice, watch a moving screen, or read light literature, these are conducive to the relaxation of the body, soon sleep will overtake you and sufficient blood will flow to the brain; the next organs to be flooded with blood are the regulatory organs: heart, lungs, kidneys, skin and endocrine glands.

Unless totally exhausted, rarely does one fall asleep in the standing position. In sleep the body is immobile; if uncovered and motionless, body temperature rapidly lowers; wear adequate clothes to cover from head to toe. In cold weather, cover with two wool blankets and/or a down comforter. Because blood must first be brought to the head before regulatory organs fill up, place a small down cover, the length of two pillows near the face and neck. Covering the neck rapidly brings on sleep. The head and neck are usually poorly covered during sleep.

Silence is important. The bedroom must not face a highway or be near a noisy train. Never place a bed under a window, regardless of how airtight closed it is. The best place for a bed is the most sheltered corner of the room preferably in an alcove like our forefathers had.

How to Live a Long Life

What if despite all previous precautions one yet cannot fall asleep?

In order to fall asleep and sleep soundly, one must have:
1. Daily fresh air and sunshine
2. An empty rectum
3. Tighten the body
4. Two hours of fresh air is recommended. Walk a mile a day.
5. The rectum contracts when it is full, it tells you to evacuate. Make sure you have a complete bowel movement and that the rectum is totally empty because when the rectum is full of feces, blood remains in rectal capillaries.
6. Tighten your entire body into a tight tremolo and soon sleep will overtake you. Tightening is shivering; like yawning, tightening brings blood to all internal organs. Birds twist their head before sleeping; twisting the head stimulates the breathing center, when breathing deepens, sleep is induced.

If you have difficulty falling asleep in the flat position, put a couple of pillows under the head for better breathing. Tenor Enrico Caruso slept surrounded by pillows. Newborn babies and terminally ill people have difficulty sleeping.

To help you fall asleep: wear a knitted undershirt, underpants and wool socks with a long-sleeved wool garb; cover with a fur blanket over a wool one; wear a fur vest; a wool or fur bonnet; don't expose any part of the body; wear gloves if necessary. Warmth induces sleep.

If I awaken in the middle of the night and can no longer sleep?

Many people drink a glass of milk, chat or listen to music. One woman prepared oatmeal to eat. Don't. Don't speak or eat. Actions divert blood to active regions, preventing blood from flowing to regulatory organs. The stronger the action, the more blood is diverted the more difficult it will be to resume sleep. Drink water and urinate. Read a little light literature; tighten body slowly several times and soon sleep will be induced.

Sometimes one word spoken out loud will keep you awake for the rest of the night. Speech is a higher manifestation of life, requiring muscles and bones, using up blood. To rest peacefully, refrain from speaking.

Awaken someone healthfully

On television we have often seen people pour a bucketful of water to awaken someone. Others are shaken up from their sleep, and family members shout from afar. These drastic awakening measures drive blood suddenly away from heart, lungs, kidneys, skin and endocrine glands. It can trigger a heart attack. In the Diary of Lady Nijo, one day, to awaken her terminally ill father, Nijo shook him very vigorously. The old man awoke, lifted himself, opened his eyes and dropped back, dead. Awaken gently to prevent regulatory organs from being jolted by shock. Avoid the one who awakens you in a start: he/she wants to destroy you. If you hate someone, scream in his ears.

The most healthful awakening method is to stroke the skin with a feather or blow on the skin until the person opens the eyes. Gentle awakening diverts very little blood from regulatory organs. Relaxation of a large part of the body makes blood available to the regulatory organs: this is the mechanism of sleep, A large part means primarily the digestive system, the skeletal muscles, or the sense organs.

Anything affecting the remaining five systems can awaken us: a noise or bright light, an overfilled rectum or bladder.

Understanding a nervous breakdown

A nervous breakdown is a collapse of the sleep mechanism—the total inability to sleep. Excess activity can bring on a nervous breakdown: physical, mental or sexual. Of the three types, the worst and most dangerous is the sexual over-activity: we know of two cases.

A sexual over-activity breakdown is characterized by a constant ringing in the head. The man who experienced it said that at first he cried and cried. He was nervous for a long time and lost all his teeth. At the very end, he ate nothing but jello, then he fasted till he fell asleep. Another woman was given electric shock treatments and from a beautiful woman, she became a wreck.

Physical and mental breakdowns are easily cared for. Do not panic when a loved one has experienced a sexual nervous breakdown. Total body inactivity is recommended, and in a short time, sufficient red cells will form to fill the regulatory organs, and sleep will recur. Some fasting may be required toward the end. Never subject an insomniac to electric shock treatments. A person who cannot sleep is very weak, indisposed. In sickness nothing is better than bed-rest. A liquid or semi-liquid diet restores the condition to normal.

What recourse when one has slept badly? Required sleep

Stop working the following day. Light foods, beverages, activate body functions. Take a long walk in fresh air and sunshine. Sleep will be deep. The idea is to prevent further destruction of red blood cells. A little work, move around slowly, are sufficient to induce sleep the next day. Darkness, solitude, silence and warmth will easily restore sleep.

Required hours of sleep

Children need more sleep than adults, see the following table:

Table 2
Sleep required at different ages

	Hours
Newborn	18 - 20
Growing children	10 – 12
Adults	6 – 9
Aged persons	5 - 9

(From Best and Taylor, **The Living Body**, p. 574.)

Older people sleep less. This may be caused by over-clogged blood vessels. If blood vessels could be prevented from clogging, older people would sleep like youngsters, maintain youth and live indefinitely. Birds hop about continuously, using their whole body for every action. As a result birds require much rest.

Understanding coma

Bears fill themselves with salmon, become comatose and spend the winter sleeping. If bears were to eat normal quantities of food, they would not hibernate.

The physical and chemical properties of blood present three ranges. A normal range of values is when blood properties vary very slightly and the brain functions normally. The second range of values is between lower normal and lower critical and upper normal and upper critical where the body suffers hypothermia or fever, respectively. The third or last range of values lies between lower critical and lower lethal and upper critical and upper lethal values where the body assumes a comatose lifelessness.

Keep a comatose patient very warm. The patient must drink water and must urinate continuously. Soon a comatose patient will emerge from his coma.

Daily regulations to follow upon awakening

Get up slowly and yawn. Remain seated for awhile. Do not speak for the next hour. Eat a light breakfast if you must go to work. Eat anything you wish if you stay home. Go about chores slowly. Keep regular with some stool evacuations at the slightest urge, it will maintain youth and health indefinitely. Listen to your body: never deny yourself a nap when rest is desired.

Now that the sleep mechanism is understood, it isn't difficult to see how the body ages. Aging is most feared by young and old people. In 1956, Dr. Alex Comfort stated that by the year 2,000, 44% of the western world's population would be over 75 years of age. Growing old is natural and inevitable, but to retain one's faculties in old age is what we hope to achieve. Senility is an increasing problem, and homes for the aged abound with incapacitated seniors—waiting for the final release. Aging in senility is not a hopeless condition; a better understanding of the aging process can prevent its devastating effects. Because it is invisible, the aging process has been impossible to unravel, let alone to find the elixir of youth.

Understand the threefold aging process

The first aging action occurs when blood is driven through the tiny capillaries of an active organ. As soon as blood is driven through the active organ simultaneously inactive organs are depleted of an equal amount of blood.

When an area is depleted of blood, metabolism lessens and changes occur. Scientific data indicate that changes occur in all regions of the living body: muscles become less elastic, bones lose density, connective tissue calcifies, body flexibility decreases, fingers and toenails become brittle.

Organs that manifest the most changes are: the reproductive system, sex organs, digestive system, sense organs, regulatory organs, skeletal system, brain. When depleted of blood supply, wastes accumulate, organs change. The larger the size of the active organ, the greater the depletion of blood from other organs, the faster aging will occur. Therefore, moderation is recommended in physical work, mental and sexual activities, primarily in large capillary areas. Though eyes and ears are small in size, very bright lights and loud noise/music are detrimental; after a day's work seek a quiet spot.

The second aging action is the functional impairment of the regulatory organs. During the eight active hours of the day, blood driven away from regulatory organs, lessens the regulation of blood's physical and chemical properties. Older people tire faster, are more susceptible to extremes of heat and cold and have less sensitivity to pain. Sleep is marred by frequent waking bouts, with consequent hypertension, arteriosclerosis, irregular heartbeat, labored breathing, defective kidneys, etc.

The third aging action is a decrease in the number of tiny blood vessels of active organs. In fast and heavy work, in order to deliver oxygen more rapidly, red blood cells force themselves through tiny blood capillaries, bursting their walls into many tiny pieces. A reduction of an organ's tiny blood vessels impairs vital processes, reducing nutritive and eliminative functions. Consequently, body movements are affected: speech slows down, movements become difficult, resulting in total immobility.

The threefold aging action is in accordance with the scientific theories:

The theory of wear and tear maintains that continued use leads to worn out or defective parts (diminution in number of tiny blood vessels).

The accumulation theory states that certain substances accumulate in body cells, decreasing cellular efficiency (accumulation of wastes as blood is driven elsewhere during the day).

The cross-linking theory states that connective tissues supporting and binding organs and structures become rigid with age, causing loss of elasticity necessary for smooth functioning of body parts (lessened eliminative function of cells with accumulation of wastes).

Selye's stress theory maintains that every bit of stress leaves the organism with some residual impairment that accumulates over a lifetime until body reserves are depleted (impairment of regulatory organs).

The immune theory of aging contends that changes were found in the immune system which is a function of the regulatory organs, it is in accordance with the present aging process. There are many ways to delay the aging process.

Combat the first aging action, never perform two actions simultaneously

Slow down all activities. Do not walk fast; run short distances. Do not raise the voice or shout. Perform sex sparingly and slowly. Eat slowly and sip beverages. Do not allow loud music or noise to bombard the ears. Do not expose eyes to blinding or blinking lights. Do not use vigorous action in different parts of the body simultaneously: when standing at work, avoid loud music. If you must stand, eat light, etc. Do not sing and dance at the same time. Do not sing and accompany yourself simultaneously. Do not drive and listen to blasting music simultaneously. Do not speak on a cellular phone when driving. Do not deal with too many people daily. Be silent.

Combat the second aging action, balance actions

Balance an action by the opposing action: eat three times, defecate three times. Stand half an hour, sit a half an hour. Speak ten minutes, remain silent ten minutes, etc. Rest between work. Lean your head back occasionally. Take a nap. Keep silent as much as possible. Sleep eight hours daily. When active in one direction, do not allow a strong action in other directions.

Combat the third aging action, avoid all strenuous movements

Do not hit a ball with a bat, play tennis, or lift heavy weights. Weight-lift 5 pounds for women, 10 pounds for men. Avoid loud, continuous speech. Do not sing opera as a profession. If obliged to sing, do it sparingly. Avoid a bare bulb light. Enjoy silence and nature. Silence preserves ear capillaries. Avoid jobs requiring your energy. Avoid working in several areas in a day: sex, travel, creative work, concentrated food, etc. Do not allow external substances to penetrate the body directly: injections, powerful Ultra violet rays, X-rays. Avoid long massages. Do not donate blood.

Be active before age 50 and semi-retire after. Thereafter, avoid a public life. Avoid working fast in three large capillary areas simultaneously. Avoid excess bouncing movements. These are conscious means to combat aging. External conditions surrounding our existence can age us rapidly. For example:

Cold floors can age you prematurely

Many homes have wood floors, cement tiles in bathrooms and vinyl tiles in kitchens. Rooms have tile floors in some countries in Europe. Gravity causes living organisms to be attached to the ground either by a root or by feet. Cold reaches the body from the ground, tile or cement floors cause cold to invade the body rapidly. This building trend must stop. Cement or tile floors can cover bathroom floors. Housewives spend hours in the kitchen therefore, only vinyl tiles should cover kitchen floors. All other rooms must have wood floors.

Wearing fur, leather and wool can prolong lives

Clothing is a life preserver. Animals are covered with fur because they are weaker than man. When weak, fur should be worn—around the house or outdoors. Leather and suede are tight: they preserve body heat efficiently. It is foolish to be against using fur as clothing. If we cannot use fur, we should not eat meat. It is less cruel to use animals' fur than to eat their flesh. The fur trade is what lured the first Europeans to settle in Canada.

Today, most people wear cotton; some wear polyester or other artificial fiber. Vegetable and artificial fiber do not protect against loss of body heat, perhaps this is the reason man is stricken with many illnesses today. We should wear wool and silk. The finest knitted wool can be found today. Children should learn to sew so that they can make their own wool clothing. Even in the hottest summer, the finest wool fabric against the skin will maintain health and prolong life. At 60° and under, wear wool. At 70° and above, wear silk.

An apartment can cause aging

In most cities, living quarters are either exposed to the sun or in the dark. Most apartments don't have both amenities. An apartment should have a sunny and a dark room. One elderly woman lived in a pleasant apartment with sunny and dark rooms. The landlord advised her to move to another apartment where all rooms were exposed to sunshine all day long. She died soon after. Some burrowing animals only come out in the dark, shunning daylight. Humans need light but also darkness.

Excess food and aging - processed foods

Excess proteins, minerals and carbohydrates ingested are stored in body cells and accumulate as wastes; externally indicated by wrinkles, stiffened gait, cantankerous movements: a warning of excess foods ingested. Beware of corn grits, molasses, fat-back, preserved meats, salted fish, cheeses, etc. Avoid canned foods and eat fresh foods, meats and dairy. Read the contents on packaged foods, containers and bottled juices. Avoid foods with chemicals or with a long shelf-life.

Chapter 13
Steer around digestive disturbances and live a long life

Soon after birth, an infant begins to suck milk—to eat because he is hungry. These cramp-like cravings of the stomach's smooth muscle are not continuous. Weak at first, they gradually become more vigorous with increasingly shorter intervals between them, culminating in a supreme degree of activity where a spasm grips the smooth musculature. History relates the misery of the human mind and body when stranded on the ocean, desert or mountain top. Hunger has driven people to cannibalism, to murder, even suicide. Yet some people never experience hunger pangs, reports Dr. Walter Cannon. To him, hunger indicates a need of nutrients affecting some region of the brain, a stimulus for gastric contractions or hunger pangs.

Hunger explained
Dr. Cannon reports that hunger pangs intensifies when blood sugar concentration reduces by 25%. Starches give a false sense of fullness, and when omitted from the diet, true hunger occurs. Hunger has a protective function. Physiology cannot explain its occurrence. Dr. Cannon coined the term homeostasis, the constancy of physical and chemical properties of the blood, comprising water, calcium, body temperature, pH, etc. Hunger is the nervous system's call for supplies to maintain constancy in the internal environment.
Deep hunger pangs: Deep sleep, the regulator of physical and chemical properties of the blood, maintains powerful hunger pangs. The opposite is also true: a light sleeper experiences slight if any hunger pangs.
Appetite explained: The thought of some delicious food stirs appetite. Specific appetite is an instinctive need for a missing element: drinking water from iron-rich streams, Indians suffering from dysenteric diarrhea scrape chalk from canyon walls. Appetite is man's search for natural sources of medication.
Understand thirst: Thirst is felt when mouth and throat are dry and saliva flow reduced. Salivary glands warn against dehydration and thirst is nature's reminder. Thirst signals a reduction in blood volume, affecting total water content. The body contains large quantities of water, 75% in body, 92% in blood. Daily work destroys red blood cells, reducing total blood volume, affecting total water content. Intake more fluids than solids at all times. Our five liters of blood must be maintained.

The loss of hunger pangs
Some people live for years without true hunger pangs. External signs indicate the power of hunger pangs. The mouth being the digestive system's opening, when

corners of mouth turn markedly upwards strong hunger pangs are present; slight hunger pangs are indicated by straight corners. When corners of mouth turn markedly downwards no hunger pangs are experienced.

The corners of a healthy person's mouth always turn sharply upwards.

Teeth: their growth and maintenance

Teeth enable proper food digestion. At different periods of life appear two sets of teeth. In a human embryo the earliest evidence of teeth appears at around the 7th prenatal week of life; the successional permanent teeth appear at about the 16th week; the germ for super-added permanent teeth appear at about the 17th prenatal week. Temporary teeth resemble the permanent set, but are smaller. The neck is more marked, roots of molars are smaller, more diverging than the permanent set.

Temporary and permanent teeth: The first set of temporary teeth appears in early childhood. There are a total of 32 teeth; at about 6 years of age 20 milk teeth are replaced by a permanent secondary set. An X-ray of upper and lower jaws of a four-year old indicates the position of temporary and permanent teeth. When calcification of different tissues of a milk tooth is sufficiently advanced to allow it to bear pressure subjection, a temporary tooth erupts.

As temporary teeth gradually fall out, they are almost immediately replaced by permanent teeth; once detached, bone cells absorb a temporary tooth's root. Under the loose crown of deciduous teeth, permanent teeth take their place. One Chinese girl never lost her temporary teeth and was always very beautiful, chewing with two sets of teeth. In her twenties she fell deeply in love and decided to improve her looks by removing all her temporary teeth. Alas, it affected her chewing power and soon she became an old woman. Never remove teeth; the more teeth you have, the better the chewing power. Crocodiles grow new teeth—not humans. Once a tooth is lost, there is no chance of growing another. If a tooth's crown is lost, leave the root alone. It may still serve well, allow chewing and retain the space it occupies. Extract only if pain is felt.

Tooth structure: Each tooth has three parts: 1) a crown or body projecting above the gums; 2) the root or fang concealed under the gum; 3) between root and crown, a constricted portion or neck. It is firmly implanted in a depression lined with periosteum also covering root up to neck. There are eight incisors, each with one root. Lower incisors are smaller and flatter. There are four canines. In each jaw, two canines flank four incisors. Larger than incisors, the canine's crown is large, the root oval, longer and more prominent than in incisors. There are 8 bicuspid teeth, two on each side of a canine. Behind bicuspid teeth lie molars. The largest teeth, there are 12 molars, six in each jaw. Upper molars have three roots, lower molars, two roots. The first molar tooth is the largest of the dental series. The third molars are wisdom teeth appearing late in adolescence.

A long section through a tooth. A long section through a tooth reveals a central chamber resembling the crown, extending through the root, opening by a minute orifice at the apex, the apical foramen. This chamber's soft, vascular sensitive dental pulp contains blood vessels and nerve, no lymphatics; surrounding its periphery a layer of columnar epithelial cells. These are odontoblasts, dentine-forming cells. Underneath them lie innumerable capillary loops of blood vessels and nerve fibrils. Odontoblasts are important columnar connective tissue cells; they become active when decay sets in, producing another layer of secondary dentine. This indicates the futility of filling cavities, for given the opportunity, teeth are able to protect themselves. New dentine forms in three days, and a painful cavity will disappear.

Chemical composition of a tooth: It has three distinct structures: 1) Dentine forms a tooth's larger portion. 2) Enamel covers the exposed part of the crown. 3) A thin layer of cement covers the root's surface. Dentine is composed of 28 parts organic matter, 72 parts inorganic matter: phosphate and carbonate with calcium, traces of fluoride, calcium phosphate, magnesia and other salts.

Enamel forms a thin crust from crown to neck. It is the hardest and most compact part of a tooth. Resting on dentine, enamel is a collection of tiny hexagonal rods, 1/5,500 of an inch in diameter. Devoid of nutritive canals, enamel is composed of 96.5% inorganic matter, 3.5% organic matter, thickest on the grinding surface, thinning down towards the neck. From tip to neck, a thin layer of cement covers the entire root. Cement resembles bone.

Preparation and growth of a tooth. Milk teeth require two years of preparation. Permanent teeth require five years preparation. The last wisdom teeth erupt at around age 20 or beyond, thus requiring more than 20 years of preparation. Due to this lengthy preparation, no machinery must touch a human tooth, neither to fill cavities nor for cleansing purposes.

Growth requires good food and relaxation. For optimum growth, a child and adolescent must not overwork physically or mentally.

When all 32 teeth are weak and wobbly, dentures become a necessity. Acrylic dentures have been available for about 50 years. Dentures are one of the greatest advances in applied dentistry, allowing the enjoyment of food. When obliged to wear dentures, make certain they are a perfect fit. One woman with new dentures made weekly visits to her dentist for a year. Perfect fitting dentures require no powder or paste to hold them in place. Paste or powder used to secure dentures will eventually be swallowed. Do not use them. If you wear a partial denture, remove it when at home. Partial dentures lessen normal blood flow to good teeth because it is tight near surrounding teeth, weakening them, with the eventual loss of your own teeth by extraction.

The difference in man's chewing power

For food to turn into chyme in the stomach, chewing, salivation and swallowing are not essential if food is introduced in a proper state of division. Unless a liquid or baby food, nutrients are rarely finely divided. Solid food requires chewing, with coordination of teeth, tongue, cheeks, palate and floor of mouth. Chewed by teeth, tongue and cheeks push the bolus, subjecting it to cutting and grinding. When thoroughly mixed with saliva, pressing against the hard palate, the tongue pushes the food bolus into the pharynx.

People chew in different ways. In 20-85% of chewing strokes, teeth make contact. With crooked teeth chewing is poorly executed. At molars, the human jaw exerts a force of 75-200 lbs. At incisors, 30-70 lbs. per square inch. For the same meal, the speed of jaw movement varies. One person might chew 100 times, others 700 times. For good digestion, chew sufficiently. A physiology professor cautioned to chew each mouthful of food 80 times. The more the fibers are finely ground, the better the digestion. If badly chewed, large particles of foods are swallowed.

How food should be chewed

There is a chewing cycle of opening, closing and shutting off phases. When sufficiently chewed on one side, the food mass is broken up with unequal muscle activity. Depending on the consistency of food, chewing movements may be vertical, side to side, front and back, with individual variation in jaw movements both between individuals and races. When deliberately done on one side, food is chewed longer, then thrown to the other side and back and forth. Chewing on both sides at once divides the force and does not grind to a proper state of refinement. Force concentrated on a small surface increases pressure. Chewing is very important as saliva mixes with dry food, easing the bolus' passage through organs of deglutition. Thus never dip bread, cookies in milk or coffee. Prior to swallowing, dry starches must mix well with saliva: the first step in the digestion of starches.

If many teeth are lost, chew in any way provided the bolus is finely ground for swallowing. One woman with both upper and lower dentures is yet unable to use them; she removes both dentures before eating, and chews with her gums. Her foods are so poorly ground for digestion even her external appearance has drastically changed.

The mouth: its external appearance

A look into the mouth shows a hard palate on the roof, ending in a soft palate hanging behind, soft arches and two prominent bodies: the tonsils. On the mouth's floor lies the tongue. Intimate adherence of periosteum and mucous membrane forms the roof of the mouth. Along its midline, a linear ridge ends in front with a small papilla, the termination of nerve filaments.

Divided into two symmetrical halves by a fibrous septum, the tongue's surface is covered by a layer of mucous membrane, its fibers running in all directions. At its base, a muscle firmly ties the tongue to the U-shaped hyoid bone. Five nerves and arteries from three vessels supply each half of the tongue. The tongue has serous and mucous glands. Due to its innumerable muscles, it has the ability to make the most complicated movements to enounce different consonantal sounds. The tongue's surface indicates the state of health. It may have a heavy coating, or in pellagra, be fiery red; in pernicious anemia it is smooth and burning. Normally it is evenly colored, finely granular. It is often the seat of ulceration by jagged teeth. In cancer, part of the tongue may be removed. Alter the diet before you let that happen.

The mouth, its salivary glands. Three large paired glands in the mouth produce saliva: the parotid, submandibular and sublingual glands. The largest parotid, 1/2-1 oz, lies immediately below and in front of the external ear. Five arteries pass through the gland. The parotid secretes a thin, watery fluid containing serum-albumin.

Lying on three muscles under the jaw, the submandibular salivary gland weighs 8-10 grams. It has two inch-long ducts with thin walls. This gland secretes a fluid of a mixed variety containing mucin and serum-albumin.

The smallest of the three glands lies under the mucous membrane of the mouth's floor. The sublingual gland is in close contact with the lower jaw's inner surface. Shaped like an almond, it weighs about 4-5 grams and secretes a ropy fluid: mucus.

Function of saliva: Always hypotonic, saliva contains water. Daily, a total of 0.5-2 liters of saliva is produced. Weakly acidic when secreted, it becomes weakly alkaline in large quantities. Ptyalin, its most important enzyme, initiates digestion of starches, splitting cooked starch into maltose. Salivary glands are sentinels, warning against dehydration. Saliva keeps mouth moist, rinses it clean, with a disinfecting action. It dilutes foods, providing a solvent for some of its components. To ease swallowing, food becomes slippery with mucus. Sour and bitter substances stimulate saliva secretion, it is prevented by sweet and sapid foods. Sympathetic stimulation produces a thick, slimy mucinous juice. Parasympathetic secretion stirs a watery flow from glands. In fever, sudden penetration of food in the mouth causes intense pain as blood rushes to vessels of salivary glands; it is a warning that dilute foods are indispensable otherwise fever will rise.

Saliva: its chemical composition: Chemically saliva comprises 0.2% salts, sodium, potassium chloride, sodium bicarbonate, acid and alkaline sodium phosphate, calcium carbonate and phosphate, potassium sulphocyanate and two gases: carbon dioxide and oxygen. Submandibular and sublingual glands mainly secrete ptyalin, maltase, serum albumin, serum globulin, urea and mucin. For optimum saliva flow, intake much fluids daily or whenever thirst demands. From the mouth, chewed food now penetrates the pharynx.

The pharynx: its description

Comparable to an apartment where all rooms open into a foyer, the pharynx has openings from ears, nostrils, mouth, esophagus and larynx. Funnel-shaped and flattened in front, about 12 cm. long, it tapers from a 5 cm. width at the skull's base, to 2.5 cm. where it joins the esophagus. From within, it is three-layered: a mucous layer with salivary glands, a muscular layer for swallowing, a connective tissue layer attaches it to surrounding structures.

Firmly attached to the skull's base, jaw, tongue and pharyngeal cartilage, four muscles dilate the pharynx and propel food down the esophagus. The attachment is sufficiently loose to allow it to glide when swallowing. Through the pharynx pass foods and air but foods have the right of way and air is shut off from lungs, thus when swallowing, one cannot breathe.

The pharynx, its three parts. The longest section, the oral pharynx extends from tonsils to epiglottis, a flap at tongue's root. From Eustachian tube to soft palate extends the nasal pharynx. From epiglottis to beginning of larynx extends the laryngeal pharynx.

A row of tonsils encircles the pharynx's inner wall. Tonsils are masses of lymphoid tissue to fight off infection. They must never be removed. Like sentinels, they guard the body from bacteria. Breathing through the mouth bypasses the nose's filtering function and bacteria or dirt can penetrate the pharynx, the tonsils then become very active, ingesting foreign particles. Inflammation of tonsils warns of either toxic foods or bacteria in the system. A light diet will alleviate the condition. Adenoids encircle the nasal pharynx. Adenoids are lymphoid glands and must never be removed.

Chewed food can voluntarily be controlled and expectorated as long as it does not touch the palatine arch at the tongue's base, and the back of throat or tip of soft palate where stimulation of involuntary muscles cannot prevent swallowing. At times, rapid expectoration may drive the bolus forward.

Some young people play around catching grapes or cherries with their mouths. Do not play with your mouth. Once a small fruit lodged in a young man's throat; unable to swallow or spit, he choked to death.

How food is swallowed

When a bolus is of a refined size, temperature and wetness, the message is conveyed to the brain, indicating the correct moment to swallow. When swallowing, breathing stops. At the back of the tongue the wall rises, muscular pillars of palate contract, preventing passage of food into nose. The soft palate rises, lifting the larynx upwards and forwards, the epiglottis descends and vocal cords contract. The pharynx dilates to receive the bolus of food from mouth. The stylo-pharyngeal muscle draws the sides of pharynx upward and outward, carrying the tongue forward, increasing the transverse diameter. The esophageal sphincter muscle opens and food moves from mouth to esophagus, the bolus passing quickly into the esophagus. These oral and pharyngeal stages take a fraction of a second. Between swallows, the esophagus is limp, both upper and lower sphincters, closed. Liquids pass directly into the stomach; esophageal muscle's action propels solid food.

How food should be swallowed. Take your time in swallowing; the bolus requires a few seconds to reach the end of the esophagus. Liquids take one to two seconds and gulping may cause discomfort as the tube retains fluids. Usually a deep breath allows a wave to reach the sphincter, clearing up the difficulty. Hurried swallowing causes irregular contractions of muscle fibers with defective propulsion of fluid down the tube, eventually curling the esophagus; older people could be affected.

The stomach does not allow foods to pass rapidly down the cardiac sphincter for in a given quantity of hydrochloric acid, a definite proportion of food can be digested perfectly. Excess food remains in the stomach, passes into bowels in a crude state, causing pain and disease. The cardiac sphincter closes on a bolus, preventing passage of all other foods into the stomach. Eat and drink slowly. A paunch is a sign that food is gulped down too quickly.

The esophagus: its description

Connecting pharynx and stomach, the esophagus is a 10-inch-long tube slightly to the midline's left. Vertical, with a half to one inch diameter, its two important flexures correspond to the neck and chest. The esophagus lies within the mediastinum, a space containing heart and other viscera except lungs. It pierces the diaphragm and expands into the cardiac region of the stomach.

Resting on the spinal column, the esophagus has three coats: outer muscular coat, inner mucous coat and in between, a fatty layer, loosely connecting former layers. Voluntary striated muscle forms two thirds of muscular coat, involuntary smooth muscle the lower third. In this way, food passes quickly down the upper two thirds, slower down the remaining third. The inner mucous coat is tough, thick above, pale below, folded into many longitudinal pleats, allowing esophagus to stretch when distended with food. Studded with tiny papillae, its surface is covered by a layer of epithelium, thickening toward the stomach. In the mucous layer many racemose glands open through a long duct; most numerous, they form a ring near the cardiac orifice.

Food descends the esophagus: When the upper sphincter opens and swallowed food enters the tube, a contractile wave appears, moving toward the stomach. Waves of 2-6 cm. require 10 seconds to reach the end of the tube. Each wave has segments of 10-30 cm. Circular muscle contractions propel food down the tube, slowly progressing toward the stomach. Once filled with food, reflex relaxation of cardiac sphincter relaxes stomach, preventing a pressure rise.

The stomach: its position and make-up

In the abdominal cavity the stomach lies behind the liver, in front of pancreas, left kidney, left adrenal, spleen, colon and mesocolon. Shaped like a jJ, attached to both curvatures, layers of peritoneum firmly hold the stomach in place. At each end, valves prevent entrance of food. The greater curvature begins at the upper fundus with its cardiac sphincter and ends at the pylorus. The stomach's four coats are: an outer serous coat, a muscular coat of three types of fibers: longitudinal, straight and circular, a third fatty coat and an innermost mucous coat.

Circular fibers are mostly at pyloric sphincter, oblique fibers are limited to stomach's cardiac end. A third fatty layer connects previous layers, supporting blood vessels before their distribution to mucous layer.

Gastric glands: their location

The mucous membrane has many folds, obliterated when stomach is distended. Covered with numerous shallow depressions or alveoli, $1/100$-$1/200^{th}$ of an inch in diameter, gastric glands open at bottom of alveoli. Around 35,000,000 tubular glands with a delicate basement membrane are present. Covering gastric glands is a layer of epithelium with three kinds of cells: parietal cells produce hydrochloric acid, chief cells form pepsinogen, mucous cells secrete mucin or gastric mucus.

Stomach varies in size: About 4 1/2 ounces in size when empty, the stomach has a capacity of five to eight pints, pear-shaped when full. Cylindrical when empty, it lies on back of abdomen but when distended, pushes the diaphragm upwards, the fundus expands, contracting the chest cavity. No other organ in the body alters its position and connections as frequently as the stomach. In fever or overfeeding, the stomach's inner coat becomes red or dry, pale and moist, losing the smooth, healthy appearance with almost complete suppression of secretions.

How food is digested

Propelled by esophageal contractions, food initiates reflex relaxation of cardiac sphincter, momentarily inhibiting peristalsis. Blood flow increases through stomach capillaries, the mucous surface brightens and peristaltic movements appear. Foveolae discharge a clear, transparent fluid, proceeding forwards as more food enters stomach.

Starting near the cardiac sphincter, peristaltic contractions mix foods. At about the stomach's mid-part, waves begin as a ring of contraction, slowly progressing towards the pyloric end; at three contractions per minute, becoming deeper as they move onward; strongest waves are manifested towards the pylorus, at the larger curvature. The active stomach rejects food that cannot be mixed further with gastric juice, nor will it admit liquid food rapidly through the esophageal sphincter.

Called chyme, the food is a homogeneous, pultaceous grayish substance of a sweetish, insipid taste, slightly acidic, it resembles rich cream if you eat butter, meat or oil, chyme is like gruel when farinaceous foods and vegetables are ingested. Churned by peristalsis, in alternating contractions and relaxation, three kinds of waves occur: 20 second waves mixing by mild pressure; peristaltic waves of three per minute and finally antral propulsive waves creating constant agitation in stomach.

Food revolves from right to left, then from left to right and lastly from right to left, counterclockwise. From esophagus to pyloric end of stomach, revolutions are completed in one to three minutes. As chyme continuously passes through sphincter into duodenum, its volume steadily decreases. The consistency and size of food bolus determine evacuation of food from stomach. Particles of food sufficiently fine to fit through the diameter of the pyloric exit pass through the gate. Crude food cannot pass. Solids, lipids, solutions deviating markedly from isotonicity empty at a slower rate than isotonic saline solution.

When the last particles of chyme are expulsed from stomach, no more juice is secreted until more food is introduced. The stomach is seldom entirely at rest but after expulsion of the last particles of chyme, it becomes quiescent. Generally a meal of bread and milk leaves the stomach in two hours. Large pieces of meat, cheese, raw meat are digested with difficulty. Strong tea, coffee, wine, beer are injurious, raising stomach's temperature.

Digestion, factors affecting its rate

Gentle exercise eases digestion but severe and strenuous exercise retards it. Immediately after a meal, the stomach rapidly empties itself; with time the process slows down. Fear, anger, fright, fever, excitement suppress gastric secretions completely or diminish them considerably; food remaining 24-48 hours in the stomach, aggravates the condition. Sharp, pointed, red eruptions filled with pus, small crusts and abrasions may appear on the mucous membrane. They do not delay or impede peristalsis but when the condition is permanent, they prevent digestion. No gastric juice is secreted when the mouth is dry and the pulse is rapid. The stomach is healthy when the tongue is clear and pinkish.

Gastric juice produced: Daily around 2-3 liters of gastric juice are produced, consisting of water, inorganic salts, hydrochloric acid, mucin and enzymes.

The digestive tract, its most common diseases

Gastric and duodenal ulcers are the digestive tract's most common diseases. Some diseases affect gastric juice secretion: cancer of stomach, pernicious anemia, chronic inflammation of stomach, chronic arthritis and gall-bladder inflammation.

Powerful external stimuli affect digestion. Refrain from excess work, heavy sports, sex and bright lights, loud noise or music. Total muscular relaxation immediately brings on a flow of gastric juice. To relax stomach muscles, lean the head back when chewing. If overworked adopt isotonic feeding.

Good digestion. Digestion is most effective in an acid environment of pH 1.4-2.5. A pH of 11 and above inactivates enzymes digesting proteins. In duodenal ulcer, the pH is very low, about 1.3 or 1.7 and the stomach digests itself, more acid than bicarbonate is formed. When weak or ill, avoid fats in food. Fats raise intestinal pH, in turn affecting stomach pH.

Normal body temperature is very important. Lukewarm foods empty quickly from stomach. Hot foods remain longer but hot and cold foods rapidly assume normal body temperature. Digestive enzymes are permanently abolished at 60° C. (140° F.). When feverish, light foods are imperative and for good health, the quantity eaten is more important than the quality.

The stomach has as much hydrochloric acid as bicarbonate in blood plasma, neutralizing some of the acidity. The sole alkaline product in gastric juice is mucin, acting as a buffer to prevent excess acidity.

Various enzymes in gastric juices act on protein, changing it to proteoses and peptones. One enzyme coagulates milk, another splits fat. Mucin, a stomach mucous membrane, prevents injury by particles of food and action of hydrochloric acid. To produce gastric juice, a good blood flow is necessary. Factors that reduce blood flow to digestive system are: excess noise or loud music, talk, people, crowds, lack of fresh air. Dine in a quiet spot or alone.

Hydrochloric acid (HCl) is formed

The formation of hydrochloric acid is baffling. The action of water on a nonmetal in the laboratory produces HCl. In 1892, C. Contrejean said that salt in the body manufactures stomach's hydrochloric acid. In salted frogs, hydrochloric acid was found in the stomach until the moment of death. A lack of oxygen or low oxygen pressure in blood slows down hydrochloric acid production; also, metabolic poisons and salt depletion affect HCl production. Eat at least one level tablespoon of salt daily in soups or sprinkled on foods.

The small intestine and its various coats

Similar to the stomach, the small intestine's four coats differ in the mucous membrane's appearance: it is thick, very vascular at its upper end, paler below. Two inches below the pylorus are many large folds. Each fold with its two layers of mucous membrane bound by sub-mucous tissues, project into the small intestine's lumen. Even when distended, intestinal folds are permanent. Large at the beginning, they tend to disappear at the ileum's lower part. Folds retard passage of food down the intestine, providing more extensive absorptive surface. Also present are tiny, highly vascular villi, imparting surface with a velvety appearance. Short and leaf-shaped in the duodenum, villi are large and tongue-shaped in the duodenum and the jejunum. The ileum has few villi, a total of 50-

90 villi in a square line; in lower intestine, 40-70 villi, a total of about 4 million villi. Also present are simple follicles or tiny tubular depressions of mucous membrane with a tiny circular aperture. Other structures found are duodenal glands and Peyer's patches, aggregations of solitary glands, most numerous in the ileum. The small intestine has about 100,000,000 glands.

The small intestine: Attached to the spine by a fold of peritoneum, the small intestine extends from the pyloric end of stomach to the opening of the large intestine. About 20 feet long, diminishing in size from beginning to end, it may be divided into 3 parts: the duodenum, jejunum and ileum.

The duodenum: The shortest duodenum is the widest and most fixed part of the small intestine. About 10 inches long, it encircles the head of the pancreas, forming a C-shaped curve. It has four portions: the superior, descending, transverse and ascending divisions.

Beginning at the pylorus and ending at the gall bladder's neck, the superior portion is 2 inches long, almost completely covered by the peritoneum. Three to four inches long, the descending portion extends from the neck of the gall bladder to the 4th lumbar vertebra, the head of the pancreas lying on its inner side. Three or four inches under the pylorus, the common bile duct and pancreatic duct enter the duodenum. The transverse portion is 2-3 inches long. About 2 inches long, the ascending portion rests on the diaphragm and touches the left kidney.

The jejunum: The jejunum represents 2/5^{ths} of the small intestine. Between jejunum and ileum there is no line of demarcation. The former is wider, 1 1/2 inch in diameter, thicker, more vascular and of a deeper color, with large, thick folds and villi.

The ileum: The ileum represents 3/5^{ths} of the remaining small intestine. Due to its numerous coils and convolutions, it is named ileum from the Greek word meaning to twist. Narrow, with a diameter of 1 1/2 inch, the ileum's coats are less vascular, its small folds scarcer with larger and more numerous Peyer's patches. The ileum opens into the inner side of the large intestine.

Digestion in the small intestine: As soon as chyme passes through stomach's pyloric sphincter, the intestinal wall is distended and between villi, glands begin to secrete intestinal juice. The duodenum is the main secretion site. At a pH of 8.3-9.3, intestinal secretion is alkaline, mixed with secretions of pancreas and liver, containing also sodium and chlorine ions.

Now called chyle, the food mass is subjected to three kinds of movements; peristalsis or constricting movements from stomach downwards, rhythmic contractions of 1-2 cm. wide at rhythmic intervals of 15-20 cm. Alternating contraction and relaxation of about 8-10 times per minute last several hours; segmenting movements constrict and relax over and over again. These movements knead the mass, bringing them constantly in contact with fresh absorptive surfaces, increasing blood and lymph flow into intestinal wall. To aid digestion further by a to and fro motion, pendular movements of 11-12 per minute, decrease to 8-9 per minute at terminal ileum, constrict the intestinal wall, displace intestinal contents down the bowel for short distances. At 3-4 per minute, villi's swaying movement propulses the mass towards intestine's tail. Kneading is faster toward the upper part of small intestine, slowing down near the rectum.

When another region is grossly distended, small intestine's contractile activity is inhibited. When overloaded with food, digestive movements become sluggish. Changes in emotional states also cause detrimental alteration in small intestine's activity. In about four hours, food reaches the small intestine; another eight hours will transfer it to the large intestine. Intestinal motility is controlled by the parasympathetic nervous system. During sleep or when relaxed, sympathetic nerves become active. Intestinal motility ceases and absorption begins in the small intestine, no wonder he who sleeps a great deal will gain weight.

Other secretions aiding digestion

Two other secretions in the small intestines aid digestion: pancreatic juice and bile from liver. The pancreas secretes as follows: when chyle enters the intestine, intestinal mucous membrane's prosecretin is converted into secretin. Diffused into the bloodstream, secretin stirs pancreas to secrete pancreatic juice, a watery fluid, high in bicarbonates. It is nature's antacid, says L.R. Johnson. Daily 1.5-2.0 liters is produced. It is isotonic with blood plasma, with a pH of 8-8.5.

The pancreatic duodenal mucous membrane also secretes pancreozymin, a juice rich in enzymes, sodium bicarbonate and water to digest proteins, starches and fats. In digestion, pancreatic secretion is extremely important.

The liver produces bile, a yellow-brown to green alkaline fluid with a bitter taste, containing bile salts, bile pigments and cholesterol. Bile salts emulsify intestinal fats, help pancreatic enzyme's fat-splitting activity and assist digestion of proteins and starches. To form bile, the liver uses constituents of blood from remains of dead red cells, to produce bilirubin and biliverdin. Daily, an adult produces 600-800 cc. of bile, at pH 7.8-8.6. Between meals, bile is stored in the gallbladder, a pear-shaped pouch with 50 cc. of fluid capacity, lying on the liver's undersurface. Its cystic duct joins liver's hepatic duct, forming the common bile duct that joins the pancreatic duct before both enter the intestine from a chamber, the ampulla of Vater. Bile directly from liver is less concentrated than gallbladder bile where much water is reabsorbed.

A diet of too much fat may shuttle bile and pancreatic juice back into the liver, with gall bladder inflammation or pancreatitis, both organs sharing a common duct. Normally this does not occur. Under stress conditions, all foods turn into carbohydrates while overwork, fear, fright, sadness, extreme happiness, creative bouts, heavy sports, raise intestinal pH, affecting digestion.

Effects of excessive bile pigments

Blood contains some bilirubin pigment. If excessive, skin, mucous membranes and whites of eyes, stain yellow with resulting jaundice. This occurs when liver is unable to use all of blood's pigments. The excess decomposition of red cells produces greater oxidation of hemoglobin, forming more bilirubin. Work destroys red cells that decompose faster when doing heavy work, fast movements, constant activity, bright lights, loud noise/music. These actions tear up red blood cells as they rapidly pass through tiny opened blood capillaries. Do not overwork.

In the human body, cholesterol is excreted as follows: liver cells convert cholesterol into two primary bile acids: cholic acid and chenodeoxycholic acid, in the ratio 2-1. The acids conjugate with glycine or taurine, forming sodium and potassium salts in alkaline bile. In the distal ileum, salts are metabolized by bacteria, of which 20% form secondary bile acids deoxycholic acid and lithocholic acid. In the distal ileum 90-95% of bile acids are reabsorbed and returned to liver by hepatic portal vessels. Six to ten times every 24 hours, about 2-4 grams of circulating bile acids form a bile acid pool, passing around hepatic portal vessels. In daily feces 0.6 g. of bile acids is excreted and replaced by new synthesis. Sometimes bile cholesterol precipitates, forming gallstones, crystals with a tendency to increase in size. The gall bladder can store bile solids secreted during 10 hours. Bile pigments and constituents are excreted in feces, assuming a dark color. The darker the feces, the greater the consumption of fats, in turn changing urine's color.

The small intestine. Food absorption

Absorption is the process by which substances from the body's surface are taken into the intestinal epithelium's interior. It occurs in the small intestine with 2.8 meters of absorptive tissue: 30 cm. in duodenum, 120 cm. in jejunum and 130 cm. in ileum, a total of 200 square meters of absorptive surface. Many cells in the small intestine absorb and excrete into its lumen. Absorption occurs when it predominates over excretion.

Foods must be decomposed to be absorbed; only then can they be used to build body tissues. Digestion protects the body from foreign proteins, carbohydrates and fats. Proteins are digested into amino acids, carbohydrates into monosaccharides, fats are converted into glycerin and fatty acids. For optimum absorption, blood flow through intestinal mucous membrane is essential. Oxygen deficiency inhibits absorption—fresh air is indispensable. Water is most important, diffusing through intestinal mucous membrane. To move substances by diffusion some fat is required in the diet, as cell membranes are high in lipid content.

In the duodenum, glucose is more rapidly absorbed than fructose. In the absence of sodium, sugar absorption ceases. Carried by villi's lymph vessels, fatty acids and glycerol enter larger lymphatics, penetrate bloodstream then brought to tissues and fat depôts. Absorption of most amino acids and carbohydrates occur in the presence of salt. Absorption of amino acids and simple polypeptides occurs by physical diffusion and osmosis. Fat-soluble vitamins are only absorbed in the presence of fat. Absorption of iron and calcium depends on hydrochloric acid in gastric juice. To prevent over-absorption, do not let fecal masses remain in the tract for many hours, a major cause of obesity as most people defecate once daily.

Diffusion and osmosis. Diffusion: A solute diffuses across a membrane separating two solutions of different concentrations until both sides of the membrane reach equilibrium. **Osmosis:** A solvent is transported through a semi-permeable membrane until concentrations of both sides are equal.

The small intestine leads to the large intestine extending from end of ileum to anus. About 5 ft. long, the large intestine represents 1/5th of the entire digestive tract. Very large at the beginning, diminishing gradually in size until it dilates just above the anus. The large intestine comprises the caecum, colon and rectum.

The large intestine. The caecum

The ileo-caecal valve leads into the caecum. It has an upper semi-lunar segment forming the ileo-colic valve, a lower caecal semilunar segment forming the ileo-caecal valve. These segments are reduplications of the small intestine's mucous and circular smooth muscle layers. The longitudinal muscle continues from small intestine. From valve to anus, the large intestine comprises the caecum, ascending, transverse and descending colons, rectum and anal canals.

The large intestine. Its internal structure

Similar to the small intestine, the large intestine has four coats: on the outside a shiny serous coat, a muscular coat underneath, a sub-mucous or fatty layer and an innermost mucous layer.

Derived from the peritoneum, the serous coat invests almost the entire large intestine. The muscular coat has longitudinal and circular fibers. Without forming a uniform layer, longitudinal fibers are collected into three flat bands producing sacculi, characteristic of the caecum and colon. When sacculi are dissected out, the tube can be lengthened, losing its sacculated character. At the sigmoid flexure, longitudinal fibers are more scattered, spreading out on lower intestine and rectum, forming a layer completely encircling this part of the gut. Circular fibers form a thin layer over caecum and colon, mostly at intervals between sacculi. In the rectum, circular muscle fibers form a thick layer constituting the anal sphincter.

The fatty layer connects muscular and mucous layers.

In the caecum and colon the mucous membrane is pale, smooth, without villi but with many crescentic folds thicker in the rectum, of a darker color, more vascular and loosely connected to muscular coat. When the rectum is contracted, the mucous membrane is thrown into two or three folds, shaped like a half-moon, containing circular fibers of gut. When empty, these folds overlap one other. They sustain the weight of fecal matter, preventing its urge toward the anus where its presence demands a feeling of discharge.

In the mucous membrane net-like tissue, simple follicles and solitary glands impart a cribriform or sievelike appearance, opening up onto the surface by minute orifices.

The large intestine, its solitary glands. Solitary glands are most abundant in the caecum and vermiform appendix; they are irregularly scattered over remaining areas of large intestine. Similar to those of small intestine, they are larger, 0.7 mm. long instead of 0.1 mm. In the submucosa, tens of thousands of lymphoid granules are scattered, especially in vermiform appendix. Similar to the small intestine, innumerable villi impart a soft, velvety appearance to the large intestine's inner surface.

The anal canal: a general view: Projecting into the rectal lumen are shelf-like transverse folds and the anal canal is pervaded by a series of permanent longitudinal folds or rectal columns. In the anus, the thickened circular muscle layer forms the internal sphincter. On the anal canal's exterior lies a sphincter of voluntary muscle. Innumerable rectal folds increase the power to accommodate large fecal masses.

Blood supply of the large intestine: Ramifying between muscular coats, the large intestine's arteries give off large branches. In the sub-mucous tissue, arteries divide into smaller vessels and pass to the mucous membrane. The superior hemorrhoidal branch of the inferior mesenteric artery supplies the rectum. About five inches from the anus, it divides into two branches running down on either side of the rectum to the urethra. Splitting up into six branches, the vessels pierce the muscular coat, descend between it and the mucous membrane. Vessels anastomose with other hemorrhoidal arteries, forming a series of loops around the anus. The anal region is thus extensively irrigated to enable the sphincter's expansion during stool evacuation. Veins follow a similar route. Due to its extensive blood supply there is never a need to operate on an anal tumor for given properly prepared food, the anal sphincter will expand without fail.

The large intestine, its food masses. In six hours' time a meal passes through the small intestine. Through the ileo-caecal valve the material intermittently flows out. When a peristaltic wave constricts the ileum, the ileo-colic sphincter relaxes. Automatically the aperture opens and contents pass into the large intestine. The ileo-colic valve prevents food residues and bacteria from backing into the small intestine. Villi reabsorb electrolytes, water-soluble vitamins and the mass becomes dryer. Fats are excreted in the stool. The colon's permanent bacterial flora breaks down carbohydrates and protein, the former by bacterial fermentation, the latter by putrefactive bacteria. Carbohydrate fermentation produces acid end products: lactic acid, acetic acid, alcohol, carbon dioxide and water. Poisonous amines are produced when protein putrefies: indole, skatole, histamine, tyranine, forming hydrogen sulfide and methane gases.

In a well-balanced diet, fermentation and putrefaction processes are in equilibrium, putrefaction is inhibited by acid from fermentation. When the balance is upset, either fermented stools or putrefied stools form. This may occur in cancer or other illnesses where blood flow is extremely slow.

The colon. Its six sections. The vermiform appendix protrudes from a blind sac jutting out two inches from the ileo-caecal valve. A blind, fingerlike structure about 3-4 inches, sometimes 9 inches long, the appendix is held in position by a fold of peritoneum from the mesentery. Its internal structure is similar to that of the intestine.

The caecum leads to the ascending colon, passing upward along the outer border of the right kidney, forming the hepatic flex. About 8 inches long, it extends as the transverse colon to the liver's right lobe, making an impression on the spleen. This is the longest part: on the outer border of left kidney it forms the splenic flexure and descends as the descending colon about 6 inches long.

The descending colon forms the sigmoid flexure, leading to the rectum. About 8 inches long, the rectum passes downward, backward to the level of the third sacral vertebra and has a backward and a forward curve, terminating at the anal orifice. The rectum is capable of great distention. In men it lies in front of the coccygeal tip behind the prostate gland, in women, behind the vagina. The anal canal is about an inch long. Ascending, transverse and descending colon form the figure of a giant "n" in the abdomen, lying in front of the mass represented by the small intestine. The entire large intestine is invested by peritoneum where blood, nerve and lymph vessels pass.

The colon: its main function. The colon has no digestive function and only serves as storage for feces. Fecal matter moves from ileo-caecal valve to anus in 18-24 hours, as follows: non-propulsive and rhythmic segmentation kneads or wrings colon contents. About 3 or 4 times daily, propulsive peristalsis occurs. Beginning at the caecum, mass contractions sweep over the entire colon to the sigmoid flexure, pushing colon contents into the rectum. Separated by long intervals of time, propulsive peristalsis involves simultaneous contraction of 8-10 inch segments.

The pelvic colon and lower part of descending colon are fecal storehouses until aroused by the desire to defecate. Food residues remain in the large intestine for about 12 hours. In the sigmoid colon before passage to rectum, some remnants of a meal are retained for as long as three days.

Stool evacuation

From about age two, the nerve center for defecation is voluntarily controlled.

Stimulated by mass movements of the colon, rectal pudendal nerves and stretch receptors mediate the urge to defecate by conducting impulses to sacral region's reflex center of spinal cord. Impulses to defecate are carried by parasympathetic fibers, relaxing internal anal sphincter's smooth muscle. This sphincter's three circular smooth muscles prevent continence.

In defecation, several groups of muscles participate: anus, rectum, diaphragm, perineum and abdominal walls. Muscles set up colonic waves, inducing anal sphincter's relaxation. Beginning at the caecum, mass contractions sweep over entire colon to sigmoid flexure, pushing contents into rectum. This is the gastro-colic reflex, often occurring after a meal. Respond promptly to the call for defecation for it may cease, feces remaining in rectum for long periods, impairing the reflex's efficiency.

Pain, fear, fever, fright, bright lights, loud music, noise, the lack of air and various mechanisms of a nervous nature inhibit the act of defecation. Violent emotions lead to dysfunction of the alimentary tract: crying, anxiety, pain and suffering, surgical operations, supreme muscular exertion, any critical condition, excitement, sadness, fright, may impede defecation, blood being diverted to the large brain where much blood is needed. Creative work may inhibit the act of defecation, thus singing, speaking, writing, knitting, crocheting, composing music, etc. For smooth bodily functions adopt a quiet life far from commitments and social activities.

Feces and what they represent

Before converting into feces, intestinal contents may remain one or two days in the large intestine; the mass is residues of food ingested the previous day. Food residues are a festering ground for bacterial growth and the colon's interior is a perfect place for their propagation. From a balanced diet, of the 100-200 grams of feces daily eliminated, 30-50% is bacteria; yeast and fungi are also present, the remaining 70-75% is water. Neutral fat, free fatty acids, soap and sterols make up 5-25%. Cholesterol is 1/3 of the fatty material. Feces have 0.5-1.5 grams of nitrogen compounds; the brown color of stool is due to products of bilirubin reduction.

Feces have a high concentration of potassium, much higher than chyme in the small intestine, calcium, magnesium and sodium salts. Gases represent 100 ml. of fecal content: such as swallowed air, the rest is produced in the colon. Some foods produce more gas: beans, cauliflower, onions, cabbage, pork. Gases comprise 15% oxygen, 5-10% carbon dioxide, 60% nitrogen. Other gases with characteristic smell are products of hydrogen sulfide fermentation, organic acids, indole and skatole, ammonium hydroxide and mercaptan. Also present are acetic and butyric acids. In 24 hours, feces expel 500 ml. of gases. The pH of feces is 7-7.5 thus basic, although it could be 5-7, forming fermented products. Cellulose is a large part of feces. When fasting, feces are still being formed, containing desquamated mucous cells and bacteria, weighing 7-8 grams. The color of feces indicates certain anomalies. When much fat is eaten, feces are black. Remove fats, and the coloration will be a normal brown. Grey feces indicate fermented products: remove carbohydrates and fats from the diet. Liquid feces indicate excess of concentrated foods. Dry feces indicate excess dry foods eaten. Use daily fecal color and consistency to regulate health.

Importance of defecation

Many people do not realize the importance of ridding the body of fecal masses. One woman allows feces to remain in her system for a week. When bacteria act on unabsorbed amino acids, large intestines form powerful poisons—extremely toxic when injected into the bloodstream. These poisons are alanine, tyrosine, histidine, ethylalanine, histamine and tyramine. Normally the body disposes of poisons, but in slow digestion they diffuse into the bloodstream through the colon's innumerable villi. The retention of poisons in the blood accounts for odorless or strongly fermented feces.

A man who suffered from a motorcycle accident had great difficulty healing a large hole at his ankle. We inquired about his eliminative functions, he admitted defecating once every three days, which explained why the wound healed with great difficulty. Another man revealed that his wife died of cancer: she was unable to move her body from the feet up. Finally, when she was unable to swallow, she died. We inquired about her daily regularity. Thinking for a moment, he said she spent very little time daily in the bathroom. With cancer, two or three stool evacuations daily are imperative.

One defecates when there is the urge roused by the passage of feces into the rectum, always empty prior to defecation. Be sensitive to rectal contraction, at the first contraction, evacuate. Feces retained for a long time in the colon prevents normal flow of colon contents, inducing over-absorption in digestive tract, loading the blood with impurities. In turn, kidneys will overwork, leading to kidney problems or inflammation. When kidneys' regulatory activities are impaired, healing processes slow down. Blood remaining in digestive organs seriously impairs regulatory functions. After defecation, blood immediately returns to regulatory organs for processes of repair and growth. Frequent stool evacuation is comparable to sleep and those who frequently rid the body of stools give the body a deep rest several times daily. Retaining feces for several days promotes absorption of waste products.

Circulation in the alimentary tract represents the largest regional blood supply. One third of the total cardiac output flows to digestive viscera, thus more blood flows to these organs than to any other organ-system. During digestion and absorption, blood flow to mucous membrane of active hollow organs is at its maximum: several milliliters of blood flow to every gram of tissue. The pancreas or liver receives 0.5 ml. per gram of tissue. The outer coat of hollow organs alone receives 0.1 ml. per gram of tissue. Frequent bowel evacuation is of the utmost importance. There is danger of collapse and sudden death when the fecal mass is retained for a long time in the colon. A duckling raised in an apartment could not defecate for an entire week: it died in increasingly greater convulsions. Man's entire efforts to prepare meals and cook, to exercise, have only one purpose in mind: to ensure continued regularity of body functions.

During a lifetime waist size indicates the state of health. A small waistline is indicative of good health. As it thickens to over 30 inches in women, all sorts of problems will assail the body. Do not let your waistline thicken and as soon as it reaches 30 inches, alter the diet.

Constipation, its causes. Constipation is the inability to evacuate stools with ease. Three factors induce constipation: too little fluids in diet, excessive absorption of water in colon, a contracted colon. If the urge to defecate is allowed to pass, the mass of feces accumulates, remaining for long periods in the colon. Eventually the call for defecation ceases, resulting in constipation. Strong emotional states prevent colonic motion, others are excess travel, social activities, crowds, public performance, work, activities, noise, music, singing, shouting, creative work.

Shoes affect daily regularity. Humans were meant to walk barefoot and shoes are unnatural. When barefoot, the pelvic and sacral regions are in a normal position. Heeled shoes tilt the pelvis, throwing the viscera off their normal position. Pointed toes or high-heels stir constipation, difficult defecation with eventual degenerative diseases. Wear comfortable shoes with space for toe movement; in shoes, feet should feel as if barefoot.

Some foods cause constipation: breads, cakes, cookies, cereals, raw foods, rice, large pieces of meat, dry, deep-fried and fermented foods. For regularity, make it a routine to exercise daily: walk long distances, work on the floor. When exercising do not exaggerate.

Some tips to promote good elimination

Air must circulate in the bathroom. Dress up adequately and comfortably but not excessively: at temperatures of 60-70° F. wear a thin wool dress or a cotton dress with a mohair sweater. In hot weather, wear a silk dress. In winter, a wool dress is important. Warm feet provide strength to push and Dr. Marten's leather shoes are excellent for cement floors. Do sweeping, slow, giant counterclockwise movements around with legs and arms holding a 5 lb. weight. Jump up and down 30 times. Climb imaginary stairs. A straight-edged toilet seat is more relaxing than a round seat. Improvise one. Use a wooden toilet seat not a soft padded plastic seat. Because the rectum is more to the left side of the abdominal cavity, let body weight rest on the left buttock. A chamber pot may prove to be useful. Silence and darkness induce a rapid movement. Lean head or body. Hold onto a bar. Concentrate.

Never use a quart-sized enema but introduce two squeezes from a child-sized enema syringe; soften tip with cocoa butter. Mornings after breakfast and evenings after the bath are the best times to defecate.

Tighten up the abdominal region and massage the body if needed. Peristaltic movements are slow and slow motion massage stimulates the intestines. Fill a little plastic bottle with very hot water, as hot as bearable, and hold it against the abdomen, the spine, legs, thighs, etc. Let the heat cause a slight burning effect. It will stimulate defecation even under the worst conditions of health. Breathe deeply and drink some hot water if necessary. One man brings a mug of coffee to the bathroom during daily stool evacuation.

From antiquity, the Chinese practiced moxibustion. Cones made of powdered leaves of the plant Artemisia Vulgaris were placed against the back of the body, along the spine. When cones burned down, blisters were left on the skin. This treatment raised body temperature and increased the red cell count. Modern man does not want to be covered with small blisters, and holding a plastic bottle filled with very hot water simulates moxibustion. It raises body temperature and provides the strength needed for stool evacuation.

For the final push, grab a bar. If weak, push or bend your ankles outward as though affected by the Sign of Babinski and push. Shift body weight from one buttock to the other. Push down with the palm of both hands. Hold onto a bar and twist your body slightly to the left and to the right. Massage your back. Do the same for the other side. S-shaped muscles have great power to push. Twist the body. Turn body articulation counter-clockwise simultaneously. Pull the head up, backwards and around, counter-clockwise. Pull the head slowly backwards, do the same with arms. Head and arms pull the rectus abdominus muscle—most responsible for a good stool evacuation. Any position is good, provided one achieves a movement. Our digestive system is 30 feet long. What can one do to rid a mass from an extra long winding tube? You shake, beat, press, bend, knead it, etc. Think of all the things you can do and imitate. Our body follows the laws of physics: when a bag is very full the upright position is best. When adequately full, the seated position is good but when very empty as when fasting, squat on a potty. Observe cats and dogs defecating and imitate.

The most important factor is a good diet and careful preparation of foods, sufficient liquids, ripe fruit, cooked vegetables will prompt anyone to evacuate. Regardless of color, smell, brown, black or gray, liquid or solid, most important is to rid the body of the fecal mass, and anything done to achieve a movement is acceptable.

Some artificial stimuli used to induce regularity

Pills and laxatives induce mass movements but distend the colon. Laxatives irritate the delicate mucous membrane, stirring ulcer or tumor formation. Eat delicate foods and avoid fibrous foods. When acids accumulate during digestion, damage occurs and they will digest the stomach. A chronic ulcer can be initiated by an episode of local ischemia (lack of blood). In hemorrhagic shock, the total gastric blood flow was reduced to less than 10% of control values. Avoid laxatives.

A level tablespoonful of Kosher salt in three glasses of very hot dilute soup or water, will ease constipation. Always accompany meals with a soup or light beverage. Avoid dry foods, they induce constipation. If constipated one day, intake only liquids the following day. Do not let constipation continue for any length of time.

The digestive system: its large glands
a. The liver

The liver is the largest gland of the human body, weighing 3-4 pounds, slightly larger in men. It represents 1/36th of man's total body weight.

Situated under the diaphragm, in the upper right part of the abdomen, the left lobe extends above the stomach. Shaped like a wedge, its base to the right, the thin edge to the left, a fold of peritoneum divides it into two unequal parts. Five fissures on its under and posterior surface, divide the liver into 5 lobes arranged like the letter H. They are the right, left, quadrate, caudate and Spigelian fissures. The largest is the transverse fissure for passage of the hepatic portal vein, hepatic artery, subdivisions of common bile duct, lymphatics and nerves. Five ligaments connect liver to diaphragm's undersurface. Five vessels supply liver, all branches of the hepatic artery, the hepatic vein.

The substance of the liver: The liver is composed of hepatic lobules held together by an extremely fine fatty tissue with branches of hepatic veins, ducts, arteries, lymphatics and nerves, the whole structure invested by a serous and fibrous coat. Liver lobules are arranged in cords of cells exposed to blood on one side, to ducts on the other.

Functions of the liver: The liver has several very important functions.

1. As blood passes through intestinal wall, foodstuffs and occasionally poisonous substances are added to it. Laden with these materials, blood immediately passes through liver. Acting as a filter, the liver removes poisonous substances and bacteria. Within sinusoids, purified blood is immediately discharged into the hepatic vein, enters increasingly larger vessels and returns to the heart by the inferior vena cava.

2. The liver is the only site producing ketone bodies. In pathological conditions, liver contains large deposits of fat. When the liver cannot deal with excessive amounts of fat or in diabetes and anemia, ketone bodies form.

3. The liver converts sugar to glycogen. Glycogen comprises about 10-15% of the liver's wet weight. When the body requires sugar, glycogen is discharged back into bloodstream.

4. After liver cells cleanse blood, the liver produces bile, an excretion. Bile is

discharged into channels of progressively increasing size forming the hepatic duct, leaving the liver to enter gall bladder.

Composition of bile. Gall bladder bile is thick, viscid, of a yellow color, sometimes brown or greenish, comprising mostly bile salts, bile pigments, cholesterol and any of these may be found in gallstones. The production of bile is continuous and during digestion, it passes to gall bladder where it is stored and as needed, intermittently flows into duodenum. Pancreatic pancreozymin released into the bloodstream stirs gallbladder to contract, expelling bile; Oddi's sphincter relaxes and bile passes into small intestine.

Indigestion is the most common symptom of gall bladder disease.

The hepatic duct is 2 inches long, the pancreas cystic duct is 1 1/2 inch long. Both join as the common duct, 3 inches long. Before opening into the duodenum the common duct expands into the ampulla of Vater.

The most common liver disease is hepatitis or liver inflammation where gall bladder infection spreads into bile and passes into liver. It can also spread into the head of pancreas, causing pancreatitis. Both are cured with great difficulty. No need for alarm. Adopt an isotonic diet immediately and all inflammation will gradually subside.

Every 24 hours only 0.6 g. of bile is excreted in the feces, replaced by new synthesis of the same amount of bile acids.

Jaundice: The excess destruction of red blood cells causes jaundice. Dead red cells stir production of liver's bile salts: biliverdin and bilirubin. Gallstones are formed when the liver cannot dispose of an overload of dead red cells. If a gallstone lodges in the common bile duct, obstructing passage, bile cannot reach the duodenum, is absorbed and jaundice results; 90% of all gallstones is composed of cholesterol. Calcium bilirubinate comprises the remaining 10%. In jaundice, do not work to exhaustion. The following represents work: excess stimuli striking the body: music, noise, excess activity done by the body: dancing, speaking, working; foreign matter penetrating the body: food, injections, pills, hours spent before a computer etc. Remove excess activity and the condition will soon subside.

b. The pancreas. Like salivary glands, the pancreas is a racemose gland with an alveolar arrangement of cells. Alveoli are drained by a system of ducts.

Comparable to a human or dog's tongue, the pancreas resembles a hammer. About 7 inches long, it lies behind and below the stomach, body and tail directed left, head fitting into the duodenum's curve, tail touching the spleen.

The internal structure of the pancreas: The pancreas has many lobules. About 3 1/2 inches below the pylorus, its ducts convey pancreatic fluid to the duodenum. At rest, the gland contains many zymogen granules, furnishing enzymes of pancreatic juice. During the secretory process, cells discharge zymogen granules into the alveolar cavity.

Pancreatic juice: Pancreatic juice is a clear, colorless fluid with an alkaline reaction composed of water with sodium bicarbonate, sodium chloride and three important enzymes: trypsin, steapsin and amylopsin.

In the small intestine's lining, acid chyme from partially digested food forms the hormone secretin. Absorbed by blood, secretin is carried to pancreas and liver, stimulating cells to secrete. The first pancreatic juice is poor in enzymes, stirring the duodenum to liberate a second hormone, pancreozymin and pancreas secretes a juice with many enzymes.

External signs of a lack of pancreatic secretion

The absence of pancreatic juice is indicated by large quantities of undigested fats and protein in feces. Excess food and alcoholic beverages cause acute inflammation of pancreas with death occurring within 24-48 hours.

Pancreas may be affected by tumors either benign or cancerous. Severe pain in the upper abdominal region indicates acute pancreatic inflammation. There is no reason to despair. When in pain, immediately alter the diet. Never continue to eat ordinary foods when abnormal signs appear (see chapter on cooking).

In dire cases, the pancreas is surgically removed. One can survive for a while but cancer soon takes over the liver and other organs, causing death. The best course to follow is to alter the diet. One cannot survive without a pancreas. Pancreatic trypsin converts proteins into peptides. Amylopsin converts starches into maltose. Steapsin splits fats into fatty acids and glycerin. Without these enzymes foods cannot be properly digested and death will ensue.

Chapter 14
Some notions about foods and how to assess nutritional requirements for a long life

Eating is one of the greatest pleasures of life. Preparation of foods enabled man to develop from a primitive hominid to modern man with a large brain, and freed him from chewing needs, allowing hands to perform delicate tasks. Only since the use of fire has there been recorded history.

Better preparation of foods stirs longevity

Better preparation of foods gradually increased life-span but longevity is not an indicator of progress unless man learns to live better. Today, there are more sophisticated illnesses. Functional disorders are due to faulty nutrition, additives and excess food causes autointoxication. Women are the greatest contributors to human progress. Around 4,000 years ago women planted sticks, baked, fermented beans and bread, reaped and stored grain, spun flax, etc.

The industrialization of nations relegated food preparation to restaurants and fast food places, leading to malnutrition. Prepared foods contain additives, artificial color/flavor deceive appearance. Commercially prepared foods are sickly sweet, stirring drug addiction, drugs being an inferior carbohydrate. Indulgence in sweet foods stirs cruelty: Eliogabalus, a cruel Roman emperor of the 2nd century is a good example. In Roman times cookies and sweets were a large part of the diet.

Food should not add vitamins for minute quantities are present in all fresh foods. Many young girls are unable to conceive. Is it caused by fast foods?

Food digestion

Digestion is oxidation. Food preparation and cooking is pre-digestion. Asians are renowned for their intricate preparations and fast cooking time. Exposure to air at preparation, is a primary process of food oxidation, which eases digestion. Last century, Dr. William Beaumont observed the digestion of food from a hole in Alexis St. Martin's stomach. He noticed that meats were the last items to leave the stomach. Meats should be carefully prepared, finely cut and marinated before cooking.

Starches constipate. Do not serve two starchy foods at once: rice and beans, bread and potatoes, rice and corn, etc. Starches must be cooked several times. The Chinese make a delicious bouncy rice cake called Bok Tong Go. Gently steam a few slices then place some thin Cheddar cheese slices above and turn heat off. When cheese is melted, serve. This rice cake is easily digestible and can be bought by the pound in Chinatown.

Pound cooked rice with a pestle until sticky like glue, then serve with vegetables and meats or cook again in a recipe. Cooking starches twice is a way to ease digestion.

Fruits are a good source of carbohydrates. The drier the fruit, the higher the carbohydrate content. Tropical fruits even as juices are hard to digest. Fruits are high in water content but if you eat many fruits, avoid other starches. Nuts are also a good source of carbohydrates however, their hardness indicates a high mineral content. They should be eaten sparingly or mixed in recipes.

Vegetables are high in minerals. Eat green vegetables sparingly. Chlorophyll is not a part of man's body make-up. If you enjoy carrot juice and other vegetable juices, dilute it by half, with water. Nature did not intend man to drink fruits and vegetables.

Cereals are carbohydrates. Choose ones that do not contain many additives. Fibrous cereals coarsen facial and body skin. In extreme nervous tension, fibrous foods scrape the digestive tract, causing ulcer or cancerous growths. Of course all foods contain fibers except for liquids.

All fats are indigestible. Saturated fats are better. If saturated fats are detrimental to man then avoid milk and milk products. Cheeses can be used to make delicious recipes—use sparingly. Be wary of milk products for excess calcium in the blood shrinks the body with bone degeneration. Avoid bottled, boxed fresh juices and other foods with added calcium. Mixtures of foods are superior. If separated in three portions: meat, vegetable and starch, combine them in the mouth and chew them together prior to swallowing.

Additional tips in preparing foods for health

Claude Bernard states that digestion is putrefaction. Putrefaction does not necessarily give rise to toxic substances causing food poisoning: Limburger cheese, fish eaten by Eskimos, the 1,000 year Chinese duck eggs. Chemical putrefaction is different from natural air-exposed putrefaction. Cooking hastens oxidation, softens food fibers and eases digestion or putrefaction.

When preparing foods, use fire with care. Vitamins, proteins are easily destroyed and food loses its value. Observe the following.

When mixing foods, cook each item separately for a short time then combine together for a second or two. Never allow smell of food to reek across apartment or outdoors. Warm up foods over medium low heat. Cook meats separately; combine with cooked vegetables or meats. Undercook foods to keep for use in a recipe.

Tenderize large pieces of meat, criss-cross with the back of a butcher knife. Marinate meat overnight in sauces, peanut butter, sugar or jam, salt, curry. Pat cornstarch on before cooking. Cook over low heat. When a knife pokes in with ease it is cooked. Be careful with fish and seafood. When hard and flaky, fish or shrimp is overcooked. Seafood and fish require a few minutes of cooking time. When a knife pokes through the fish, it is done.

Before cooking, remove skins of fruits and fruit-like vegetables.
In pastry baking, use half the given amount of sugar. Toast bread.
Make your own dough. Boil some water and pour it over raw flour.
Roll dough with a broomstick size rolling pin.

Make an interesting dough with a mixture of cooked, pounded rice, two potatoes, egg, vinegar, salt and flour, lard.

In indirect cooking, steaming, baking, boiling, use medium high heat. To warm up pastry or to toast bread, use direct low heat. When aroma is perceptible, remove from the heat. For oven roasting meats, render the fat over high heat then lower heat and add seasonings to cook inside until aroma is perceptible in the air, or if a knife pokes through with ease. Some people prefer roasting meats with all seasonings over the lowest oven heat. The result is good.

When preparing coffee or chocolate milk, dilute milk with water, by three-quarters. For each cup use a few drops of percolated coffee, a dash of cocoa, a small teaspoonful of honey.

Nutritional requirements. Carbohydrates

Carbohydrates are not essential dietary constituents. They may be formed from some amino acids and the glycerol portion of fats. Carbohydrates supply half of man's energy yet blood normally contains less than 0.1% at all times. Excess carbohydrates will be stored.

Whether a fat, carbohydrate or protein, food derived from these sources represents stored or potential energy. When digestive enzymes reduce food to its simple constituents, the latter are absorbed in the small intestine. Carbon and hydrogen are oxidized in body cells, liberating energy for muscular work to maintain vital functions: heartbeat, breathing, speaking, excitability of nervous tissue, manufacture of hormones, etc. When food intake exceeds energy needs, the body will store food as carbohydrate in the form of glycogen and fat. When energy value of food is less than body's requirements, body will draw on stored energy. Though the liver stores energy as glycogen, the actual circulating carbohydrate is about 0.1%.

Carbohydrates contain carbon, hydrogen and oxygen. A monosaccharide, glucose is the most important single carbohydrate in physiology. Glucose, fructose and galactose are immediately absorbed monosaccharides. All three have a similar formula with different positions of hydrogen and oxygen atoms.

Three important disaccharides are sucrose (beet, cane, maple sugars), maltose (malt), lactose (milk). They are different kinds of hexoses. When ingested, intestinal enzymes split them into their monosaccharide constituents.

With whole-meal bread, stools become softer and bulkier, however whole-meal cereal contains phytate and fiber. By combining with minerals, phytate interferes the absorption of calcium, iron and zinc in the gut. In India, children develop rickets and adults are affected with osteomalacia. Fiber and whole grain cereal are to be eaten sparingly.

High sugar consumption causes dental caries. Addiction to sugar aggravates or brings on diabetes: when absorbed, blood sugar rises, similarly blood glucose level; to burn sugars efficiently, the pancreas beta cells secrete insulin. High blood sugar level and reduced secretion of insulin stir diabetes where beta cells cannot produce sufficient insulin to cope with increased carbohydrate contents in blood; blood sugars remain high, leaking into urine.

Excess insulin production causes low blood sugar, with weakness, tremor, faintness, followed by unconsciousness, convulsions, even death. Body glucose derives not only from ingested food. Protein digestion yields amino acids, forming glucose. In starvation, glucose is produced from body protein. Diabetics are usually fat and must limit their sugar and starch intake. Years of indulgence in sweet and starchy foods lead to diabetes. Honey, the best sugar, is a simple sugar, requires little digestion. Other sugars are complex sugars.

Foods high in carbohydrates are barley, buckwheat, flour, breads, cakes, icings, candies, cookies, corn meal, lentils, pasta, pies, canned fruit in syrup, popcorn, pizza, dried fruit, creamed soup, rice, sugars, cereals, potatoes, wheat flour, white enriched flour, bread flour, pastry flour. Potatoes and sweet potatoes are good starches high in water content. Avoid excess starches and the desire for pastries, alcohol or drugs, will diminish. Drugs are lower grade carbohydrates.

Muscle contains glycogen from blood glucose. When muscles contract, muscle glycogen breaks down into glucose, forming lactic acid, ultimately re-synthesized into glycogen and in part oxidized to carbon dioxide and water. Heavy sports raise blood's normal 0.1% content in blood, causing diabetes. Long distance walking, household chores are excellent exercise.

Fats

Fat is not really required in the diet. On a fat-free diet, essential lipids: lecithin, cephalin, sphingomyelin and the cerebrosides cannot be synthesized. Some required essential fatty acids are linoleic, arachidonic acids; animal fats: pork, chicken and duck fats are good sources of saturated fat. The cheapest source of energy, fats supply twice as much energy per gram but fall within the normal carbohydrate value of 0.1% in blood.

Fats comprise 11-18% of man's body weight. Made of carbon, hydrogen and oxygen, when a molecule of a triatomic alcohol, glycerol, combines with three molecules of a higher fatty acid, either palmitic, stearic or oleic acid, a neutral fat forms. In the triglyceride molecule, depending on which fatty acid, the following fats form: tripalmitin, tristearin, triolein, respectively. Animals' fatty tissue is composed of connective tissue deposited with a mixture of neutral fat, chiefly triolein, some tripalmitin and very little tristearin. Intestinal enzymes hydrolyze triglycerides into their constituents: fatty acids and glycerol. In the presence of a base, fat is decomposed, fatty acids forming soaps.

The body contains sterols, steroids, phospholipids or phosphatides. Sterols are a secondary alcohol combined with fatty acids: waxy substances known as steroids. Hormones of sex glands, adrenal cortex are composed of sterols. The human body contains cholesterol as cholesterol esters. First isolated from gallstones, cholesterol is an important bile constituent chemically related to cholic acid, Vitamin D and the sex hormones. Nerve sheaths, brain tissue and skin contain cholesterol. Brain, muscle, liver, milk, eggs have phospholipids. Lecithin, cephalin, sphingomyelin belong to this class of substances, and when hydrolyzed yield fatty acids, phosphoric acid and a nitrogenous base.

Food and carbohydrates form animal fat. Fat is stored energy the body draws upon when needed, as during a fast. Fatty acids ingested must recombine with glycerin to produce the body's characteristic fat with the proper mixture of the three types of neutral fat. Before transportation across cell membranes, fatty acids must initially be transformed into phospholipids.

Fats are saturated or unsaturated. Saturated fats hold all the hydrogen they can. Unsaturated fats can hold more hydrogen. The body cannot synthesize certain unsaturated fatty acids, i.e., linoleic acid, the most important essential fatty acid required by humans. Saturated fats are directly converted into the body's own saturated fats. Unsaturated fats must first be saturated then converted into the body's saturated fats, a double duty to perform.

For cooking use a little saturated fats and avoid unsaturated fats altogether. The softer and more fluid the oil, the greater the degree of unsaturation. Deep fat fried foods are the most preferred foods. Wipe them repeatedly to remove fats. Fried foods are difficult to digest, causing catarrh with expectoration—a dangerous sign. Deep fried foods induce a terminal state quickly.

The more fats eaten, the more absorbed, the more cholesterol penetrates the bloodstream. From fatty foods the liver manufactures cholesterol. All fats consumed to excess develop atherosclerosis, manifested by fatty streaks underneath the lining of arteries. Heavily clogged blood vessels risk heart attacks. The International Society Commission for Heart Disease recommends that fat from all food sources be limited to 33% of man's daily caloric intake. In extreme illness avoid fats altogether. Data prove that already in their twenties some young people have clogged arteries.

When a person is sick, the liver accumulates large quantities of fat. Fats are emulsified by bile from the liver; bile activates pancreatic steapsin, accelerating its action; bile dissolves insoluble fatty acids, assists in the absorption of fats and reduces intestinal putrefaction by stimulating peristalsis. The glycerol portion of fats forms glycogen, contributing to the glucose supply. The liver contains 100 grams of glycogen but is able to store up to 400 grams. Liver is a reservoir and glucose may be drawn from it if blood sugar level falls below normal.

Proteins: Proteins comprise 7% of man's blood. Our normal daily requirement is about one gram per kilogram of body weight. At 200 lbs. about a quarter pound of protein daily is sufficient. The best proteins are from animal tissues: eggs, milk, liver, meat. Plant proteins in cereals and vegetables are inadequate.

Proteins are the chief constituents of muscle, gland and nervous tissue, many hormones, enzymes and blood. A protein molecule's basic elements are carbon, hydrogen, oxygen, nitrogen, sulfur and phosphorus. The body's nitrogen, sulfur and phosphorus depend entirely on proteins. These basic elements are combined in a protein molecule, linked together as amino acids. Some 23 amino acids have been discovered of which the simplest is glycine.

Proteins contain 50-1,000 molecules of amino acid combinations, strung out on a chain. Many proteins have 15 varieties of amino acids and can reach to over 200 molecules. The size of protein molecules varies in different proteins. Egg albumen's molecular weight is 200,000, other proteins are over a million. Their shape varies: globular in albumin, long and fiber-like in myosin of muscle, tendon and ligaments.

Repair and growth processes depend on dietary protein content. Peptidase, an intestinal juice, breaks down proteins into their constituent amino acids, are absorbed into the bloodstream and carried to body tissues. Each tissue chooses the amino acids it requires, rejecting others. Animals are able to manufacture some amino acids. The human body is unable to make 8-10 essential amino acids. In nutrition, proteins are not of equal value. Those resembling body proteins are of the highest nutritive value. They are of animal origin, i.e., fish, eggs, milk, meat. Gelatin and maize are incomplete and do not maintain growth and nitrogen balance in the adult. Gliadin of wheat, horlein of barley, legumin of peas lack certain essential amino acids. They repair body protein but cannot support growth in the adult. Young animals fail to grow on a diet of these proteins.

Lactalbumin of milk, ovalbumin of eggs, proteins of meat, glutenin of wheat contain essential amino acids, also whole egg, lean beef, horsemeat, halibut, haddock, soy bean, navy beans, defatted peanut, sunflower seeds, barley, buckwheat flour, cheddar cheese, meal, corn, whole milk, oatmeal, unpolished rice, whole rye, whole wheat. Consume sparingly foods high in protein and fat such as milk, cheese and meat. Some cereals contain protein but for sufficient amino acids, large amounts must be consumed. Organ-meats: sweetbreads, kidney, liver, gizzard, balls, etc contain many cells high in nucleoprotein content with purine derivatives. Deamination of purine derivatives forms uric acid. From adenine and guanine, ammonia is split off and oxidized by tissue enzymes. Uric acid is a nitrogenous compound present in urine and blood. When deposited in tissues as sodium urate crystals, uric acid produces gout or painful arthritis. Gout aggravates when large quantities of organ meats are ingested, which can cause mental deterioration.

A diet high in protein causes osteoporosis with loss of bone density and brittle bones. Growing children and lactating or pregnant women require more protein. A person weighing 150 pounds should eat two ounces of protein daily. If too little, add more but do not double the amount.

For antibody effectiveness and to restore depleted tissues and bone marrow, proteins must be of high quality. Proteins produce phagocytic cells to engulf and digest bacteria. An antibody is a serum globulin, its synthesis depends on the diet, particularly on high-quality proteins. A lack of protein causes personality changes. Heat-coagulated proteins are easier to digest than raw proteins. From digested protein, almost 58% of amino acids form glycogen to be stored in the liver and returned to blood as sugar.

Water: Water is the most important required inorganic substance: 92% of blood is water, body tissues contain 65% water. The adult daily requirement is 21-43 ml. of water per kilogram of body weight. At 70 kilograms at least 1,750 ml. of water per day are required, of which 650 ml. are from liquids, 750 from solid food, 350 ml. from oxidation water. A 5% water loss causes impairment of performance. A 10% loss is severe dehydration and a 15-20% loss causes death. A large quantity of a hypotonic solution results in water intoxication with impaired performance, headache, nausea or convulsions. Several glasses of dilute juices, a few cups of light coffee or cocoa, two bowls of broth daily can keep you on the safe side. At the first sign of thirst, drink a mouthful of water. It is better than drinking several glasses of water.

Calcium: Calcium is required for bone and teeth growth, to clot blood, to form milk when lactating, and calcium paracaseinate curd in digestion. Pregnant women and children require more calcium than adults. The ingestion of cocoa, spinach, rhubarb causes calcium deficiency due to their high oxalic acid content. Oxalic acid combined with calcium forms insoluble calcium oxalate which the body cannot absorb. Milk and milk products are high in calcium. The daily calcium requirement is one gram for growing children, 0.7 g. for adults. Bone degeneration may occur when excess calcium is consumed.

Salt: Salt or sodium chloride is required because blood is salty and this saltiness must be maintained throughout life. The buffer systems in blood and tissue fluids are sodium salts, i.e., sodium bicarbonate and sodium phosphates. Sodium bicarbonate produces the proper pH for enzyme action of saliva, pancreatic and intestinal juices. It assists elimination of carbon dioxide in lungs and acid products in kidneys. For adults, the minimum daily requirement of sodium chloride is about

10 g., for children, 1.7 g. Use Kosher salt freely on foods and avoid iodized salt.

Phosphorus: Phosphorus is essential to form bones, teeth, and milk. Organic phosphorus compounds such as phospholipids, nucleoproteins and casein, phosphate buffers, esters of phosphoric acid oxidize carbohydrates. The ratio of calcium to phosphorus in the diet should be about 2 to 1. Many foods contain phosphorus and a deficiency is unlikely. Daily intake of 1.3 g. of phosphorus is adequate for children and/or adults.

Magnesium: Magnesium is a constituent of blood plasma. A deciliter of blood plasma contains 2 mg. of magnesium. In a normal diet, do not worry about magnesium in blood.

Potassium: Potassium is a constituent of animal cells. With sodium, it relaxes muscles. Potassium salts are found in red blood cells, sodium is present in blood plasma. Daily requirements of potassium are 1.5 g. for children, 3 g. for adults. In a normal diet, do not worry about potassium. Excess potassium can be detrimental to the heart's pacemaker action.

Iron: Iron is required to form hemoglobin of red blood cells. In anemia, there is deficiency in iron. Symptoms are tiredness, headache, diminished performance, impaired skin growth, hair and nails. Frequent blood donation, menstruation, gastrointestinal bleeding cause chronic blood loss. Work reduces blood. Beware of activities done by the body, materials penetrating the body, striking the body. Avoid donating blood.

Normally, the body requires from 10-15 mg. of iron daily; it increases during menstruation, pregnancy and lactation. Chief sources of food iron are meats, eggs, beans, spinach, peas, wheat and oatmeal. In a newborn infant sufficient iron is present to last about six months, after which meats provide additional sources of iron. The adult body stores 4-5 g. of iron of which 800 mg. can be mobilized at any time.

Fluorine: Fluorine is supposed to prevent dental caries. A daily allowance of 1 mg. is safe, but 5 mg. is toxic, causing osteosclerosis.
Iodine: Iodine is essential in the development and function of the thyroid gland. Iodine deficiency causes hypothyroidism and simple goiter. Iodine has been added to some table salts: a dangerous practice as many have developed thyroid tumors from consuming iodized salt. Seafood and crops grown in coastal regions contain sufficient iodine to meet daily requirements of 150 micrograms. The body stores 10 mg. of iodine.

Copper: Copper is required for iron absorption. Copper deficiency leads to anemia and disorders of pigmentation. About 100-150 mg. of copper is stored in the body; do not be concerned about daily requirements of 2-5 mg. Copper is probably needed as a catalyst to form hemoglobin which contains no copper. The daily requirement is very small, and ordinary diets provide sufficient copper.

Do not tamper with minerals. Normal blood contains around 1% of minerals, the body 5% — very little. Careful cooking preserves all minerals in foods.

Trace elements with acknowledged physiological function are iron, fluorine, iodine and copper; overdoses disturb body functions. Do not tamper with trace elements. A good diet provides the required vitamins and minerals. Dissolved in water, in and out of body cells, minerals combine with chloride to form electrolytes. Between water, cells and the medium without, a movement of electrolytes occurs constantly. To maintain life, this transfer of electrolytes is essential for all vital processes.

Vitamins

Besides minerals in foods, some essential chemical substances promote growth, cure some diseases, and maintain overall health. They are vitamins, present in minute quantities in natural foods. In 1906, Sir F. Gowland Hopkins of Cambridge University said that no man can live on a mixture of pure protein, fat and carbohydrate. Therefore, the body requires minute quantities of vitamins without which a living organism cannot flourish.

Vitamins are in the body's enzyme systems. They must be supplied for the living body cannot manufacture them. In a well-balanced diet, vitamin supplements do not benefit and can be detrimental to health. Some people leave a trail of odor from vitamin pills. In children, vitamin over-dosage stirs over-activity and nervousness.

Vitamins are either fat-soluble or water-soluble.

The fat-soluble vitamins

Vitamins A, D, E, and **K** are fat-soluble vitamins. They are formed from carotenoids in the body, and provitamins in food. Vitamin D is synthesized from provitamin B4 in a photochemical reaction when the sun's ultra-violet light acts on skin.

The water-soluble vitamins

The B complex vitamins are water-soluble. They are Vitamin B1 or thiamine, Vitamin B2 or riboflavin, VitaminB3, nicotinic acid or niacin, Vitamin 6 or pyridoxine, Pantothenic acid, Choline, Inositol, Para-amino benzoic acid, Vitamin H or biotin, Folic acid, Vitamin B12, Vitamin c or ascorbic acid.

Folic acid is a complex molecule composed of a yellow pigment called pteridine, para-aminobenzoic acid and glutamic acid. Many plant and animal tissues contain folic acid, especially plant foliage but yeast, soybeans, wheat, liver, kidney and eggs are good sources. No specific requirement is established for man but to cure macrocytic anemia with red cells of gigantic proportions, 100-200 mg. were given. It is beneficial in the treatment of anemia.

Vitamin B12, similar to Folic acid, is useful in the treatment of anemia in humans and animals, especially pernicious anemia. It is closely related to the animal protein factor essential in growth and lactation. Vitamin B12 and Folic acid increase hemoglobin and red cell count. Vitamin B12 has a therapeutic effect in nervous symptoms of anemia. With a molecular weight of 10,000, higher than that of other vitamins, Vitamin B12 is a red, crystalline compound containing cobalt. Liver, milk and beef extracts are the best sources of B12. The daily requirement has been established at 5 micrograms and minute quantities are therapeutically effective.

Vitamin C or ascorbic acid is found in paprika, citrus fruits: lemons, oranges and grapefruit, tomatoes, raw cabbage, strawberries, green leafy vegetables also in cereals, meats, eggs, milk. Cooking destroys a large amount of ascorbic acid and boiling 30 minutes destroys 70-90% in cabbage and vegetables. A deficiency of ascorbic acid causes scurvy with weak teeth, swollen gums, bleeding and a tendency to bleed to death. Early symptoms of scurvy are weight loss, anemia and fatigue. In severe cases, gums swell, bleeding readily, teeth loosen, bones become brittle, breaking easily. Ascorbic acid's essential function is to form and maintain the intercellular substance cementing cells together, of great importance in capillary walls, cartilage, bones and teeth. A diet lacking in ascorbic acid results in loss of intercellular substance with structural weakness of capillary walls, bones and teeth.

The daily allowance is 75 mg. In large doses, Vitamin C does not reduce frequency of colds, may even be harmful, precipitating the demineralization of bones. It may stir kidney stones, reduce fertility in women, and interfere with liver function. A daily dosage of 1,000 mg. completely saturates tissues and larger doses are excreted in the urine.

Fat-soluble vitamins can be stored in large quantities, sometimes several months. The same for water-soluble Vitamins B12 and folic acid. All other vitamins are stored in limited quantities and must regularly be replenished.

There is no need to take vitamin supplements if one has sufficient sunshine, does not overcook foods and some fresh fruits daily. Two hours daily of sunshine and air are imperative. To assess the carbohydrate content of many common foods here are three tables compiled from a list available only to physicians and pharmacists in Italy.

Table 3
Carbohydrate content in 100 g. of various food groups

Food	Carbohydrate
Fish and sea food	0 - 1.1 g.
Meats	0 - 5.9 g.
Eggs, milk, milk products	0.7 - 6.1 g.
Beverages: coffee, coca cola, lemonade, tea, wine	0.8 - 12.0 g.
Fresh vegetables and beans	4.1 - 10.6 g.
Fresh fruits	6.4 - 22.2 g.
Potato, corn	7.7 - 22.1 g.
Fresh nuts	20.7 - 45.6 g.
Condensed milk, milk powder	38.2 - 52.0 g.
Dried fruits	66.5 - 77.4 g.
Dried nuts	78.0 g.
Grains, bread, pasta, cereals, flour, rice, soy and other grains	48.7 - 80.4 g.
Dried vegetables and beans	58.2 - 82.6 g.
Tapioca	86.4 g.
Marmalade, honey, sugar	70, 82.3, 99.5 g.

Oily products and alcoholic beverages are not included in Table 3 for it is believed that oils and alcoholic drinks do not contain carbohydrates. This is erroneous for fats are esters of fatty acids and glycerol, a polyhydric alcohol, and carbohydrates are derivatives of polyhydric alcohols. Thus carbohydrates may be classed as alcohols and vice versa. The fermentation of sugars produces alcohols.

Due to the concentrated nature of fats and alcohols, 100g of the latter have a 500% carbohydrate content, perhaps even higher. In illness or when older, avoid fats and alcohols like poison.

Table 4
Alcohol content and caloric value in 100 g. of common alcoholic beverages

Beverage	Alcohol content	kcal
Beer	3.6 g	47
Wine	8.8 - 12.5 g	80 - 120
Rum	35.1 g	248
Whiskey	35 g	245

TABLE 5
Lipid content and caloric value per 100 g. of some commonly used fats

	Lipid content	kcal
Butter	81 g	716
Mayonnaise	78.9 g	718
Margarine	78.4 g	698
Vegetable oils	99.9 g	883
Lard	99.0 g	901
Cod liver oil	99.9 g	901

A killer diet consists of corn grits, molasses and fat back.

Chapter 15
How to cope with external signs of illness

Some illnesses are indicated by marks on palms of hands, reported a recent magazine article. Though one cannot trust such diagnoses alone, many external indices do reveal declining health or the oncoming of a serious illness. The following passages analyze many of these signs.

Detect illness by pulse and breathing rates

In ancient and modern China, the pulse is an important diagnostic tool. Simultaneously taken with breathing, pulse rate determines varying states of health. Modern western medicine measures pulse rate alone per minute. Simultaneously taken with inhalation, pulse rate assesses the total amount of blood flowing through heart and entire regulatory organs. Two pulse beats to an inhalation denotes perfect health and optimum blood flow through regulatory organs.

At three pulse beats to an inhalation there is slight fever. Blood flow through regulatory organs is adequate but upon the slightest exertion, excitement, sudden fright, blood flow rapidly decreases through regulatory organs with serious disturbances.

Four beats to an inhalation indicate approaching death. Blood flow through regulatory organs is much reduced.

These measurements must be taken only upon awakening, not under any other circumstance for upon awakening the slightest effort will change pulse rate. At a rapid pulse, the heart pumps harder to bring blood to remote parts. Blood vessels are clogged, their lumen slightly reduced. Alter the diet and the condition will rapidly improve. You may be terminally ill when pulse is four beats to an inhalation. Do not be frightened. Get hold of yourself and gradually eat an isotonic diet or feed yourself in a yet lower proportion. You will survive.

How to cope with changes in breathing rate

Breathing is either normal or labored. Breathing rate is normal at 8-26 inhalations per minute. Imperceptible breathing indicates freely flowing blood with excellent digestion and regulation of body fluids. At 1-8 inhalations per minute. one is in a state of coma. There is high fever at 25-40 inhalations per minute and above. This is a quick way to assess the state of health. When breathing rate is seriously impaired, alter the diet immediately. At high altitudes, a few deep breaths with a pause are inhaled, followed by renewed deep breathing. Oxygen is decreased at high altitude, and is a threat to health. Do not live in high risers. People at work in high risers manifest bad temper—they cannot be blamed.

At a pH under 7, blood is acidic and breathing deepens. Others are affected by spasmodic attacks of wheezing, shortness of breath, hiccuping. Avoid breathing in chemicals, i.e., domestic and garden aerosols. Remove pets from apartments. Avoid forceful exercise, emotional factors: drugs, excess travel, too many people around, too many objects in the apartment. Improve breathing with small meals, the last meal before 6 PM. Avoid fried foods, cereals, sugars, and carbohydrates. Keep regular several times daily.

Breathing problems affect those living in walk-ups. Many run up several flights of steps. When climbing stairs, walk up slowly and lock knees at each step—it won't be tiring.

How air is brought to blood

To reach tiny air sacs where exchange of gases between blood and lungs takes place, air must pass through nostrils, pharynx, larynx, trachea, bronchi, terminal bronchioles, alveolar ducts and atria. Air literally passes through 23 generations of branching before it reaches a total of 750 million alveolar air sacs in both lungs. 280 billion pulmonary capillaries surround tiny air sacs allowing great contact between blood and air spaces.

Within air sacs, two membranes separate blood from inhaled air. Due to their thinness, alveolar and capillary walls do not hinder the free exchange of respiratory gases: oxygen and carbon dioxide. To transfer gases, a surface area of 70 square meters with a thickness of 0.1 micron is available. Every minute 5-10 liters of blood flow through alveolar membranes. At rest, 250 ml. of oxygen are required per minute, but in heavy exercise, 20 times this amount are needed, up to 5,500 ml. per minute. Today, in hermetically closed gymnasiums, workplaces, homes, man does not obtain much oxygen—a good reason for heart attacks.

What happens to air before it reaches the lungs

Air passing through the nose is air-conditioned and filtered by nostrils' hairs. It is subjected to maximum turbulence by contact with mucous membranes in twirls of turbinate bones.

At 600 times per minute, fine cilia sweep the passing air outwardly, filtering out microscopic particles of dirt and bacteria. Mucous membrane's blood vessels humidify and warm up inspired air. Filtered air passes unchanged through pharynx, and tonsils guard entrance of bacteria, fighting them off before air passes into larynx. From larynx down through trachea, primary bronchi, bronchioles and terminal respiratory bronchioles, inspired air in lining of tubes is filtered by the upward sweeping cilia. The anterior third of nose, part of pharynx and terminal respiratory units distal to respiratory bronchioles are not ciliated. Occasional nose blowing or coughing dislodges foreign materials from respiratory tract.

The alveolar lining provides a final cleansing. Its macrophages engulf the last remnants of inspired foreign particles and bacteria before air comes in contact with the bloodstream. Passing single file through capillaries that surround each alveolus, red cells are in contact with alveolar space for less than 0.3 second as carbon dioxide is delivered to alveoli and oxygen is picked up by hemoglobin.

Preserve good breathing

Breathing in humid air liquefies mucus, easing coughs and nose blowing. If humidity is a problem drink beverages daily. Warm air contains more water vapor than cold air, loosening mucus. Secretions liquefy, airflow increases to ease coughing and eliminate foreign particles. In cold weather, do not stay outdoors longer than necessary. An hour or two is the maximum, and a brisk walk is better than standing without movement.

In lungs, air is never completely expired. Lung capacity is 2,500-3,000 cc. of air, when forced to expire fully, 1,000 cc. of air is expired. In breathing, 500 cc. of air moves in and out of lungs, about $1/10^{th}$ of total volume of inspired air. When breathing in, not all is fresh air, 150 cc. are from respiratory passages, indicating that blood is not continually oxygenated by fresh air—all the more reason for living/working quarters to have fresh air at all times. To ensure circulating air, leave windows open two inches even in the coldest weather. Avoid lacy curtains for fabrics occupy space, pick up dirt and dust, and reduce the available air. Keep curtains, draperies and rugs, to a minimum. Too many things around the house are detrimental—donate to thrift shops.

Extremely dangerous are too many plants in the apartment. Each plant is a living organism, breathing in oxygen, exhaling carbon dioxide reducing the amount available for humans. Keep only three or four plants around the house. One woman has 150 plants in her apartment. Her complexion is dark. Keep few or no pets in the apartment. Lower animals breathe in much oxygen, especially dogs and cats.

If the amount of free oxygen in systemic capillaries is abnormally low, a person can suffer from anoxemia. Shallow breathing and diseased states stir anoxemia: influenza, pneumonic conditions, with the following symptoms: frequency of heartbeat, increase in blood pressure, feeble breathing and pulse.

External signs of anoxemia are: bluish lips, tongue and face. In extreme cyanosis, lips are either black or leaden gray. In slight cyanosis, lips are a pale purplish red. Advancing anoxemia dulls the senses and intelligence, affecting the memory and powers of judgment. Irrational fixed ideas, uncontrollable emotional outbursts, muscular incoordination, loss of power in limbs with eventual paralysis may also occur.

When short of breath, prop up in bed during sleep. The horizontal position easily induces anoxemia. The breathing center is in the brain. To maintain good breathing, wear a hat. Increasing brain temperature increases breathing rate. Never tie hair up in braids; the tightness decreases circulation to brain. Permanent waving straight hair increases warmth to the head. Never sit on metal or any cold furniture. Keep silent as much as possible. Too much talk prevents digestion: acid from stomach rises to the nose causing a stuffed nose. To prevent illness for a lifetime, try to perspire during sleep—perspiration eliminates toxicity in blood.. Never undress suddenly after heavy perspiration. A high school student played ball vigorously; after the game, he undressed totally. He died the next day. If you suffer from breathing problems, never travel by air and eat light. Sleep propped up by six pillows. Avoid alcohol, it decreases pulmonary function. Keep feet warm with lined boots. Wear fur or cover with fur at home if necessary. There is nothing like fur in cold weather.

Ripley's **Believe It Or Not** relates the case of a Frenchman who wore 15 pairs of stockings every single day of his life. He died at the age of 50.

Cope with snoring

Snoring is almost beyond help, but there is hope. One snores at night during sleep to digest the heavy foods ingested. Avoid large pieces of meats, and eating vegetables and starches separately. Sandwiches are better. Foods presented in separate portions quickly induce a terminal state. Foods should have the consistency of stuffing but without so much bread.

Snoring will be less pronounced if you eat the last meal of the day four hours prior to bedtime. Once we met a Chinese girl who seemed like a living skeleton: eyes sunken deep in the orbit, facial skin covering a thin layer of muscle. This could only be attributed to her coming to the U. S., unaccustomed to the food, her body gradually changed and with time, her appearance. This should be a warning to avoid large steaks, chops, etc. Mixtures of foods, balls, croquettes, ravioli, dumplings, egg rolls, strudels, etc. are better.

Cope with coughing: When noxious fumes, dust or other particles, irritate air passages, a sudden expulsion of air from lungs induces a cough as mucus backs up, stopping up air passages. Cold air brings on a cough. Beware of draughts and avoid sitting between door and window. Fried foods cause formation of catarrh. Catarrh stirs expectoration which can shorten life. Stay away from carbohydrates and fats.

Cope with changes in heartbeat: A man's heart beats 70 times per minute but among the healthy, 60 or 75 is not unusual. The heartbeat's sound is the opening and closing of heart valves. In exercise, emotional excitement and high environmental temperatures heartbeat accelerates. Abnormal conditions increase heartbeat: hemorrhage, surgical shock, fever, hyperthyroidism and certain disorders of the heart.

It is believed that the faster the heart beats, the more blood flows through the heart. This is an erroneous concept. Test it as follows: press an empty pump several times in a row, then press a full pump only a few times. A slow pulse rate per minute indicates optimum blood flow through the heart. A Chinese woman once had a heartbeat of 59 per minute. She never did strenuous exercise beyond her daily household chores and lived to 89 years. Napoleon was known to have a very slow heartbeat: 62 or less per minute. He had a tremendous capacity for work and could fall asleep anywhere. He never required much sleep and was ready for work after a catnap. Aside from administrative functions, he led troops to 40 wars. A young man had a high pulse rate even in the horizontal position. He was exempt from military service.

According to the quality of our formation, our heartbeat will either be slow or fast. A slow heartbeat is better, a fast one usually means fever. Physiology cannot explain fever. Fever warns of a menace to the body's defensive mechanisms: in fever, there is rapid proliferation of white blood cells. Proteins of blood plasma may be coagulated. Change to a dilute diet.

If blood from the digestive system is not sufficiently cleansed by the liver, blood passing from liver to heart is loaded with toxins, raising body temperature. To prevent further accumulation of toxins, adopt a fruit diet. When feverish, do not expose large areas of the body—water evaporates quickly. No need for alarm as long as body regularity is maintained. To lower temperature in fever, many cultures adopt dancing or shaking. Learn ballroom dancing or take long walks, drink a lot of fluid to alleviate a feverish condition.

Cancer is characterized by constant slight fever. Do not be too concerned. Be careful with carbohydrate intake. Except for pure liquids or gelatine, all foods contain carbohydrates—some contain more. Be selective with foods and feed yourself scientifically. If you have a sweet tooth, fresh fruit tarts, mildly sweet, are excellent. Oils and fats produce carbohydrates, use these sparingly: cream, whipped cream, butter, sour cream, fats, oils, cream cheese. Alcohol is pure carbohydrate. You will avoid inferior carbohydrates if you eat less carbohydrate rich foods.

Avoid a heart attack

Overexertion precipitates a heart attack. In heart failure, the heart propels less blood than the circulatory system demands. Even at rest, a heart attack can occur but overexertion is the chief culprit. The first warning signal is pain in the head. Headaches, intermittent or constant means that the heart is the next organ affected. Understanding the heart can help prevent heart attacks.

The heart lies in a very protected position in the chest. Directly behind the sternum, it is cuddled between both lungs. A soft padding of thymus gland and fatty tissue separates heart from sternum. Behind the heart passes the windpipe and behind the windpipe, the esophagus.

A double pump open at both ends, the heart is hidden from view by its ingenious shape. Less than a pound in weight, the fist-shaped heart lies within a strong fibrous, double-layered bag, the pericardial sac, enclosing the heart completely to an inch and a half above the exit or entrance of large blood vessels. The pericardial membrane loses itself on the external coating of blood vessels. Three strong ligaments firmly tie the pericardial sac to the top and bottom of the sternum and to the central tendon of the diaphragm which separates chest from abdominal cavity. Thus tied to sternum and diaphragm, the heart is ensured of shock from body movements; pointing slightly to the left, out of the sternum's way, the apex is the only vulnerable region. In the heart, two powerful layers of muscles lie between two outer and inner protective coats. Double-layered muscles are attached to fibrous rings surrounding entrance to ventricles and large arteries, preventing blood from backing into auricle. Four chambers divide the heart into a venous right side and an arterial left side. Two large veins penetrate the right auricle, the superior and inferior vena cava, carrying impure venous blood from upper and lower parts of body to the heart, respectively. From right auricle, blood enters right ventricle, then pumped to lungs through pulmonary artery. In the lungs, carbon dioxide is given off to the millions of alveoli and oxygen is picked up. At low pressure, four pulmonary veins immediately bring oxygenated blood from lungs to the left auricle.

From left auricle blood enters left ventricle and at high pressure, is pumped out through the inch-wide aorta whose branches bring oxygenated blood to the tiny end capillaries of all body parts with a combined surface of 1,000 square meters. When oxygen is delivered to body tissues, blood picks up wastes and flows back to the heart through tiny veins, then larger veins to the superior and inferior vena cava and empty into the right auricle. And the cycle continues.

At each ventricular contraction blood is sucked into the auricles and simultaneously pumped out through the aorta and pulmonary artery at a speed of 0.4 meters per second, to reach capillaries at 0.5 mm. per second, speeding up as it reaches the large veins on its way to the heart.

Weakest at the left auricle, heart muscles are extremely powerful around the left ventricle where muscle fibers entwine themselves around the right ventricle, penetrate the vertical septum in middle of heart, surround left ventricle and terminate on the fibrous ring where they originated. Some heart muscles are S-shaped, with powerful ridges. At each contraction these muscles wring blood out from the left ventricle, propelling blood into the aorta.

Arising from base of aorta, paired coronary arteries supply heart tissue, thus ensuring heart muscle with the purest blood. Veins accompany arteries, draining into the right auricle. The vagus nerve and nerves of the sympathetic ganglia, control coronary vessels and ensure a continuous supply of the purest blood to heart muscle despite opposing bodily activities. Though well supplied by blood, heart muscle is extremely sensitive and heartbeat increases when sensitive nerve endings are stimulated. Bright lights, loud noise, strong odor, stroking skin, fright, anger, emotion, hasten heartbeat immediately, decreasing blood flow through the heart. A 60-year old Chinese woman was having a violent discussion with her son — she fell backwards, fainted and died.

At the entrance of the superior vena cava lies the heart's pacemaker. It is a mass of small fibers where venous blood penetrates the right auricle. These node fibers set up impulses propagated throughout muscles of right and left auricles, converging next on the atrio-ventricular node, cross the fibrous rings, propagating down a two-pronged, fork-wise direction along inner walls of both ventricles, to reach the heart's apex. Impulses ensuring continuous heartbeats always follow this direction for in the heart's hollow cavities, there are only connective tissues. Impulses travel at two meters per second and reach the tip of ventricles at one meter per second.

The quality of venous blood affects excitatory pacemaker fibers. For a normal heartbeat, potassium, sodium and calcium ions seem to be the most important. When these ions increase or decrease in concentration, arrhythmia results. Excess potassium ions are especially dangerous. When potassium ions diminish, pacemaker activity dominates. Calcium salts harden and stiffen blood vessels which become brittle. Fats are equally dangerous, affecting the inner lining of blood vessels as a soft, fatty material replaces the inner lining, later depositing lime salts. This is atherosclerosis, the chief cause of cerebral hemorrhage and coronary thrombosis.

Plain table salt is most important. Blood tastes salty and this saltiness must be maintained. It is safe to ingest a level tablespoonful of salt, daily, sprinkled on foods, soups, etc. Troubles will arise if not enough salt is ingested. Advised by her physician to avoid salt, an older woman began to experience extreme difficulty with daily regularity and shortly after, died. Another elderly woman intakes some kind of salt substitute and her appearance is ragged.

For optimum heart function, avoid foods high in calcium and potassium and use Kosher salt on all foods. Kosher salt contains no tricalcium phosphate nor silicon dioxide, a kind of powdered stone. Kosher salt can be purchased in any good supermarket. Foods high in potassium are cereals, grains, rice, soy products, flour, hard or dried vegetables: carrots, roots, cocoa, chocolate, nuts, mushrooms, beans, wheat germ; all dried fruits and tropical fruits. Foods containing less potassium are meats, fresh fruits and fresh, fruit-like vegetables. Understand that foods are medicine for man in a dilute form. To serve us well, proper cooking techniques must dilute foods further.

Because the heart's covering is tied to the top and bottom pieces of the sternum and to the diaphragm, if you want to live 100 years, do not over-exercise by jogging, running or violent sports. From a normal weight of 350 grams in heavy sports, the heart's size can increase to 500 grams. Further exertion cannot enlarge it more and death can ensue. Rest and relaxation can resume original heart size. Each heart beats only so many times during a lifetime. Sports forces rapid beating and will shorten life. Long walks, light household chores are better. Every body movement is work: pumping blood, looking at objects, listening to sounds, moving around, the orgasm, muscular contractions, etc. Do not give your body more activity than necessary. Try to save energy, especially with advancing age.

Exercise alone is not the culprit for heart attacks. Indulgence in sex is dangerous. As in heavy physical labor, much energy is expended at the climax, said Masters and Johnson. Analyze your daily activities to ascertain that no large capillary areas have been overactive: the head in mental work, muscles and bones, the 30 ft. digestive tract, the uterus in pregnancy, the sex organ etc. Train rides, air travel, incessant talk are equally detrimental. Creative activity is overtaxing and no one could advise great composers of the past to refrain from composing. Only a better knowledge of the living body can prevent similar occurrences in the future.

Today most people with a weak heart undergo a heart by-pass or receive a transplant. Heart transplant patients live a year or so; a maximum of 10 years with heart by-pass surgery. By altering the diet one can live indefinitely.

Continued function of the heart depends on kidneys' smooth eliminatory functions. Only a better understanding of kidney function can prevent kidney transplants, dialysis, etc.

The myth of high blood pressure

A reading of systolic and diastolic pressures measures blood pressure. Systolic blood pressure indicates the pumping of blood into arteries. Diastolic pressure represents the lowest pressure of blood before the next beat. During a lifetime blood pressure varies. A newborn infant's blood pressure is 40 mm. Hg, 100 mm. at 12 years of age, 120 mm at 17 years of age, rising about 0.5 mm. each succeeding year.

The following indicates why one cannot trust a blood pressure reading. Blood pressure rises after sexual intercourse. It rises drastically in muscular exercise or when suddenly frightened, in great happiness or after a meal. Blood pressure rises when standing up suddenly from the seated position. Also when rising from a crouched position.

A blood pressure reading can be trusted only if taken upon awakening from a good night's sleep and in the horizontal position. The following maintains the body's blood pressure: A change in blood viscosity, changes in total blood volume or change in elasticity of arterial vessel walls. These factors interact with one another to maintain blood pressure at a fairly constant level. Don't worry if the blood pressure is a little on the high or on the low side. More important is maintaining normal blood composition with a good diet.

External signs indicative of weak kidney function

Facial signs may indicate kidney disease. Puffiness around eyes, a distended abdomen, swelling of face, ankles and thighs, elbows and forearms. Facial skin more brown than usual, becoming pallid and dry. Cramps, aches and pains when walking, jerky movement of limbs are other signs. The smell and color of urine are immediate indicators of the function of kidneys. Do not put colored deodorants in toilet bowls; urine color should be observed daily. If one voids little and urine color is white, there is serious kidney trouble: no poisons are leaving the body. If urine is colorless and voiding frequent, the danger is less. Scientists assert one can survive if only $1/10^{th}$ of kidney nephrons is functional.

Frequent urination with burning pain may denote kidney stones. Frequent urination night and day indicate weak kidneys. Pain in kidneys may be due to the ingestion of concentrated foods and intense difficulty in rising is a sign of kidney inflammation. Urine frothing persistently indicates excess protein in the system. Excess fruits, starches, honey and sugar causes sweet urine. The worst type of kidney disturbance is the inability to form and to void urine. This is an extreme condition probably due to a tumor.

Many people today have kidney problems. They are advised to either undergo dialysis treatment or to await a kidney transplant from a donor who, with a single kidney left, will eventually experience kidney trouble. A single kidney will definitely cause troubles. One woman, born with only one kidney, lived 65 years. A better understanding of kidney structure should help avert artificial help and enable one to live a lifetime in greater freedom.

What one should know about kidneys

Most important regulatory organs, kidneys preserve blood's constant composition, maintain the heart's pacemaker ability and ensure purified blood throughout the body.

Bean-shaped, fist-sized structures, kidneys are about 4 inches long, 2-2 1/2 inches wide, an inch thick. On both sides of the vertebral column, at waist level, kidneys face each other at the hilus or concave side. Kidneys receive blood from renal arteries, two short, thick vessels branched off from the abdominal aorta. Sometimes two arteries to each kidney are not unusual.

Entering the hilus, the artery divides into anterior and posterior vessels from which five segmental vessels arise, fanning out into smaller vessels supplying five or six pyramidal shaped funnels. Vessels decrease in size, ending as tiny arterioles entering millions of tiny filters or glomeruli where blood is sieved, forming urine. The renal artery brings impure blood to kidneys. It is the afferent artery. Blood leaving kidneys flows in the renal vein, containing purified blood. It is the efferent artery.

Tiny afferent arterioles entering millions of tiny filters are known as glomerular tufts where blood is sieved by three sieves of increasingly smaller size. They are 1) the glomerular capillary walls; 2) the basement membrane between tuft walls and Bowman's Capsule; 3) the lining of Bowman's capsule. A glomerular tuft contains both afferent and efferent arterioles. Tiny vessels fit into Bowman's capsule like the tip of a glove. About 50 tiny parallel capillaries bent into short loops form a compact mass in the capsule.

Much like a kitchen sieve, Bowman's capsule extends into a series of tubules: proximal tubule, Henle's loop and distal tubule. From tubules urine is collected into five or six cup-shaped collection tracts called minor calyces. These join at the apex and at the hilus, enter the ureter. One foot long, thick as a lead pencil, the ureter varies in size throughout its length. Along the ureter, peristaltic contractions propel urine, entering bladder at the rate of 1-5 jets per minute. Wrinkled when empty, the bladder fills up slowly with collected urine.

In women, the uterus separates bladder from rectum. As it expands and contracts, the bladder's slippery covering slides along other structures and organs without friction or irritation. The bladder can contain as much urine at its capillary capacity allows. When no more blood flows to bladder capillaries greatly distended by urine, voiding becomes imperative. Rhythmical contractions of bladder's detrusor muscles lead to the urgency to urinate. The frequency of urination may be used as a measure of degree of blood vessel clogging. In general the more frequent the desire to urinate, the more blood vessels are clogged. As a scientific measurement, it must be standardized.

Two sphincters control the voiding process. When muscles contract, both sphincters relax and voiding is made possible. Before discomfort is felt, a pint or pint and a half collects in the bladder.

The path taken by sieved blood

Sieved of its impurities, blood leaves glomeruli via the efferent arterioles. These tiny vessels entwine around proximal and distal tubules before converging into the renal vein and carries purified blood back to the heart. During the course of their descent along the tubules, efferent arterioles absorb the body's required substances: sodium, potassium, chloride, calcium, magnesium, phosphate, amino acids and vitamin C. Most important is the re-absorption of water and salt.

Principal functions of kidneys

The kidneys' principal duty is to maintain blood plasma's and body fluid's constant chemical composition by differential excretion of substances. Kidneys allow us to take in more than necessary and excrete what is required, allowing freedom of excess by ridding the body of unwanted materials. Kidneys secrete and excrete incessantly 60 minutes an hour, 24 hours a day for life, clearing blood plasma of end products of metabolism: urea, uric acid, creatinine produced in quantities too large to eliminate from blood in other ways. If not removed, poisons would gradually viciate the body proper and lead to death. Also excreted under hormonal control are physiologically essential substances.

Other functions of kidneys

Besides excretory properties, kidneys secrete a hormone: renin, formed by juxtaglomerular cells surrounding afferent arterioles prior to entrance into Bowman's capsule. Renin produces a most powerful vessel constrictor raising arterial blood pressure. Renin also releases aldosterone from adrenal cortex. Aldosterone increases absorption of sodium in renal tubules. The following conditions produce adrenaline in blood and stir renin formation: fear, fright, exercising and fatigue. Other states releasing renin: low arterial blood pressure, salt loss, reduced plasma volume, blood loss or injection of adrenaline.

Kidneys produce erythropoietin, indirectly stimulating bone marrow to produce red blood cells. Also produced is prostaglandin to regulate blood flow and blood pressure. Kidneys produce the active form of Vitamin D to maintain and form healthy bone and promote absorption of calcium for the digestive tract.

What affects kidney filtration rate. Narrowing of blood vessels affects rate of blood flow into tiny glomeruli. Poisonous deposits thicken arterial walls and blood trickles through glomeruli. Avoid heavy oily foods, extremely sweet foods and alcoholic beverages. Let hunger pains direct food intake.

Filtration rate increases or decreases depending upon the use of body parts in various activities. Relaxation of body parts increases rate of flow through kidneys. Indulgence in vegetable oils prevents normal filtering processes. Concentration of substances rising above critical level saturates the tubular mechanism and prevents their excretion at a maximal rate and beyond that point. Kidneys cannot dispose of all wastes in the bloodstream, a warning to avoid excess consumption of any substance, food, drugs or medicines.

Some causes of kidney disease

All types of illnesses can cause kidney failure: diabetes, hypertension, cancer, repeated sore throats, heart failure, gout. Painkillers and drug abuse, steroids such as cortisone trigger kidney problems. Thrombi or clots eventually clog up kidneys. Toxic chemicals and drugs lead to acute renal failure. Avoid compound painkillers containing phenacetin and caffeine and strenuous activity: physical overexertion, loud music, loud noise, heavy foods, indulgence in sex, hollering, singing, strong emotion, continuous activity. These decrease glomerular filtration rate. When preparing for final medical exams, a young man exerted himself mentally to excess and had blood in his urine. With advancing age, a decrease in the number of functioning nephrons reduces glomerular filtration rate, leading to eventual renal failure. The injection of foreign substances in the sick and weak decrease glomerular filtration rate and may cause death.

Avoid laxatives and cortisone therapy. Gastrointestinal disorders lead to nephrosis. When kidneys fail, modify the diet immediately. Read a book about dieting in disease. Foods high in calcium cause kidney stones: proteins, chocolate, cocoa, tea, rhubarb, spinach, beets, cheeses, milk products, milk, ice cream. Much liquid intake can pass out a kidney stone. A man during 50 years grew a 14-pound kidney stone.

Always observe color of urine. If it is yellow with a distinctive smell, kidneys are functioning normally. If it remains white for long periods of time, poisons are not leaving the blood. Time to reduce drastically carbohydrates and fats. If urine froths, excess proteins have been ingested. Reduce the latter.

The diet to follow in kidney malfunction

Eat little protein, very little starches and increase the liquid intake. Several cups of dilute coffee or cocoa: much water with a dash of milk, a dash of coffee or a little cocoa and honey. Dilute fresh juices, dilute soup should comprise the diet.

Clothing is very important. Men are well protected by long pants but their hairstyle works against health. Let hair grow to the shoulders. Women keep hair long but are too flimsily clad. Use wool-lined boots in cold weather, wool-lined slippers in the house, leggings or stockings. Preserve body heat. Sleep with a wool dress above a cotton undergarment. In illness nothing equals preservation of body heat.

One terminally ill woman began to experience difficulty walking. Advised to wear sheepskin-lined booties, she did as told and to her great surprise, she was able to walk without pain, even run. Warm shoes radiate much heat throughout the body, preserving body function. Today many shoes are made like clogs. These are dangerous footgear. Our heels maintain body weight and must be kept particularly warm.

When affected with kidney disease, patients are advised to perspire, forcing skin to remove poisons. Induce intense perspiration in the sun. Dress adequately and remain in the sun until heat gradually raises body temperature and perspiration drips. It is an excellent way to maintain health and prevent illness in cold weather.

Do not eat grapes' skin and seeds; pigeons won't eat them neither should man. A man had a small tumor on his back. He eats everything in grapes or melon: pits, skin and watermelon seeds. His face is mottled with dark spots.

Skin sensitivity

Your skin is the only externally visible regulatory organ. Other regulatory organs are indicated by breathing, pulse, heartbeat and urine.

Skin informs us of all sorts of dangerous substances. Its thickness acts as a barrier between the interior of the body and the outside world. Skin stretches, gliding as we move about.

Skin is sensitive and reacts to various stimuli. Wrong foods cause skin to develop eruptions. When subjected to pressure, heat, cold or solar irradiation, skin breaks out. Drugs like cortico-steroids and antibiotics may cause psoriasis. Skin is sensitive to clothing, and wool itches on bare skin. Some detergents cause eczema. Some noxious products may provoke violent allergic body reactions. Certain abnormalities can be diagnosed and solve medical problems.

What skin reflects

Skin reflects the function of endocrine glands. When the thyroid gland is removed, skin is thick and leathery with sparse, dry, lusterless and brittle hair. In deficient thyroid secretion facial features are coarse with thick and puffy skin, sparse and brittle hair, reduced sweating and sebum secretion. Eyebrow hair is lost, head hair is tough and unyielding, nails become brittle and grow slowly. Hyperthyroidism is indicated by warm, sweating skin with vitiligo and alopecia, premature graying of hair and nailplates separate from nails.

In Addison's disease, a destructive condition of the adrenal cortex, skin becomes bronze or dirty gray mottled with pale, depigmented regions next to overpigmented areas. The mouth's mucous membrane tends to become strongly pigmented.

Hypersecretion of the adenocorticotrophic hormone is indicated when face and trunk become obese. The face is round with fat, piling up on the neck.

Extreme obesity and dwarfism in a growing child indicates deficient secretion of pituitary gland's anterior lobe. In an adult man, fat distribution acquires a feminine character, mostly concentrated on hips, thighs, chest and skin becomes like a woman's, soft and smooth. In atrophy of anterior lobe, skin becomes dry, sallow, wrinkled and gray with sparse hair.

Skin also reflects liver function. In acute hepatocellular damage, skin turns yellow. In cirrhosis of bile, skin assumes a greenish-brown tint. In portal cirrhosis there is hyperpigmentation of skin, nails' shape changes and acne may develop. Pimples, boils and carbuncles indicate end stages of disease affecting pancreatic islets of Langerhans—diabetes.

General structure of skin

In all animals with a backbone, skin has two layers, epidermis and dermis. From skin's surface to where dermis merges with fatty layers under skin, its thickness varies from less than 1/25th of an inch (1 mm.) on eyelids to 1/8th of an inch (3 mm.) in regions between shoulder blade, on palms of hands and soles of feet. Under the dermis lies the hypodermis carrying major blood vessels and nerves to skin. The hypodermis contains many fat cells. An extension of the dermis, the hypodermis is 10 cm. thick in the abdomen.

The epidermis

Ridges in the epidermis increase the number of dividing cells and areas of contact between epidermis and dermis. Several layers thick, the epidermis is maintained by cell division of the lowest cell layer. From top to bottom, the five layers of cells in the epidermis are: clear layer, granular layer, prickly layer and germinal layer above a basement membrane. Epidermal cells receive nutrition from tissue fluids diffused through prickly layer's intercellular spaces.

Cell division takes place in germinal layer. As new cells form, they are forced upwards by newly dividing cells underneath. Affected by environmental temperatures, daily regeneration replaces the entire epidermis, cell division lasting 60-90 minutes. Pushed upwards, cells change in shape. Irregularly shaped in prickly layer, cells are spindle-shaped in granular layer, they appear as a homogeneous line in clear layer and become flattened out without a nucleus in horny layer where there are 10-20 layers of flat, dead, dry, keratinized cells continually and imperceptibly shed as microscopical flakes.

In the epidermis, other cells are present. Each square millimeter of skin has around 1,000-3,000 pigment cells. The pigment melanin is formed in specialized organelles called melanosomes and remains as insoluble, fine granules. Melanin is derived from phenylalanine via tyrosine by a series of reactions catalyzed by enzyme tyrosinase. In fair-skinned peoples, pigment cells are present in deepest cells of germinal layer. In darker peoples, they are found throughout germinal and prickly layer, extending into granular layer. Other cells in the epidermis are keratinocytes, Langerhans cells and modified cells.

The skin's components. Five components make up skin of which the most important is collagen, synthesized by fibroblasts, long, flat, spindle-shaped cells with long processes. Collagen fibers are bundles of strong, tough fibers, very flexible but non-elastic. Made up of 1,000 amino acids, disorder in collagen formation causes skin to tear easily with poor healing power; 71.9% of skin is collagen forming a fine top layer and a coarser deeply placed layer. Abnormality in intermolecular cross-linkage of collagen fibrils changes skin's physical properties and metabolic stability. Skin's collagen performs best in the 2nd and 3rd decade of life, decreasing in quality yearly by 1% after the 2nd decade.

Elastin is the second component of skin. The major stress-resistant element in skin, these long and thin elastic fibers produced by fibroblasts make up 0.6% of skin's dry weight. Collagen and elastin are embedded in a matrix of loose ground substance, the third component of skin. Composed of mucopolysaccharides, proteins, water and dissolved substances, ground substance has an important function in regulating the diffusion of material through the dermis.

Keratin is skin's fourth component, forming the epidermal top layer, synthesized by keratinocytes whose protein is transformed into the tough, chemically inert protein, keratin. It toughens skin's surface, rendering it waterproof and maintains skin's flexible resistance to mechanical stress. Continuously shed and replaced from below, keratinocytes are clear, scale-like cells without nuclei. Outer layers of skin and nails contain keratin.

The fifth and last component of skin is the pigment melanin formed by germinal layer's melanocytes. Other important cells in skin are histiocytes, a type of white blood cell migrated from bloodstream into surrounding tissue. As mature cells called histiocytes or tissue macrophages, they become stationary. In inflammation, these cells multiply and form walls around foreign bodies, dissolving them. Mast cells are other skin cells. Every millimeter of skin contains 7,000-12,000 mast cells, increasing in number in skin ailments, i.e., dermatitis etc. Large in size, about 10-15 millimicrons in diameter, in inflammation, they release granules.

In skin's tissues the five main components bind other structures together: hair, glands, sense organs, blood vessels, forming a supporting framework. There are no hairs or sebacious glands on the palmar surface of hands and soles of feet, but many sweat glands are present. Ridges, grooves are dermatoglyphics, characteristic and unique to each individual.

The dermis

Separated by a thin layer of cement substance from the epidermis, the dermis has two layers, a papillary layer and underneath, a reticular layer.

The papillary layer is so-called due to its millions of tiny, fingerlike processes fitting into sheath-like sockets in the overlying epidermis. Each square millimeter of dermis has around 40-140 papillae. Papillae are connective tissue containing sweat glands, sebacious glands, lymphatics, vascular loops and specialized nerve endings of 11 types.

The reticular layer is dense with collagen fibers, the principal dermal constituent. It is a tough, elastic fibrous protein secreted by fibroblasts. To ease inflammation, gel, wandering cells, fibroblasts and mast cells are also present.

The hypodermis. Underneath the dermis, the hypodermis is a fatty layer, a deep extension of skin, with connective tissue and many fat cells. Some regions of the body have no fat in the hypodermis: skin of eyelids, penis and scrotum.

Though not a part of skin proper, the hypodermis carries major blood vessels and nerves to skin.

Mucous membranes

A different type of skin, i.e., mucous membrane, lines respiratory tracts and genitourinary tracts. Mucous membrane has three main parts: an epithelial layer of cells upon a basement membrane, a layer of connective tissue and a submucosa of loose connective tissue with vessels, nerves and glands. Mucous membranes secrete a slimy material: mucus made of protein produced by epithelial cells: mucin. As mucin accumulates in cells, these distend and burst, liberating mucus.

Lips and entire digestive tract have an additional muscular layer under the second mucous layer. Erectile tissue covers tips of breasts with a nipple surrounded by a darkly pigmented circular areola. Both lips and nipples do not secrete mucus.

The chemical composition of skin

A kilogram of fat-free skin has 694 g. water, 53 g. nitrogen, 45.7 g. collagen, 79.3 mEq. sodium, 23.7 mEq. potassium, 71.4 mEq. chlorine, 14 mEq. phosphorus, 3.1 mEq. magnesium and 9.5 mEq. copper. Skin contains textural fats, mostly sterols and phospholipids, 367 mg. of cholesterol after age 14. In children, hair fat is three times higher than in adults. Subcutaneous lipids are 0.2 % cholesterol and 19.6% skin lipids. The various components of skin form a supporting network for skin's various appendages: hair, sebacious glands, sweat glands, sense organs (see chapter 12) and blood vessels.

Hair

An adult human has 5 million hairs, 0.1 million or 100,000-150,000 in the scalp. On head, chin, armpits and pubic area, hair is thick, coarse, dark and large. Hair is of the vellus type, short, pale and fine on the face, trunk and limbs.

Hair is continuously shed and renewed by alternating cycles of growth, rest, dedifferentiation and renewal of hair follicle growth and its associated structures. Hair grows for about three years but only three or four months on chest. On scalp, hair generally grows 0.4 mm. per day. Different varieties of hair have an average life of 4 1/2 months for downy hair, 3-5 years for long scalp hairs. The number of hair follicles do not vary after birth but their appearance and the number of hairs vary.

Hair diameter varies from 15-110 or 40-120 microns. Hair is composed of the following constituents: 65-95% protein, water, lipids, pigment and trace elements, though hair filaments are dead, thin flexible shafts of highly keratinized epithelial cells. Lustrous hair depends on deep sleep. Hair appears lifeless with poor sleep, excess work. Poor quality of hair is noticeable in the elderly, where body fluids are insufficiently regulated. The accumulation of excess nutrients in body tissues detrimentally affects hair growth. Vegetable oils cause hair to be lifeless and shaggy.

How hair is formed

Arising from epithelium, hair penetrates deeply into skin's subcutaneous tissue as follows: a root of epidermal follicle turns in like a glove's finger, forming hair instead of a horny layer. The follicle's deepest portion is enlarged, enclosing a vascular papilla projecting from dermis into bulb. Immediately above and around this papilla, a layer of cells is hair's germinative matrix. Along its axis, a human hair fiber is divided into three distinct zones. Buried within the dermis, forming a swelling, the first zone lies around lower end of root or bulb. Synthesis and orientation occurs in this first zone. Keratinization occurs in the second zone projecting beyond skin's surface, along hair's shaft. The third and last zone emerges from skin and is composed of dehydrated cornified cells and intercellular building materials.

Close to the bulb's neck lie delicate strands of erector muscles so hair can become erect, roughening skin as in goose flesh. About midway from the root, lobulated sebaceous glands empty into upper part of hair follicle. These glands are found mostly in scalp hair, facial hair and hair of front, back and upper chest. Sebaceous glands secrete sebum, waterproofing hair. Endocrine glands control the activity of sebaceous glands. When glands function poorly, sebaceous glands' secretion also changes.

Dark and curly hair

Darkness and curliness are dominant genes, the result of regulating the body at temperatures of 80° F. during the first 20 years of life. Dominant genes become very prominent after sleeping for generations in tropical climates. Normally dark hair is maintained by optimum body temperature. Extreme stress, fright, worry, change hair color. The night before her execution queen Marie Antoinette's hair turned entirely gray. High temperature inactivates body enzymes. They are necessary to catalyze the series of reactions leading to dark hair formation. In slight fever, hair becomes colorless (albino) or gray (old age). Hair on the head is a sign of strength as shown in the story of Samson and Delilah. Nature endowed us with hair to protect very delicate parts of the body.

Loss of hair

Rapid body movements stir loss of hair. Do not gulp food down rapidly. Sip your drinks, pick at foods. Excess sex can stir complete baldness. Starches, sugars, alcohol, cured meats stir loss of hair.

Nails

Similar to horns, claws and animals' hooves, human nails are modifications of skin and derive from the epidermis. Nails extend from the white, moon-shaped area at nail plate's base, (the lunula), up to tip of finger, growing over and beyond it.

Human nails are densely compacted, highly cornified dead epithelial cells containing remnants of degenerated nuclei. They are plate-like, translucent, keratinous structures growing from proximal epidermal matrices called nail roots. The nail's root is embedded in skin, the dermis is the nail-bed. The shiny exposed part of nail is the epidermal clear layer. The cuticle at nail's base is the epidermal horny layer. The cuticle prevents bacteria from penetrating the body. It must never be cut away. The cuticle overlaps the moon-shaped lunula.

Nails grow by multiplication of germinal layer's outer cells. From one finger to the other, growth rate varies, averaging 0.1 mm. daily. The middle finger's nail grows quickest, then index and ring fingers. Nails of thumb and little finger grow slowly. The dominant hand shows a faster growth rate.

Growing parts of the body indicate the state of regulation of body fluids. Brittle, ridged nails indicate ischemia. Clubbed nails indicate pulmonary osteoarthropathy and thyroid acropathy. Changes in nails accompany liver cirrhosis. Long and thin nails indicate a proneness to lung and chest disease. It is more pronounced when nails are ridged. Too short nails without half moons indicate weak heart action. There is possible nerve disease when nails are flat and sunken into flesh. A deep furrow across nail indicates illness of nervous system while very narrow nails may indicate spinal illness. There is a tendency towards paralysis when nails appear very flat and shell-like.

Because nails grow incessantly, they are true thermometers of overall health. Newborn babies have flat nails. Overall strength is indicated when nails show no strain in later life. Nails shaped like a bird's beak indicate restless growth and illness will manifest early in life. A peaceful life is recommended for these people. The best type of nail is medium-sized with a distinct lunula not excessively large and not curved like a beak, according to Cheiro.

Nails allow hands to work. Once a woman kept fingernails 10 cm. long on one hand, crippling herself for life. Fingernails must be at level with the fleshy part of fingers to allow proper bathing.

Painful toenails: With advancing age in-grown toe nails may cause intense muscular pain. Do not panic, let the toenail grow beyond the toes fleshy part and do not cut nails' sides. Soon the pain will subside.

Sebacious glands

Sebacious glands open into hair follicles' necks. About 0.2-4 mm. in diameter, these multi-lobulated glands have short ducts. When sebum forms, at the gland's edge, germinative cells proliferate. As cells mature and move toward gland's center, little droplets of lipid progressively accumulate in their cytoplasm. Cells finally burst open, liberating the lipid material, diffusing upward in the hair follicle, impregnating hair and surrounding horny layers of skin.

A mixture of triglyceride, fatty acid, wax, ester squalene and cholesterol, sebum forms a film on skin's surface. Skin becomes pliable delaying water loss from epidermal horny layer. Sebum also delays absorption of foreign substances dangerous to the body and protects skin from exogenous infections.

On scalp, face, front and back of chest, sebaceous glands are most dense. Beginning in intrauterine life, sebum secretion decreases at onset of puberty. Changes in sebum secretion is associated with endocrine, metabolic and immunological disorders. Sebum secretion depends on pituitary, thyroid, gonads and renal glands. Acne is the main disease affecting sebaceous glands.

Sweat glands

Around 2 million apocrine and eccrine sweat glands are present in skin's dermis, with a total tubular length of 13 km. or 8 miles.

Mostly found in skin of armpits, genital area, nipple area, perineal and pubic regions, apocrine glands are sparsely found in external auditory canal and eyes' ciliary bodies.

Multi-lobulated, branched and blind tubular structures, apocrine glands are 0.02 mm. (1/15th of an inch) in diameter. Two-cell layered with an inner epithelial lining and an outer myoepithelial layer of contractile cells within lower dermis, the gland's secretory portion lies in a ball-like structure.

Ten times larger than those of eccrine glands, tubes of apocrine glands join with the pilo-sebacious unit of each hair follicle pouring the secretion slightly above sebacious gland, forming the apo-pilo-sebacious unit.

Except when decomposed, producing a characteristic body odor, apocrine sweat is odorless. Apocrine sweating is under neural and emotional control. Fluorescent in ultraviolet light, it has proteins, is turbid and milky, drying like glue, forming a light-colored plastic solid. It is hypotonic, freezing at 0.1- 0.48° C at pH of 5.5-7.0, containing 6-10 mg. of iron in each ml. of sweat.

Eccrine glands are all over the body surface. A young adult has around 120 ± 10 glands in a square centimeter of skin. At ages 73 -77 eccrine glands decrease in number to about 104 ± 20 glands in a square centimeter. The ratio of eccrine glands to hair follicle is 0.3 -1 on face, 3 -1 on body surface. In lower dermis, not joined to hair follicles, a fairly straight duct leads eccrine glands to the epidermis, coiling upwards as it reaches horny layer, opening in a tiny sweat pore.

Eccrine sweat contains sodium and potassium, has no proteins, a pH of 4-6 and shows no fluorescence in ultraviolet light. When emotionally affected, eccrine glands are stimulated to sweat. In psychic stimulation, palms of hands and soles of feet sweat. Other areas sweat by heat stimulus. Sweat contains urea, salt and sodium.

Heat acclimatization increases sweating and sweat's sodium concentration decreases. Sweat is hypotonic but in heavy sweating, much salt is lost. In prolonged sweating, secretion declines as sweat production shows fatigue.

Sweat has some bactericidal effect and inhibits proliferation of microorganisms. Excess sweat loses this power, encouraging bacterial growth, but skin's horny layer prevents penetration of bacteria. Tight membranes of sweat glands prevent water penetration. Sweat's acidity is important against bacteria and fungi. Bacteria more readily invade body parts that do not sweat. Sweat is composed of water, propionic acid, acetic acid, caprylic and caproic acids, salt, lactic acid, citric acid, ascorbic acid, urea and uric acid, which explains sweat's acidic nature at pH 3.37.

Heavy sweating eliminates wastes rapidly from bloodstream. Emotional sweating is hard work, involving the entire brain. In this tendency abstain from public performance. Light foods are recommended.

Blood flow through skin

Arteries penetrating deep connective tissue provide skin's blood flow. Blood supplies the dermis alone. To prevent body temperature from falling too low on nose, ears and cheeks, blood vessels form three plexuses of capillaries, branching and joining with each other. Under dermis, the first plexus forms networks between fat cells, the second plexus is in dermis' deep layer, with branches to sweat glands, fat cells, hair follicle papillae. On the top, the third plexus directly connects small arteries and veins.

Skin's color and temperature depend on blood flow through sub-papillary venous plexus. Skin is deep in color and warm when vessels are dilated. Skin is red when blood flow through plexus is rapid. Skin is pale when plexus is constricted. When blood flow is much reduced, skin is bluish. Parallel to blood vessels run lymphatics.

The scalp has more blood vessels than the body's other regions. Head arteries are extremely tortuous, nature's way to adapt itself to such a movable region. Arteries from one side of head communicate with those on other side and a cut easily induces bleeding. It may seem terrible but one now understands why. Arrest bleeding with a sterile gauze pad and in a short while, bleeding will subside.

The sympathetic nervous system controls blood supply to skin. When relaxed or sleeping, skin receives a great blood flow. When relaxed, skin is velvety and smooth. When tense, skin appears raw. Deep sleep and a fiber-free diet improve skin.

Deal with aging skin

With advancing age, skin breathes less efficiently, carbon dioxide accumulates, preventing skin's normal cell division. A reduction in the number of dermal capillary loops lessens skin's metabolism, with abnormal tissue formation. Skin structure and function are at their optimum up to the third decade of life, declining shortly after and by the 4th decade, lines appear on forehead and lower eyelids. By the 5th decade, lines, wrinkles, furrows and depressions are more pronounced. Skin continues to atrophy by the 6th decade, becoming like parchment with more accentuated wrinkling, with possible hyper-pigmentation, lips and skin thin out with less elasticity. Hair thins out, with loss of subcutaneous fat. The number of collagen fibers decreases 1% per year in both men and women. Dark people age slower as melanin carries extra oxygen in blood.

Aging skin develops warts, excrescences and Campbell de Morgan spots, varying from several millimeters to several centimeters in diameter on trunk and abdomen. With advancing age, the horny layer dries up and cracks. Skin's protein metabolism declines, permeability is lost, skin does not retain heat, losing temperature. Aging skin contains less water, loses elasticity and produces less enzymes. With age, cholesterol content also declines.

Do not expose bare skin to sunlight. Upon exposure to radiation, skin becomes dry, leathery and thick, cutaneous elements atrophy with a loss of elasticity, excess wrinkling, known as solar elastosis. The horny layer dries up with a tendency to crack as sebacious and sweat glands atrophy, lessening their protection. Dress up adequately and perspire under the hot sun. It is superior to exposure of bare skin to direct sunlight.

To maintain youthful skin

Fresh air is very important. Keep windows open all year round and in summer months, remain outdoors at least two hours daily.

Some creams and emollients stimulate perspiration through skin but others depress it. Placental extracts, yeast extracts, pantothenic acid, white petrolatum, cold cream activate skin respiration. Preservatives, antiseptics, fatty acids, placental extracts in high concentration, 5% hydrocortisone, 3% fluorides and butyl alcohol depress skin respiration. Make sure skin has ample opportunity to breathe all the time. When skin is painted we will soon die. Do not poke holes on your skin, the only hole allowed is on the ear lobe. Do not wear too much jewelry. Use natural fiber for clothing.

Proper cooking is of great importance and this information is given in another chapter. Deep sleep is of utmost importance and whoever obtains much sleep will have beautiful skin.

How to deal with warts, moles, wens, excrescences, wrinkles

<u>Warts</u>: tie a hair around it. Every day pull it tight. It will turn black and drop off. For a <u>wens</u> which fills up with liquid regardless how much one picks at it, do the

following: grab it suddenly and pull. Blood will gush out, place a gauze pad over it and it will heal by itself.

Moles: never touch a mole, whether transparent or black in color. Moles unfortunately will never disappear. If a mole is inadvertently opened, keep it open by removing the scab formed. It will diminish in size if continued for several days.

Nail-heads: the result of excess starches in the body: never let them appear. At the appearance of a single nail-head, remove all starches from the diet and be very careful with your diet from then on.

Loose wrinkles are signs of aging. Tight wrinkles indicate illness. Both can disappear by short fasting bouts. One woman only ate juices and light coffee in the morning for a long time. She became very beautiful.

The various functions of skin

Skin heals wounds. Skin's keratin is rapidly replaced, protecting the body from bacterial invasion. An inflamed skin indicates a wound can no longer heal. To defend against bacterial invasion, pus soon forms, the combined action of white blood cells on bacteria. Once pus is cleansed out, the wound will heal.

Skin contains cholesterol and when exposed to the sun, skin naturally forms Vitamin D. The pigment melanin protects skin from excess synthesis of Vitamin D. Pigment cells form a screen against ultraviolet light.

Skin protects bacteria from penetrating the body. Bacteria cannot digest dry scales on surface of skin.

Skin is a temperature regulator. In warm temperature skin is 36°C., but a degree higher throughout the body. Under widely varying conditions, body temperature is remarkably constant. Body temperature is most normal after a good night's sleep. During the day, work, physical exertion, foods, destroy red blood cells, produce calories and raise body temperature. In late afternoon, body temperature is a degree or a degree and a half higher than in the morning.

Skin emits radiant energy, as much as a heat radiator. Daily, a third of the resting heat produced evaporates through skin i.e., about a liter of water. More heat is lost on a hot than a cold day. Long hours in the cold and cold furniture lower body temperature.

Body heat is mostly lost through bare skin. Normally 500 cc. of water is lost from skin's surface, 300 cc. from lungs, daily, representing a heat loss of 480 calories. Suitable clothing is recommended for clothing traps air spaces, preventing airflow.

Skin makes cholesterol and is the most active fat-forming tissue. To replace loss of fat in scaly layer of epidermis, skin synthesizes at least 50 -100 mg. of fat daily.

Chapter 16
Cope with problems of endocrine glands

To direct normal growth of body parts, the nervous system requires an excellent quality of blood, made possible by endocrine hormones directly secreted into the bloodstream.

Though minute in concentration, glandular hormones are catalysts and their action on tissues is profound. Blood requires an effective concentration of these substances and their secretions are more or less continuous. Hormones promote physical, sexual, mental development and to meet the demands, organ-systems modify their activity.

Hormones maintain the constancy of many physiological parameters: osmotic pressure, blood glucose level, etc. They either inhibit or accelerate cellular metabolism, control body growth and development of secondary sexual characteristics. When hormones accumulate, their action is arrested.

There are five endocrine glands: the thyroid, parathyroid, pituitary, adrenal cortex and sex glands.

The thyroid gland and the hormone

Immediately under the voice box, the thyroid gland surrounds the trachea's front and sides. Shaped like the letter U, about an ounce in weight, the gland is slightly heavier in women, enlarging during pregnancy and lactation. At gland's bottom, a band or isthmus connects the sides, the apices pointing upward and outward. About 2 inches long, 1 1/2 inch wide and 3/4 of an inch thick, the isthmus is half an inch wide, 1/2 an inch deep and covers the 2nd and 3rd tracheal rings. Its base is at level with the 5th and 6th tracheal ring. By carefully probing with fingers under the Adam's apple and surrounding it, the gland can be felt.

A capsule connected to neck muscles firmly holds it in place. Dipping into its substance, an elastic layer right under the gland, divides it into irregularly shaped masses. Brownish or amber red in color, the gland is composed of lobules of microscopic closed vesicles, masses of alveoli, round or oval spaces lined by a single layer of epithelial cells. The alveoli's tiny cavities are filled with a homogeneous thick, viscous material secreted by lining cells, containing the gland's active principle.

The thyroid gland stores sufficient hormone to last three weeks. Normally, when the demand is small, little colloid is present, but in times of need, it increases in quantity.

Thyroxine is the major macromolecule secreted by the gland's follicular lumen. Synthesized by follicular cells, a constituent of the protein thyro-globulin, it is a highly specialized glycoprotein with a molecular weight of 660,000, composed of many proteins, of which 60% is iodine and 8-15%, carbohydrate. When released into the bloodstream, they are bound to serum proteins, namely plasma albumin and prealbumin.

Iodine in the body

A halogen, iodine is a rare element present in drinking water. The human body contains 50 mg. of iodine. Large quantities of iodine, about 1-15 mg., are stored in the thyroid gland. Summer storage is greater than in winter. The iodine present in the diet is sufficient to form the hormone. Iodine is also stored in salivary glands, skin, gastric mucous membrane and other epithelial structures. The human body requires very little iodine and.too little or too much iodine can form a goiter.

Thyroid gland utilizes iodine to form thyroxine

Absorbed from the intestines as iodide, blood plasma carries dietary iodine to the thyroid gland. Concentrated by follicles with the help of a special carrier, iodine is taken up, forming the hormone. Excess chloride affects follicles' concentrating capacity.

When thyroxine level is below normal, the pituitary gland is stimulated to produce thyrotropin or TSH circulating in blood, bound to a gamma globulin. Blood flow increases through the gland and follicular cells increase in number and size. From plasma, oxidized iodide is taken up and concentrated, forming components of thyroglobulin. Thyroxin is a constituent of the protein thyro-globulin whose iodinated derivatives are de-iodized and released into the bloodstream bound to serum proteins albumin and pre-albumin, readily available to body tissues.

Thyroxine: its function: A gland associated with sex and virility, the thyroid gland has a tremendous effect in forming personality. It maintains normal body temperature and creates a thermostatic setting for the metabolic rate. It regulates body tissues' rate of oxygen consumption, creating an environment where other hormones can influence metabolic processes more effectively. Minute quantities of the hormone are effective, i.e., in 10^{-6} values.

The hormone is involved in the maturation of certain tissues, especially in brain, bone and skin. It activates the sodium pump, maintaining the electrolyte gradient inside and outside tissue cells. It helps maintain less sodium ions and more potassium ions in cells, more sodium ions and less potassium ions outside of tissue cells.

Thyroxine deficiency, its effects. Humans are affected by deficiency of the thyroid hormone in two ways: during growth and in adulthood. In growth years, cretinism can result. Cretins sit, crawl, stand and walk at a later age or not at all. This has occurred in mountainous areas in Switzerland, far from the ocean. The problem has been resolved today.

Deficiency in adulthood lessens mental and physical activity with marked thickening of skin, shrinking of the gland, a condition known as myxedema, also premature senility with bradycardia, slightly lowered body temperature and dry skin. A lack of iodine in drinking water causes hypothyroidism.

Over-secretion of thyroxine. Symptoms are opposite from those in myxedema: increased metabolic rate and heartbeat, above normal body temperature, increase in mental activity and extreme nervous irritability, rapid hair growth, protrusion of eyeballs, heat intolerance, weight loss in spite of increased appetite. Externally the thyroid gland is enlarged, forming a goiter.

Hypo and hyperthyroidism, external manifestations

Both hypo and hyperthyroidism are indicated by enlargement of the thyroid gland. An abnormal protein in blood plasma called *Lats,* may cause a hyperthyroid state. Drugs and chemicals prevent iodine from being used in the thyroid hormone synthesis. Large amounts of iodine interfere with the gland's oxidation and use of iodide. Thyroid tumors are common. Excess iodide saturates the halogen pumping system. To ensure a normal production of thyroxine, adequate protein, iodine and carbohydrate must be available. Unrestricted diets cause the gland to overgrow. Too much carbohydrate, protein or iodine can form a goiter. Avoid iodized salt.

The gland functions well with adequate sleep. Some foods activate goiter formation. Large quantities of soybeans, walnuts, impair absorption of thyroid hormone from the intestine. Drugs, salicylates and others prevent proteins in blood from binding to thyroxine. Other foods that contain thiocyanates are: cabbage, kale, kohlrabi, rutabaga, cauliflower and mustard greens; a normal consumption is not dangerous. Excess fats interfere with absorption of iodine in the diet, causing a goiter. Poor sanitation, infections, avitaminoses, increase the need for iodine and are conducive to goiter formation. Other detrimental foods are those high in calcium, the lack of vitamin A, and iodized salt.

Other factors preventing formation of thyroxine by the gland

Stress, severe illness and the intake of glucocorticoid hormones reduce the thyroxine-binding globulin and thyroxine-binding prealbumin. Overexertion affects the function of the entire hormonal system with a detrimental effect on the quantity of manufactured hormones. The skeletal musculature's conditions, functions of the gastrointestinal tract, sensory nerve receptors, including taste, smell, touch experiences, age and sexual activity affect responses to diet. Diets high in protein depress appetite and raise body temperature.

What to do about bulging eyes and goiters. Usually attributed to hyperthyroidism, bulging eyes are due to the intake of heavy food prior to retiring at night. A young Chinese girl had very bulging eyes. After several days of questioning, she revealed her habit of eating cheese before retiring at night. We cautioned her that cheese is not part of the Asian diet and should never be eaten before retiring. She decided not to eat cheese again; we advised that it can be eaten during the day, mixed with other foods. Foods eaten late at night cause heavy breathing during sleep, pushing soft parts of the body out of shape. This may explain protruding lips, deformed nasal cartilages, protruding eyes. Late dinners cause abnormal growth, and youngsters may reach seven feet during growth years. Foods for evening snacks are juices, clear soup, light coffee or cocoa.

A 55 year-old woman has a large goiter at her throat. When asked whether she used iodized salt, she was surprised but acquiesced. Warned about the danger of excess iodine, she decided never to use that salt again. She said her 20-year old daughter was also developing a tumor at her throat. She was advised to use Kosher salt. Never eat salt or other foods with added iodine.

The Parathyroid: the gland and the hormone

Embedded behind the thyroid gland, one on each side of the trachea, parathyroid glands are attached to end stalks formed by branches of an artery and a nerve. Parathyroid glands are small, ovoid, pea-sized glands, the smallest member of the entire endocrine system. Normally two or three pairs of glands are present but sometimes two to twelve small glandules may occur.

The upper pair is behind the upper poles of the thyroid lobes, the lower pair behind, a little below the thyroid's inferior lobes. Surrounded by a delicate capsule dipping into its substance, internally each parathyroid gland comprises masses of small cells arranged in a column, interspersed with numerous blood vessels.

Parathormone, the gland's hormone, is a chain-shaped protein of 84 amino acids with a molecular weight of 8,500. Once parathormone enters the bloodstream, amino acids cleave into smaller units. Parathormone secretion depends upon blood plasma's calcium concentration. When the latter falls, parathormone secretion begins. Parahormone maintains calcium and phosphate balance in the continual buildup and breakdown of body tissues. Parathormone promotes the synthesis of nucleic acids RNA and DNA of bony tissue, stimulating mitosis and cell regeneration. In excess calcium concentration, RNA synthesis alone is stimulated but normal regeneration of cells will not happen. Parathormone causes bony tissue to assimilate minerals less readily, which reduces the enzyme phosphatase; the latter prevents phosphate accumulation. Parathormone enhances calcium's rate of dissolution and increases the kidneys' rate of calcium reabsorption. To see and understand parathormone's function a better knowledge of calcium's role is necessary.

Calcium and phosphate in blood

The normal daily intake of calcium is one gram, of phosphate, 2 grams. From this ingested gram of calcium, about 7 mg. is present in 100 cc. of urine and about

79-90% remains in the intestine. A state of equilibrium is reached when the amount of calcium salts ingested equals the quantity excreted.

Plasma calcium is very important. It forms the bony skeleton, binding calcium with phosphate and carbonate. In the bloodstream, only plasma contains calcium as red cells do not have the binding quality of plasma proteins. To use and absorb lime salts in blood, vitamin D must be present. Sufficient vitamin D forms a constant quantity of lime salts in bloodstream, allowing the excretion of excess calcium through feces. Similar to a hormone, vitamin D promotes intestinal calcium absorption.

HCl and vitamin D enhance calcium absorption. Alkali, excess fats and phosphates, phytic acid in oatmeal and certain cereals hinder calcium absorption. Without vitamin D, very little calcium is absorbed. Two hours of sunshine daily, especially in the summer, provide vitamin D. Normally in a diet without milk or cheese, 0.5 g. of calcium is present. Every pint of milk contains 0.65 g. of calcium, 100 ml. of blood has 10 mg. ±1 mg. of calcium.

About half of blood's calcium is filterable, the remainder is bound to plasma proteins. In ionic form, the filterable calcium is under parathormone control. It is of greater physiological importance than non-ionic calcium.

A reduction of blood calcium to about 4-6 mg. per 100 cc. of blood results in tetanus, with possible convulsions. In latent tetanus, each 100 cc. of blood have 7-9 mg. of calcium, with characteristics of nervousness, weakness, fatigue and spasms. Blood calcium can also rise to 12 mg. per 100 cc. of blood, even 20 mg. percent, when skeletal degeneration occurs, hindering normal bone regeneration. In a medical book is a picture of a woman whose blood indicated hyper-calcemia; her body was reduced to the size and had the appearance of a soft-bodied frog! This indicates that calcium rich foods may be eaten only during growth years. In an adult excess yogurt, milk, cheese, ice cream, raise blood calcium and prevent normal bone regeneration; instead, degeneration occurs, with inability to move limbs. Ice cream, yogurt, cheese are man-made concentrated natural products and must be eaten sparingly.

About 2.5-3.5 mg. percent is the normal inorganic blood phosphate content. Phosphate is present in a variety of forms. The filterable part is in ionic form, 80% of phosphorus is stored in bony tissue, the remainder in cell protoplasm. In the small intestine, fats, a low calcium diet and acids facilitate the process of phosphorus absorption, it is hindered by diets high in calcium and basic salts. When blood is too basic, both calcium and phosphate ions become non-diffusible, non-filterable, causing eventual convulsions. The ingestion of excess fats causes blood pH to rise, becoming basic. Therefore, avoid fats, but some good quality animal fat is essential.

Sugar, carbohydrates, oils, fats, raise stomach pH, eventually affecting blood's quality. To maintain continued health, cut down on these foods. In tetanus, the phosphorus content in blood rises to 7 or 10 mg. percent. Insufficient parathormone production causes tetanus. Symptoms: hands and feet tingling, carpopedal spasms, spasms of larynx and convulsions.

Phosphate acts as a buffer in acid-base reactions. It is a catalyst and in carbohydrate metabolism, phosphorus-containing compounds are required. Phosphorus is an important element in the living body.

Insufficient parathyroid secretion. When normal production of parathyroid secretion is interfered with, parathyroid insufficiency develops. Some signs are: irritability, helplessness, convulsive attacks, mild symptoms of fatigue, gastro-intestinal irritability, muscular weakness, trophic changes in nails, skin, cataract in eyes, with possible affection of brain metabolism.

There is excess phosphate in blood, about 4-6 mg. per 100 cc. and less serum calcium, 5 or 6 mg. percent. Foods high in phosphates are nuts, chocolate, flour, milk, meats, cheeses, cereals, egg yolks, potatoes, legumes, molasses, cocoa and cauliflower. Do not eat many foods high in phosphates.

Parathyroid gland, signs of hyper-secretion. The tiny parathyroid glands can be severely overactive and enlarged. Occurring slowly, this condition is often associated with high blood calcium, about 12 mg. per 100 cc. of blood.

Symptoms of hyper-parathyroidism are nausea, vomiting, anorexia and stupor. At a high blood calcium level, regeneration of bone is either nil or abnormal. About 50-60% of hyper-parathyroid cases are affected with renal calculi. Hyper-parathyroidism is associated with increase in the gland's size.

Excess bone resorption with increased absorption of intestinal calcium with hypo-calcemia, may be caused by drugs. Other drugs cause hyper-calcemia, i.e., antacids containing calcium and absorbable alkali impair kidney function. Thiazide diuretics increase calcium excretion and transiently raise serum calcium in most patients. Avoid all drugs. After a calcium rich meal, a heart attack may occur, with ensuing death. A symptom of hyper-calcemia is bradycardia. Calcium is deposited in blood vessels and kidneys, forming kidney stones.

In high blood calcium, inorganic phosphates become indiffusible, non-filterable from bloodstream, causing extreme nervousness with eventual convulsions. Reduce milk and milk products, nuts, meat, fish, internal organs. These foods are high in phosphorus content.

Calcium regulation is affected by parathormone

Parathyroid hormone does not help control the amount of calcium in bloodstream. The thyroid gland secretes calcitonin, a polypeptide containing 32 amino acids, molecular weight 3,600. Excess blood calcium ions secrete calcitonin, lowering blood plasma's calcium concentration. Calcitonin affects bony tissues' bone-forming cells. It decreases calcium uptake from intestines, reduces stomach acidity, lowers blood plasma calcium and inhibits tubular resorption of calcium.

The thyroid and parathyroid glands, surgical operations

The parathyroid gland may accidentally be removed during an operation on the thyroid gland. As blood calcium begins to decrease, death occurs within a few days. Never operate on the parathyroid glands. More effective would be a change of diet. Once parathyroid glands are removed, animal extracts of parathormone must be taken daily forever. There is no need to remove a tumor on the tiny gland. A diet isotonic to the normal composition of blood will gradually shrink a tumor. Also effective is rubbing the area. Regardless how one discusses calcium, iodine, chlorine, fluorine, phosphorus or other trace elements and minerals, the best advice is to leave them alone and not consume much calcium rich foods or iodized salt. These two elements, calcium and iodine have been overemphasized. Traces of iodine are present in the human body, and vitamin D formed directly from sunshine is more effective than added artificial vitamins.

The pituitary gland: origin of anterior and posterior lobes

The master endocrine gland, the tiny pituitary gland's hormone affects all other endocrine glands. Connected to the brain's base by a narrow stalk, the pituitary gland sits in a small recess, the *sella turcica*, about 10-11 mm. deep, in the sphenoid bone at base of skull. Measuring a little over half an inch in its longest diameter, it weighs about 0.5 grams.

The pituitary gland has two lobes, an anterior and a posterior portion, separated by a fibrous lamina. Known as the adeno-hypophysis, the anterior lobe is larger, oblong in shape, a little concave behind where it receives the round shaped posterior lobe or neuro-hypophysis. The anterior lobe comprises 70% of the gland, it is the larger; the posterior lobe, 20%, the fibrous lamina, the remaining 10% of its weight. A layer of dura mater covers the entire gland except for a hole through which passes the infundibulum or neural stalk.

Both divisions differ in development and in structure.

As a hollow pouch, the anterior lobe arises from the embryonic mouth cavity. At developing brain's base, a down-growth of nervous tissue from the 3rd ventricle's floor forms the posterior lobe. The anterior lobe or Rathke's pouch grows upward, meeting the brain's downward growth. The adeno-hypophysis, is that portion in front of the slit, the neuro-hypophysis, the portion behind the cleft.

Functions of the pituitary gland

The pituitary is the master gland of the endocrine system, the only gland directly connected to the brain at the stalk or infundibulum. Through the stalk, the gland receives messages from brain cells, with respect to blood's hormone concentration of other endocrine glands: thyroid, parathyroid, adrenals and sex glands. When the respective hormone concentration is low, nerve cells send releasing hormones to the pituitary gland, indicating the correct time to produce trophic hormones, and stimulating secretion of a particular gland. The pituitary gland does not restrict hormone production and excess secretion has led to tumors.

The pituitary gland also produces three hormones: growth hormone, melanin-stimulating hormone and the lactating hormone. To form a particular hormone, nerve cells send release-hormones through the infundibulum to the pituitary to stimulate or inhibit its production stirring normal growth processes,

Dwarfism or gigantism. To produce the growth hormone composed of proteins, 191 amino acids are needed. Absence of these amino acids in the bloodstream inhibits growth hormone production. Excess sugar and fatty acids also inhibit its production. Growth hormone promotes endochondral ossification, the basic process by which bones grow lengthwise before puberty. Peak growth hormone is concentrated at night during sleep. Aside from homeostasis regulation, sleep repairs and restores lost energy. Stress, pain, fright, work experienced during the day inhibit growth processes. Many child actors do not grow tall. Children should not embrace the acting profession or work until fully grown.

To ensure normal growth processes

The quality of baby foods is of utmost importance. A growing infant must be given dilute fresh juice. Meats and vegetables must be deliciously seasoned. Stir-fry meats, grind and pass it through a sieve. A child should taste delicious food from babyhood. Sunshine is very important. After puberty, excess growth hormone production does not affect growth in length but bones and soft tissues may deform and thicken—acromegaly. In juveniles excess growth hormone leads to gigantism. Late meals, French fries, large chunks of meat eaten late at night stir growth processes. One young man reached the height of 2.5 meters. Eat dinner before 6 PM and growth will not be affected. In this 21st century we should be able to eradicate dwarfism and gigantism.

An 80-year old woman is bent in two. She only uses frozen vegetables. Another senior citizen cooks vegetables on her own. Her posture is perfect. Cut down the use of boxed foods, canned products, etc. Beware of contents.

The reproductive hormones: their actions

Reproductive organs, ovaries in women, testes in men, produce hormones. By the end of the third month of prenatal life, female and male hormone production come to a halt, becoming active at puberty at around age 10 in boys, 12-15 in girls.

The embryonic development of reproductive organs is set by the third month of pregnancy. Aside from puberty, reproductive hormones lead to the development of secondary sexual characteristics: beard, moustache and deepened voice in the male. In the female, sex hormones change uterine tissues preceding implantation of the egg, in mammary glands, preceding secretion of milk. Reproductive hormones are estrogens and gestagens in women, androgens in men; the most important is testosterone which control the function of reproductive glands—seminal vesicles, prostate gland, Cowper's gland in the male, maturation of the egg and the female menstrual cycle in the female.

Changes at puberty

At about 10 years of age in boys, 12-15 years in girls, sperm and egg cells respectively begin to mature. When a sufficient build-up of estrogen in the female, testosterone in the male occurs, the anterior lobe of the pituitary gland begins to produce follicle-stimulating and luteinizing hormones.

Gonadotrophic hormones are secreted into the bloodstream, they act upon reproductive organs, nourishing both testes and ovaries, respectively inducing production of sperm and egg, and testes secrete testosterone, a secondary hormone. Testosterone is of utmost importance in the development and formation of male accessory glands: seminal vesicles, prostate gland and male sexual characteristics.

In the female, gonadotrophic hormones ripen ovarian follicles, each follicle surrounding an egg. At maturation, the egg breaks out of follicle, enters the Fallopian tube. The luteinizing hormone induces follicles to rupture, releasing the egg; the developing corpus luteum secretes progesterone, preparing the uterus for pregnancy. Developing follicles generate estrogens, preparing the female tract for sperm reception. Mostly males produce androgens but estrogens are also produced in small quantities. The female also produces small quantities of testosterone. A build-up of end products of hormone action arrests further release of pituitary hormones.

Enhance reproductive powers without artificial hormones

Humans require a period of 10-20 years for maturation of male sperm and females eggs. The total number of eggs is set by the third month of prenatal life, but ovaries and testes are vital organs and do not mature until twelve years later. Exceptions do occur. The case of a girl who at five years of age gave birth to an infant, indicates that eggs could mature sooner than the ten-year waiting period.

Conditions surrounding a developing child are most important. Limit the amount of work time so that a child may relax. For optimum development a growing child must be given excellent food. At home, children must not be assailed by loud noise, rapid moving pictures on a screen, fright and emotion. They must not exercise forcefully and two hours of fresh air and sunshine daily are essential. A mother must prepare delicious fresh foods for her growing child to ensure optimum growth of reproductive organs.

Hormones being steroids, their formation requires some fat and a good quality of fat is necessary. Animal fat: pork, bacon, chicken and duck fat are excellent. The Chinese use lard in most recipes. The older one becomes the more care should be given to the preparation of foods.

The pancreas, the islets of Langerhans

Embedded in the pancreas' substance are aggregates of one or two to 200 islet cells. The human pancreas has 200,000 to over a million and a half islet cells, the tail end richer in islet tissue than the body or head. These cells have an endocrine function. Reticular connective tissue separates larger cells from the gland's exocrine portion. A narrow, clear space delineates the majority of islet cells from the exocrine portion.

Islet cells are of two types: alpha or A cells with a large nucleus and large granules, forming sharply defined groups at islet's center. Beta or B cells with smaller nuclei, richer in chromatin and basophilic granules, forming cords, interrupted by groups of A cells. Two other types of cells are also present.

Hormones of alpha and beta cells. Alpha cells produce glucagon, beta cells produce insulin and delta cells secrete somatostatin. Insulin is a proteohormone composed of two polypeptide chains arranged in parallel, linked by disulfide bridges, with a molecular weight of around 6,000. A polypeptide in the shape of a single chain, glucagon has a molecular weight of about 3,500. Insulin was the first hormone, the first protein to be experimentally synthesized.

Insulin, its functions. Insulin lowers blood glucose level: when blood glucose level rises to 0.3-0.5 percent, the pancreas produces insulin, releasing it into bloodstream. Blood sugar is built up to glycogen (animal starch), stored in liver and muscle cells, restoring the normal blood sugar level of 0.1%.

Insulin has other actions: increases cellular permeability to glucose in skeletal muscles, heart muscle and fatty tissue; lessens glucose formation from amino acids. Insulin influences the metabolism of fat, acting against the appearance of ketone bodies, preventing acidosis. The changing carbohydrate consumption continually threatens the constancy of blood sugar concentration. In exercise the variable rate of sugar oxidation increases several-fold, converting glycogen rapidly into glucose and poured into the bloodstream.

Ketone bodies. Oxidation of acetoacetic acid produces ketone bodies, normal intermediate products in fat metabolism: beta hydroxybutyric acid, acetoacetic acids and acetone. A healthy person has small quantities of ketone bodies, acetoacetic acid being almost completely oxidized to carbon dioxide and water. Ketone bodies accumulate in both blood and urine when rate of breakdown of fats increases, responsible for the acidosis and coma of diabetes. In the diabetic, the loss of a molecule of carbon dioxide converts acetoacetic acid to acetone. Acetone is exhaled in breath and excreted in urine.

Glucagon, its functions. Glucagon's function is antagonistic to insulin's. Normally it adjusts insulin's activity. Its various functions are: it promotes the breakdown of glycogen into glucose, raising blood sugar level. It accelerates liver's oxidation of fatty acids that convert into ketone bodies, enhancing storage of fatty acids as triglycerides. Glucagon assists in balancing and adjusting insulin activity and promotes sugar formation. Depending on the amount of sugar ingested, plasma concentration of the two hormones varies. The concentration of insulin and glucagon is not controlled, instead these hormones are controlling elements and maintain a constant blood glucose level. The changing amounts of carbohydrates consumed and exercise continually threaten blood sugar constancy.

Diabetes and how to control its ravaging effect

Deficiency in insulin production characterizes the diabetic. After meals, sugar is incompletely removed and blood sugar level rises. As sugar is excreted in urine, body tissue is used for energy purposes followed by weight loss and inanition. In diabetics the usual cure is to restrict carbohydrate consumption. When treated with commercially prepared insulin, degenerative diseases affect the diabetic patient, such as arteriosclerosis and cataracts. Diabetics who restrict carbohydrate intake do not require insulin administration. This is the best course to pursue.

For a sick person, of great importance are several stool evacuations daily. Destructive factors are excess work, excess physical exercise, loud noise or music, rapid moving objects. Computers disrupt normal regulation of body fluids. Reduce the number of hours spent before a moving screen. Avoid violent exercise and do not tamper with endocrine glands. Adjust the diet and modify living habits. It is a better alternative than medicine or surgery.

Secretions of the adrenal glands

Above each kidney lies an adrenal gland. Surrounded by fat, yellowish-brown in color, each gland weighs about 3-8 grams. The right gland is triangular in shape, the left, half-moon shaped. A fibrous capsule covers each gland, with processes penetrating furrows on front and base.

When cut in half, the gland presents an external firm yellow or red striated cortical region forming the greater part of the gland. The internal medullary region is soft, pulpy, of a brown or black color.

The two parts of the gland are of different origins. In early embryonic development, the medulla arises from groups of cells split off from the neural crest. The outer cortex develops from multiplication of cells closely related to those of sex glands. From the surface inwards, the cortex comprises three zones: the glomerulosa, fasciculata and reticularis. The glomerulosa's cells are grouped together. Arranged in columns, cells of the fasciculata form the greater part of the cortex. Cells of the reticularis have a loose arrangement.

The medulla's cells are arranged in compact bundles held together by strands of connective tissue. Very vascular, sinusoids are interspersed among cells, allowing intimate contact between cells and bloodstream.

The adrenal gland produces two different secretions. The cortex forms a group of hormones known as cortin. They are steroid derivatives of which 30 are not formed in any other organ. Cortical hormones are known as cortico-steroids or corticoids. Cells of the adrenal cortex have no connection with the sympathetic nervous system. The adrenal medulla produces epinephrine and noradrenaline, reinforcing the action of the sympathetic nervous system, raising the body's defense mechanisms to a high level of efficiency against dangers and rigors of the environment.

The most important functions of adrenal glands

The adrenal cortex exerts an important influence upon the metabolism of water and salts. Tissue cells have a high potassium concentration. Without the adrenal cortex, sodium and water are excreted in excess and potassium escapes from tissue cells into body fluid. Kidneys' excretion of potassium is impaired and its concentration rises in other tissues and blood.

The adrenal cortex influences carbohydrate metabolism due to a hormone different from that controlling metabolism of water and salt. The cortex of the adrenal gland is vital to a living organism and when removed, death occurs in a short time. The adrenal cortex also influences the development of sexual functions and when removed, developmental abnormalities of a sexual nature occur. Children show unusual muscular development, women become obese and masculine in appearance, with a tendency toward mannishness or virilism.

Adrenal cortex disease. The adrenal cortex may be overactive or under-active. When the gland is enlarged, hyperactivity is congenital. Hyperactivity is present when a tumor is grown which can be removed. When operating, care must be given to prevent loss of the gland's capsule. Tumor in the gland is indicated by excess excretion of epinephrine or adrenaline. Symptoms of the illness are periodic episodes of high blood pressure, heart palpitation, sweating with pounding headaches, anxiety, nausea, vomiting.

Hypo-activity of the gland is indicated by Addison's disease. Skin gradually discolors, turning gray, to end in death in two or three years. Prominent features of this condition are disturbances of water and salt metabolism. The treatment is to administer a hormone from the adrenal cortex, or a synthetic preparation combined with a diet high in salt and low in potassium.

A better alternative is to remove all starches from the diet, use salt freely in foods and raise fluid intake. Frequent bowel elimination and deep sleep rapidly restore an ill condition to normal. Alter the diet before opting for an operation on tumor. Do not tamper with endocrine glands, they are vital organs.

The function of the pineal gland

An out-pocketing of the brain's third ventricle, the pineal is a small, conical-shaped gland attached by a narrow stalk to the base of the brain. About 8 mm. long, 6 mm. wide and 4 mm. thick, weighing about 170 mg, the pineal gland lies in a depression in the brain, between the two superior colliculi; the stalk is made of a lower and an upper lamina, separated by the small pineal recess.

The gland is composed of a number of follicles lined by epithelium. Inside supporting tissue between follicles, thin-walled blood vessels are enclosed. Blood vessels may contain deposits of calcareous salts known as brain sand composed of phosphate of magnesia and ammonia.

The pineal gland is a light sensitive endocrine gland, with secretory functions of a nervous nature. It produces melatonin and to a lesser degree, seratonin and certain polypeptides with endocrine actions. Melatonin allows melanin granules to aggregate in skin's melanocytes. Melatonin lightens skin's color, inhibits secretion of gonadotropin and controls activity of reproductive glands.

Destruction of the pineal gland in youth promotes sexual maturation and pineal influence on fertility, and sexuality is lost.

A light-sensitive gland, light and sunshine affect man's reproductive capacity. One must obtain sufficient sunshine otherwise one's reproductive ability will lessen. People today live in closed quarters with little light, sunshine or air. It is time to build houses with a garden in front and a back yard, allowing the sun to shine on house and garden. Man will live close to the earth, procreate and leave sufficient offspring for a next generation. Each individual is a link to the next generation and birds indicate it to us every spring. We must listen to their silent message.

Chapter 17
How to cope with problems of blood and lymph

Blood

Blood is the body's most important tissue and to solve its problems, we must know something about it. The passage of blood through the heart ensures its continuous action. The most important fluid in the living body, blood is a tissue; it contains living cells and has specific functions, of which the most important is to convey materials from one body part to another. Each living cell carries out in its own substance, the chemical processes required for its survival. The living body's principal required materials are sugar, amino acids, fat, vitamins, oxygen, salts, hormones and water. After digestive organs convert food to a substance blood can absorb and deliver to body cells, waste materials must be disposed of. Blood conveys food to body tissues and waste materials away from body cells.

Never in direct contact with tissue cells, blood circulates in a closed system. At around 100° F. blood represents 1/20th of man's body weight and has a basic reaction. It is salty to the taste with a particular odor. In health, the chemical constitution of gases and solids in blood and body fluids, vary within very narrow limits. Homeostasis is the unvarying condition of the internal environment, a term coined by Dr. Walter Cannon. Homeostasis allows man to live a normal life in freedom, indicating the approximate constancy in concentration of dissolved substances, in temperature and pH. Homeostasis is a basic requirement for the normal cell function of the organism as a whole.

Blood, its composition. An opaque, viscid fluid, blood emerging from an artery is bright red or scarlet in color, from a vein, dark red or purple. At 120 pounds, the body contains about five liters of blood. Blood is divisible into two distinct parts, a yellow fluid or plasma and suspended red, white blood cells and blood platelets.

Plasma's composition. Plasma is a clear, faintly straw-colored fluid but after a meal with fat, the minute fat globules impart plasma with a somewhat milky appearance. Found in greatest quantity in plasma are protein and common salt. Plasma has the general nature of raw egg white diluted with 0.9% salt solution with the following normal composition:

1. 90 to 92% water
2. 7% to 9% protein (fibrinogen, globulin, albumin)
3. 0.9% to 1% salts (Na, K, Ca, Mg, Fe, Cu, etc.) Inorganic constituents
4. 0.1% sugar, urea, uric acid, creatinine, xanthine, hypoxanthine, creatine, ammonia, amino acids, neutral fats, phospholipids, cholesterol, glucose. Organic constituents.
5. Respiratory gases: oxygen and carbon dioxide
6. Internal secretions, antibodies and various enzymes

1. Water in blood: Water in blood eases the flow through tiny capillaries. Water with protein, organic and inorganic components provide blood's viscosity. Too great a viscosity would overwork the heart and reduce circulation through certain vital organs. Water maintains tissue water content by a constant exchange of fluid across walls of finest blood vessels. If body water were reduced, osmotic pressure would rise, reducing urine output, thus retaining poisons. Thirst warns us to replenish water content. The amount of water taken into the body daily or over any considerable period must equal the amount lost from body.

2. Blood plasma proteins: The chemical basis of all life resides in a watery medium of proteins. Proteins attract water. If proteins were present in cells only and not in blood, water would pass from blood into tissue cells which would swell and become dropsical. A balance of proteins in blood and body cells maintains water equilibrium. Proteins allow blood to clot and prevent bleeding. Of the 7% proteins of blood plasma 4% represents serum albumin produced by liver, 2.7% globulin from lymphocytes, 0.3% fibrinogen from liver. Serum globulin splits into alpha, beta and gamma globulins.

How proteins are formed in the body

After digestion of food in stomach and intestines, protein is broken down into individual amino acids whose molecules pierce intestinal capillary walls. Blood picks them up and conveys them to tissue cells. Protein molecules are numerous special amino acids held together with ammonia, by peptide links. Colloidal in nature, the protein fraction is a mixture of proteins of high molecular weight from 44,000-1,300,000. During transport from intestine to storage organs, proteins bind to small molecules. They are brought to needy areas to maintain constant osmotic pressure, thus regulating water distribution between plasma and interstitial fluid.

The 0.5-8 grams per deciliter of protein content provides the high relative viscosity of blood plasma. If a cell loses a protein's particular amino acid, the appropriate one can be acquired from the assortment carried in blood. Albumin is the largest plasma protein fraction. A rising albumin concentration produces a marked effect on colloid osmotic pressure; in reduced concentration, interstitial edema results.

By combining with acids and bases, plasma proteins form salts and maintain a constant pH. Plasma proteins help the clotting process and prevent bleeding. When skin is cut, blood clots as the protein fibrinogen solidifies and coagulates. A chemical process, clotting occurs as follows: the dissolved fibrinogen in plasma separates out as a spongy network of fibrin connecting edges of a wound, preventing further passage of blood cells.

Though the normal blood plasma content of protein is 7%, in disease the protein proportion varies greatly, i.e., cirrhosis of liver, nephrosis. Normally, an adult body carries 3 liters of plasma with 200 grams of protein in solution.

Functions of plasma proteins: Plasma proteins have an osmotic pressure of 25-30 mm. of Hg, important in blood volume regulation and urine excretion.

To maintain blood pressure, plasma proteins provide the viscosity of blood.

Blood coagulates due to fibrinogen.

The production of immune bodies is associated with gamma globulin. In the process of immunization, gamma globulin concentration increases.

3. Inorganic constituents

Plasma contains potassium, calcium, magnesium, sodium bicarbonate and minute amounts of iodine and iron. Phosphorus is present in both organic (40 mg.) and inorganic forms (3 mg.) per 100 cc. of blood. Potassium is relatively high in blood cells and solid tissue cells, low in plasma and body fluids. Sodium is high in blood plasma and body fluids, low in blood cells and cells of solid tissue. Serious results follow when proportions of inorganic elements in plasma, blood cells and whole blood are disturbed.

Sodium chloride or salt in blood primarily serves to dissolve proteins. Most blood proteins do not dissolve in pure water. Other salts can also dissolve proteins but produce dangerous side effects, i.e., potassium chloride arrests heart action and ammonium chloride triggers convulsions. In blood, table salt is a most important compound. The body accurately regulates the percentage of sodium chloride in blood. When salt is insufficient, kidneys cease to secrete salt in urine. Kidneys maintain proper salt balance. Normally, urine contains a considerable quantity of salt.

Heavy perspiration causes loss of several pounds of sweat in a few hours, and workers in deep mines or ships' furnaces quickly feel the deficiency of salt. Sweat is almost pure salt solution. Water alone does not replenish salt and salt concentration drops to critical levels with terrible muscle cramps in different muscles. Taking salt tablets or other salty edibles prevent cramps.

A level tablespoonful is a normal salt intake per day. Of all minerals in the body, table salt is the most abundant, responsible for blood's salinity. Mineral salts preserve the necessary alkalinity of blood and assist in forming tissues, i.e., bone. In blood plasma, blood salinity is extremely important. Between blood vessels and tissues, it is essential to the interchange of fluid, to maintain rhythmic heart action and to preserve red blood cells' life.

Through osmosis, pure water invades cells, are diluted, swell and die. Similar to red cells' salinity, they remain safe in saline plasma and osmosis occurs without harm.

Each 100 cc. of blood have 3 mg. of inorganic phosphate, 40 mg. of organic phosphate, the highest concentration of salt, lesser quantities of potassium, calcium, magnesium, sodium carbonate and minute amounts of iodine and iron. Though lesser quantities of calcium, potassium, magnesium ions are found in plasma than sodium ions, they are of value for the heart's continued function depends on a fine balance between calcium and potassium ions.

Sodium bicarbonate, iodine, iron and phosphorus are present in organic and inorganic forms. Sodium bicarbonate transports carbonic acid from tissues to lungs and maintains blood within very narrow limits, immediately on the alkaline side of neutrality. The interaction of plasma's sodium bicarbonate and red blood cells' hemoglobin maintains blood at pH 7.4. The addition of either acid or alkali to blood slightly alters blood's hydrogen ion concentration. If blood is more acidic, breathing increases, becoming violent, easing plasma's expulsion of carbonic acid and blood becomes less acidic. If blood is more alkaline, kidneys relieve the condition by excreting more alkali in urine.

4. Organic constituents: 0.1% sugar, urea, uric acid, most of the organic constituents of plasma other than protein represent waste products of metabolism: Urea, uric acid, etc. together with nutritive materials (amino acids, glucose and fats) absorbed from intestinal tract.

5. Respiratory gases in blood plasma: Arterial and venous blood contain gases. Similar proportions of nitrogen and carbon dioxide are present in arterial and venous blood but the latter has less oxygen. In red cells, oxygen is loosely combined with hemoglobin. In blood plasma nitrogen is present in simple solution. Carbon dioxide is combined in sodium bicarbonate and carbonate.

6. Internal secretions: From their origin, internal secretions are secreted into blood and brought to more or less remote areas where they assert their specific physiologic action. More than 50 different substances have been identified in plasma, many of them proteins, polypeptides, amines, amides and steroids, internal secretions, antibodies and various enzymes.

The following plasma components exert little effect on physical and chemical properties of blood: nutrients, vitamins, trace elements, amino acids, sugars, fats mostly bound to blood proteins. Sugars and fats are tissue foods and sources of heat. Amino acids are great tissue builders.

Among products of intermediary metabolism, lactic acid is most abundant. In oxygen deficiency, its concentration rises. Pyruvic acid, a key substance in the energy metabolism of amino acids and carbohydrates, is always present.

Substances to be excreted from plasma: The most important end products of metabolism are carbon dioxide, urea, uric acid, creatinine, bilirubin and ammonia. Secreted by kidneys, with exception of carbon dioxide, all contain nitrogen. When kidneys are impaired, their blood concentration rises.

The above values of blood's constituents are for normal individuals. In illness values may rise or decrease considerably.

Homeostasis is a basic requirement for normal cellular function

Homeostasis indicates the approximate constancy in concentration of dissolved substances, in temperature, in pH. As it circulates through the body, blood's composition and physical properties constantly change due to food intake and physical conditions. In health, some organs correct the changes. In disease, the correction may not occur sufficiently well to maintain constancy, thus disturbing the organism's normal function. In plasma, the concentration of dissolved substances is indicated by the osmotic pressure. Isotonic solutions have similar osmotic pressure, hypertonic solutions, a higher osmotic pressure, hypotonic solutions, a lower osmotic pressure than blood plasma; 96% of blood's osmotic pressure is due to the presence of inorganic electrolytes, mainly salt; homeostasis is critically dependent on salt intake. In hypotonic or hypertonic extra-cellular fluid, severe impairment of function results, thus, to maintain health, it is correct to feed proportionately to the normal composition of blood plasma.

TABLE 6
Some pathological conditions due to increased concentration of some blood constituents

Constituent	Pathological Conditions
Creatinine	Nephritis, Uremia
Glucose	Diabetes
Hemoglobin	Polycythemia
Oxygen Content	Polycythemia
Urea, Nitrogen	Nephritis, Cardiac Failure, Intestinal or urinary obstruction
Uric acid	Nephritis, Gout, Leukemia And Eclampsia
CO2 content	Vomiting, tetany
Chloride	Nephriis, cardiac conditions
Fibriniogen	Pneumonia, infections
Amylase	Acute pancreatitis
Bilirubin	Obstructive jaundice, hemolytic jaundice
Calcium	Multiple sclerosis
Cholesterol	Diabetes, nephrosis, biliary obstruction
Globulin	Cirrhosis, nephrosis, chronic infections
Phosphatase (acid)	Carcinoma of prostate
Phosphatase (alkaline)	Obstructive jaundice, rickets, diseases of bone
Phospholipids	Diabetes, nephrosis
Phosphorus	Tetany, nephritis
Potassium	Pneumonia, acute infections
Protein (total)	Mulltiple myeloma

TABLE 7
Some Pathological conditions due to decreased concentration of some blood constituents

Blood constituent	Pathological Condition
Glucose	Addison's disease
Hemoglobin	Anemias
Ascorbic acid	Scurvy
CO_2 content	diabetes, nephritis
Chlorides	Diarrhea, vomiting, pneumonia
Calcium	Tetany, nephritis, celiac disease
Cholesterol esters	Pernicious anemia
Phosphorus	Rickets, myxedema
Protein total	Nephoris, liver disease
Sodium	Addison's Disease, severe nephritis

From **Fundamentals of Inorganic, Organic and Biological Chemistry**, J. I. Routh, Appendix.

Types of cells in blood: the red blood cells and where they are formed

Red blood cells are circular, biconcave discs, resembling a doughnut without a hole. The biconcave shape provides a greater surface area for blood cells' various functions. Red cells do not have a nucleus.

The embryo's yolk sac forms blood. Descendants of embryonic tissue cells, basophilic cells give rise to large nucleated red cells. In later embryonic life, the liver is the seat of red cell formation, soon replaced by bone marrow, the only site of formation of both red and white blood cells in the adult.

Primitive stem cells called myeloblasts are transformed to become red blood cells. In the developmental stage, depending on the degree of maturity, red cells are called polychromatophil erythroblasts and normoblasts.

Red cells alter shape and structure

Under pressure, red blood cells change shape, adapting themselves to vessels' size. Red cells stick to one another, forming stacks or rouleaux. During the course of a day they vary in number; lowest in the morning, the count increases gradually toward midday. The number of red cells is slightly higher in newborn infants than in older children. Each cubic centimeter of blood has 4-5 million red blood cells.

The form and structure of red cells vary. In anemia red cells are nucleated. Immature red cells called reticuloblasts may be found. In blood of high salt content some red cells assume a mulberry shape. In some anemias, red cells are smaller or larger than normal. In sugar or salt solutions denser than plasma, red cells assume a stellate, crenated appearance. Solutions diluted to the same specific gravity as blood restore normal shape of both red and white cells.

Life span of red cells

A mature red cell circulates in blood 100-120 days. In tiny capillaries, any tissue may destroy red cells, but they are rapidly renewed. Each 100 ml. of blood contain 12-17 grams of hemoglobin. In warm-blooded animals hemoglobin is responsible for intense oxidation of tissues.

Rapid sweating increases red cell count. At high altitudes, the number increases but size and shape of red cells vary. In a red cell, around 60% water and 40% solids are present, mostly the red pigment hemoglobin. Normally non-nucleated, in severe anemia, nucleated red cell types may appear in the circulation. When destruction exceeds production of normal red cells, immature cells are not given sufficient time to mature and nucleated types appear. There is no need for concern. Silence, solitude, relaxation and a good diet can soon restore the condition to normal.

Blood count is analyzed by pricking the fingertip. This test should not be performed, as blood from fingertips does not reflect blood flow in the body. Self-analysis is a more trustworthy procedure. Today people have the tendency to talk too much. Emitting sound from vocal cords destroys many red cells. Animals do not speak, the only sounds produced are hissing, barking, meowing or chirping. Were animals able to speak they would soon die; a barking dog will not live long. Try to not speak, sing or hum, and you will live long. Do not indulge in seafood. The homeostasis of cold-blooded animals differs from humans' homeostasis. The cell will shrink or swell when many substances flow with water and pass through the red cell membrane. A red cell swells in an acid medium, bursting the membrane. This is known as hemolysis or laking of blood.

Function of red blood cells

Red blood cells carry oxygen to all parts of the living body and in exchange, pick up carbon dioxide, ensuring respiration in every living cell. Red blood cells contain hemoglobin, a chromoprotein of 4 polypeptide chains, each with a pigment component called *heme*. Made of the pigment porphyrin, heme is combined with iron. Porphyrin combines with various metals: copper, cobalt, magnesium, silver, nickel and iron. The molecular constitution of hemoglobin is porphyrin+iron=heme or hematin. Heme or hematin+globin=hemoglobin. Heme's chemical characteristics are: iron in the ferrous state, and 4 pyrrole groupings provide it with a superficial relationship to chlorophyll. Chemical agents easily oxidize heme to hematin where iron is found in the ferric state. With a molecular weight of 64,500, each hemoglobin sub-unit has a molecular weight of 16,000. The four identical heme groups form a porphyrin with a central bivalent iron ion, its crucial functional component.

When separated from red blood cells, hemoglobin crystallizes readily. Hemoglobin carries oxygen due to its ability to combine loosely with oxygen and in the living body, hemoglobin is oxygenated, forming oxy-hemoglobin, a reversible reaction. It is a physical process, not a chemical one. Exposed to pressure at end capillaries, oxygen is liberated by blood to body tissues. The normal concentration of hemoglobin is 15-16 grams and 20 cc. of oxygen per 100 cc. of blood.

Though normally oxygenated, in the presence of much waste material, hemoglobin becomes oxidized, forming met-hemoglobin. Normal blood contains some met-hemoglobin but when large quantities are formed, there is danger for in the oxidized state, oxygen is not released to body tissues and cells may asphyxiate.

Avoid overeating, especially dangerous are proteins and carbohydrates: fats, starches, sugars, alcohol. Often we are advised to eat foods high in iron content; all vegetables, fruits, meats, nuts, contain iron in sufficient quantities to maintain the amount required by man's blood. We are also advised to take calcium and other minerals. Beware. They are not to be tampered with.

Hemoglobin has a great affinity for carbon monoxide, greater than for oxygen and once bound to hemoglobin, carbon monoxide is released 200 times slower than oxygen. In newborn infants, blood contains 200 grams of hemoglobin per liter with individual variations, falling to 115 g./l. at a year's age, rising slowly to adult level. At 130 grams of hemoglobin per liter of blood, there is anemia in an adult. One gram of hemoglobin binds 1.39 ml. of oxygen, depending on temperature, pH, carbon dioxide's partial pressure and other parameters of importance in diseased states. The ability to bind and release oxygen to body tissues is hindered when blood is too acidic, too basic, when abundant wastes accumulate in cells.

White blood cells

Smaller than red blood cells are white blood cells or leucocytes. About 1/2,000th of an inch in diameter, in health, each micro-liter of blood has around 4,000-10,000 or 10,000-12,000 white cells.

White blood cells are formed outside of vessels in bone marrow, spleen or lymphatic glands. By ameboid movements, they find their way into the circulating blood, work their way out of blood vessel walls, then back into tissue cells where they are needed. There are three main groups of white blood cells: granulocytes, lymphocytes and monocytes.

1. Granulocytes: 60% of white blood cells are granulocytes. They are neutrophils, eosinophils and basophils.
- a) Neutrophils comprise 96% of granulocytes. With a nucleus of 2-5 lobes and granules staining with neutral dyes, neutrophils circulate for a short time in blood, averaging about 6-8 hours. Every micro-liter of blood has around 4,150 neutrophils. In acute infection, these cells rapidly proliferate. In the

body's unspecific defense system they are the most important functional elements, decomposing and phagocytosing bacteria. Pus is mostly composed of neutrophils.

b) Eosinophils comprise the remaining 2-4% of white blood cells, about 100-350 cells per microliter. Their granules stain with acid dyes and show a 24-hour periodicity: 20% lower in late afternoon and morning, 30% higher at midnight. In response to allergy, worm infestations and immune diseases, eosinophils increase beyond the normal count, engulfing foreign particles. In infectious conditions, white cells engulf bacteria faster when less solid food is ingested. A light semi-liquid diet cures an infection very rapidly, i.e., appendicitis, blood poisoning, immune disease, measles, small pox, etc. In hospitals today, after a serious operation patients are placed on a liquid diet. We would not be surprised if an isotonic diet cured paraplegia.

c) Basophil leukocytes comprise 0.5-1%, about 50 cells per micro-liter of blood. Circulating about 12 hours, cells have a bilobed nucleus with a diameter of 7-11 micrometers, in the cytplasm, large granules staining with basic dyes containing heparin.

2. Lymphocytes: 25-40% of white cells are lymphocytes, about 3,600-4,000 cells per micro-liter of blood. In children 50% of white cells are lymphocytes. Beyond 4,000 cells per micro-liter of blood, cells have proliferated. Less than 3,600 indicate lymphopenia.

The site of production of lymphocytes: The following tissues produce lymphocytes: lymph nodes, tonsils, Peyer's patches, appendix, adenoids, spleen, thymus gland and bone marrow.

3. Monocytes: they comprise 8% of all white blood cells, about 450 per microliter of blood. Originating from bone marrow they have a diameter of 15 microns and a horseshoe-shaped nucleus. Monocytes exceed all other white blood cells in the capacity to engulf foreign bacteria and other particles.

There is a proportion of one white blood cell to 400-450 red cells. Granulocytes differ in nuclear configuration and in granules.

The function of white blood cells

White blood cells are important in the body's cellular defense mechanism, guarding from all types of microorganisms. In acute infections the white cell count increases rapidly. Once outside the bloodstream, white blood cells are capable of active movement. When moving, their appearance changes, protruding fingerlike processes or pseudopodia. When a granule or bacteria is encountered, a pseudopodium is pushed out, wraps around the granule, lodging it in its own substance, engulfing it. Granulocytes move towards a chemical gradient, notably of carbohydrates. White blood cells contain many enzymes, of which those in white blood cells with multi-lobed nuclei are most important.

Some abnormal white blood cell counts

Leukemia is characterized by an enormous increase in white blood cells. A reduction in white cells is known as leucopenia. Neither condition should be cause for concern. Excess physical exercise, injections, pills, excess starches in diet, even excess proteins including seafood can raise white cell count. Foodstuffs exceeding the normal proportion in blood become foreign matter or wastes, and white blood cells will consider them as such, their cell count increases to rid the body of accumulated foodstuffs by engulfing them. After engulfing foreign materials, white cells are destroyed. From Chapter 1, we have seen that anything done by the body, acting on the body, penetrating the body destroys red blood cells. The more foreign materials penetrate the body, the more white cells proliferate to engulf unwanted substances. During a lifetime, let hunger direct food intake. Be selective in the choice of foods, especially when not feeling well. Health will be restored.

Blood platelets, thrombocytes

Blood platelets are small non-nucleated cellular bodies derived from megakaryocytes, the largest bone marrow cells. Outside of the vascular tree, the fusion of several reticulo-endothelial cells give rise to megakaryocytes. The shedding of cytoplasmic buds of megakaryocytes produce blood platelets. Each cubic milliliter of blood contains 25,000-500,000 blood platelets varying in size 1-3 microns and 0.5-0.75 mm. thick. They contain a little blue cytoplasm, their inner structure staining deeply. Platelets live from three to five days, circulating 5-11 days in blood, to be destroyed in the liver or spleen.

Platelets' cytoplasm has three types of granules: alpha, beta and gamma granules. Platelets closely stick together, an important agglutinating property, plugging up small loopholes in the blood vascular apparatus. When platelets are greatly reduced in number or completely lacking, blood tends to seep out of the circulation into skin and mucous membranes and black or blue spots appear.

Platelets have other important functions. They produce thromboplastin, the clotting factor, initiating the series of reactions forming the fibrin clot. In the circulation, platelets participate in the body's defense mechanism and aggregate around foreign particles, viruses and immune bodies including bacteria. Thrombocytes contain serotonin and histamine and enzymes involved in glycolysis. There is tendency towards bleeding when the number of platelets falls below 50,000-30,000 per micro-liter of blood.

The laking of blood, hemolysis

Certain chemical solutions prevent the retention of hemoglobin in red blood cells. Hemoglobin escapes, coloring plasma; this is known as laking. Hypotonic solutions such as distilled water added to blood, causes blood to lake. Other substances are chloroform, ether, benzene and other solvents, i.e., bacterial poisons, venom of certain snakes and specific hemolysins.

How blood clots

Normally, blood vessel linings prevent blood from flowing out. In blood, platelets and certain compounds and enzymes lead to clot formation. When a vessel is cut and blood escapes, to prevent further blood loss, capillary linings retract about the injured area. Damaged tissue cells and disintegrated blood platelets liberate thromboplastin, a lipid or fat-like compound containing phosphorus, widely distributed throughout tissues, in lungs, especially rich in the brain. Blood plasma has small quantities of thromboplastin. Blood will not clot unless free thromboplastin converts inactive prothrombin into active thrombin. To form the framework of a clot, thrombin acts as an enzyme, converting plasma's fibrinogen into insoluble fibrin deposited as fine threads. Blood clots in 5 minutes, with a variation of 2-6 minutes. Hemophilia is present when blood clots from 40-60 minutes later—a deficiency in the thromboplastin mechanism. In clotting, vitamin C is important. Without vitamin C, capillary linings cannot protect the body, blood oozes into tissues and in injury, the normal number of platelets is insufficient to plug small breaks. Eating fresh citrus fruits is very important.

The external appearance of the spleen

An external serous coat adheres to an internal fibrous elastic coat forming sheaths, giving off fibrous bands in all directions such that internally, the spleen appears like a sponge with small spaces containing splenic pulp. Due to the elasticity of fibrous tissue, the spleen is able to change its size to accommodate storage of cells. Splenic pulp is characterized by a soft mass of dark, reddish-brown color with branching cells and intercellular substance. Cells communicate with one other and one may find in its spaces more white cells and many red cells in all stages of disintegration. Due to its blood-containing properties, the artery penetrating the spleen is tortuous and large, divided into six or more branches. Veins branch out but arteries do not. Lymphatics penetrate the spleen with blood vessels. Nerves supplying the organ derive from the right and left semi-lunar ganglia and the right pneumogastric nerve.
The spleen stores blood cells: The spleen stores both red and white blood cells. A fist-sized body on the left side it is between the stomach's fundus and the diaphragm; it measures 5" or 6" long, 3" wide and 1" thick, weighing about 7 oz. The spleen is oval in shape, brittle in consistency, highly vascular and represents 0.25% of man's

body weight. The pancreas sits on the spleen's hilus where blood vessels and nerves penetrate the organ. Except at the hilum, two peritoneal folds surround the spleen completely.

Functions of the spleen. Several functions are attributed to the spleen.

Spleen is a blood reservoir. The substance of the spleen holds in its spaces a large amount of blood. Delivered to splenic pulp by small arteries, blood percolates through gaps, into spaces between splenic cells and drained by veins. Blood conveyed to the portal vein enters the liver to be cleansed. Splenic blood has more red cells than the general circulation. When the spleen contracts, the total volume of circulating blood increases. Some conditions can cause splenic contractions: emotional excitement, strenuous exercise, fright, rage, strong emotion, carbon monoxide poisoning and hemorrhage. The spleen is a very sensitive organ, and a sudden noise can cause the spleen to contract. Spontaneous rhythmic splenic contractions of two per minute produce small changes in blood volume and variations in blood pressure.

Splenic macrophages engulf damaged red blood cells.

The spleen forms lymphocytes and other blood cells.

It produces antibodies, stores iron and in some diseases, fats.

In various infections, the spleen takes up bacteria and their toxins.

The spleen is a very important organ and should never be removed. In every case where the spleen was excised, death has occurred. If you survive removal of spleen, you would not be able to cope with emergency situations where more blood is required, i.e., in surgical shock or hemorrhage.

The lymphatic system

The lymphatic system is a very important part of the body. Lymph absorbs materials from body tissues and conveys them to the circulatory system. The lymph's most important function is to remove proteins and other substances reabsorbed into blood capillaries. Lymph's second function is to drain fluid between body tissues and capillaries, and if the capillary filtrate increases in volume, to prevent its accumulation in spaces.

Where lymph vessels are found: With the exception of the skin's top layer, nervous tissue, bones, cartilage, nails, cuticles and hair supplied by blood vessels, all remaining parts of the body contain lymphatic vessels.

Not as small as blood capillaries, lymphatic vessels run alongside arteries and veins and are not as closed a system as the blood vascular system. The lymphatic system is an open system and the upper lymphatics empty into veins. Their caliber is not as large as that of arteries and veins.

Beginning as fine capillaries, lymphatic vessel walls are formed by endothelium, a continuous layer of very thin cells cemented together. Enlarged lymphatic vessels have an inner coat of endothelium, an unstriped coat in between and an external fibrous coat. With exception of lymph capillaries, bicuspid valves in larger lymphatics prevent lymph from flowing backward.

Lymphatic vessels begin at the body's periphery as very fine vessels. Arranged in two layers, under the skin, a superficial layer joins a deeper layer under the submucous fatty layer of skin. Fine vessels join, forming larger vessels, ultimately forming two large trunks: the thoracic duct and the right lymphatic duct.

The right lymphatic duct, the thoracic duct: Half an inch long, the right lymphatic duct receives lymph from right side of the head, neck, thoracic wall, right arm, right leg, right heart, upper surface of liver and empties into the right subclavian vein. The thoracic duct, 15-18 inches long, receives lymph from the rest of the body and empties into the left subclavian vein.

Lymph nodes or glands

Lymph nodes lie along the course of lymphatic vessels. Pinkish-gray bodies varying in size from small nodules to flat masses two inches long, they are found on the underside of body, at elbow, armpit, behind ear, on both sides of neck, behind knee and at the groin. Each node is divided into a cortical and a medullary region. From the surface into the node's substance, a fibrous capsule sends bundles of fibers, forming a network with intervals filled with lymph sinuses and lymph cell columns.

Each node's cortical region has rounded nodules of lymphoid tissue. The medullary region has elongated cords. At convexities of the fibrous capsule, lymph vessels reach nodes. Four vessels pierce the capsule. When leaving a node, lymph travels upward toward the heart.

Depending on its origin, lymph has different names. When lymph has not traversed a gland it is known as peripheral lymph. When lymph has passed through one gland but not through another it is called intermediate lymph. On its way to the blood, lymph is known as central lymph. Lymphatic vessels known as lacteals supply the entire digestive system. After a meal with absorbed fat, lymph from lacteals is milky white in appearance. Lymphatic vessels from digestive system transport fat away from digestive tract.

Lymph, its chemical composition. Similar to blood plasma, the concentration of lymph's constituents varies. Lymph has 3-4% protein, a lesser concentration of calcium, phosphorus, sodium, potassium, magnesium, chlorine and sugar than blood plasma. Its concentration of urea is identical to plasma.

Accumulating at a rate of about 2 liters in 24 hours, during heavy muscular work lymph increases by ten times.

Lymph, its cellular composition. Lymph contains many lymphocytes, an odd granulocyte and very few red cells. Every cubic millimeter of lymph has 1,000-2,000 lymphocytes.

Lymphocytes are formed in nodes. When a greater number of lymphocytes is required, germinal centers develop. As lymph pours into nodes, the latter filters, removing and destroying bacteria and other toxic substances. Lymph nodes defend blood against invading microorganisms. The disintegration of lymphocytes in nodes allows nodes to manufacture plasma protein. Lymphocytes are composed of globulin. Blood plasma's gamma globulin is closely associated with antibodies destroying bacteria and their toxic products. Lymph nodes are not the only manufacturers of plasma globulin and lymphocytes. Spleen, tonsils, thymus, appendix, adenoids, Peyer's patches (nodes of digestive system) manufacture plasma globulin and lymphocytes. Because of bacteria, lymph nodes are easily inflamed. Excess bacteria penetrating a node prevent the filtering process with possible inflammation. To maintain constancy of tissue fluid composition, fluid movement must be rapid and in 24 hours, a maximum of 2 liters of lymph accumulates, representing 10% of reabsorbed capillary filtrate. Lymph flow is slow in lymph vessels. When lymph vessels' smooth muscles contract, lymph is transported.

In adults, about 25-40% of white blood cells (about 1,000-3,600 cells per cubic millimeter) are lymphocytes. In children, 50% of white blood cells are lymphocytes. Lymphocytes at 4,000 per cubic millimeter, there is lymphocytosis, an inflammation. Lymphocytes may enlarge in size, assume cell division and increase synthesis of RNA, DNA, proteins and enzymes, increasing the availability of immuno-globulins and their defensive function.

In infectious diseases, lymphocytes increase in number. In syphilis, tuberculosis, a mantle of lymphocytes surrounds areas of sub-acute or chronic inflammation. The same occurs in a tumor's presence. Lymphocytes collect around parts injured by mechanical or chemical irritation. Lymph nodes may be a means of dissemination of virus particles as in HIV infection.

The adeno-corticotrophic hormone of the pituitary body controls lymphocyte disintegration in lymph nodes and antibody production. A gland of the regulatory organs, the function of the pituitary is spurred by deep sleep. Good sleep habits ensure production of more lymphocytes with improved defensive function. Today tumors, virus infections, etc., are treated with medication, surgery or high-powered rays. These treatments retard lymphocyte formation and prevent their natural defensive mechanisms. Elimination of wastes helps deep sleep.

Blood discrepancies are treated with irradiation, chemotherapy, etc. We may say that many diseases result from abnormality of blood. In infectious conditions, the blood vascular system is no longer a closed system, rapidly inducing the proliferation of dangerous microorganisms. Other illnesses are memory loss affecting brain cells. Others have difficulty walking, or to move as in paraplegia. Symptoms of all illnesses bring us to the same conclusion.

Chapter 18
How blood is distributed to all body parts

Arteries - description
Arteries distribute blood to all body parts. Veins return blood to the heart. Cylindrical, tubular vessels, arteries have three coats:
1. An internal three-cell layered endothelial coat: endothelial pavement layer, connective tissue layer and elastic fenestrated layer.
2. A middle muscular layer circularly arranged in lamellae. Very variable, a single layer thick in small arteries; in large arteries, elastic fibers unite alternately with muscular fibers.
3. An external connective tissue coat, thin in large arteries, thickest in medium-sized arteries.

To supply arteries, blood vessels and nerves form large plexuses on larger trunks. Arteries convey blood to capillaries, the tiniest vessels interposed between smallest arteries and veins. Arteries divide dichotomously into two, four, etc. Branches of arteries arise at variable angles, some obtuse, others acute or right. Where intense circulation is required, arteries branch out and communicate with one other, i.e., in the brain, abdomen and intestines.

Before penetrating the skull, arteries **describe** a series of curves, nature's means to lessen velocity of flow by increasing the extent of surface over which blood circulates. Between arteries, anastomoses are most numerous in lower limbs, especially around joints. Throughout the body, larger arterial branches pursue a straight course but where much movement is required, they become tortuous as around lips and facial muscles.

Circulation through the heart
From upper and lower parts of the body respectively, two large veins, the superior and inferior vena cava, bring impure blood to the right auricle.

A. **The pulmonary circulation:** From right auricle, blood penetrates right ventricle. Pumped to lungs through the pulmonary artery, a short, wide vessel about two inches long and 30 mm. in diameter. Positioned in front of the aorta, the pulmonary artery arises on the left side, at base of right ventricle. The pulmonary artery divides into the right and left pulmonary arteries; each divides again into two, supplying the lung's right and left lobes.

In lungs, carbon dioxide is given off to millions of alveoli. Simultaneously at low pressure, purified blood picks up oxygen and through four pulmonary veins, two from each lung, blood returns to left auricle. Pulmonary veins differ from other veins: they carry arterial blood and have no valves. In lungs, carbon dioxide is given off to millions of alveoli. Simultaneously at low pressure, purified blood picks up oxygen and through four pulmonary veins, two from each lung, blood returns to left auricle. Pulmonary veins differ from other veins: they carry arterial blood and have no valves. Pulmonary veins are slightly larger than the arterial vessels they accompany.

B. **The systemic circulation:** Oxygenated blood enters the heart through four pulmonary veins in the left auricle and at high pressure, penetrates left ventricle. Powerful ventricular contractions pump blood out through the inch-wide aorta. The aorta comprises the aortic arch, ascending and descending aorta.

1. The ascending aorta: Beginning at upper part of left ventricle, the ascending aorta is about two inches long. Enlarged slightly above its beginning, the aorta presents three small dilatations: the sinuses of Valsalva to which three semi-lunar valves are attached. The only branches of the aorta are coronary arteries supplying heart muscle.

2. The aortic arch and its branches: Extending from heart to body of 4th thoracic vertebra, the aortic arch gives off three branches supplying head, upper chest and arm: the innominate artery, the left common carotid artery and the left subclavian artery. The innominate artery divides into the right subclavian artery to upper extremity and the right common carotid artery supplying right side of head and neck.

The right subclavian artery is the largest branch of the innominate artery. It supplies the brain, muscles between ribs and mammary gland.

Both subclavian arteries continue as the axillary artery with branches supplying upper chest wall, lymph glands and muscles of the region.

The axillary artery continues as the brachial artery from armpit to elbow bend, dividing into the radial and ulnar arteries of forearm.

The radial artery supplies muscles in front of radius. It winds to back of wrist, forming the deep palmar arch crossing the palm under the long tendons.

The ulnar artery supplies muscles in front of ulna, forming the superficial palmar arch.

Head and neck arteries

The right common carotid artery, a branch of the innominate artery, supplies blood to the head and neck. The left common carotid artery arises directly from the aortic arch. Accompanied by the jugular vein on the lateral side and the vagus nerve behind, both left and right common carotid arteries proceed upward on both sides of the trachea. The common carotids supply the head and neck.

At upper border of the thyroid cartilage, each common carotid artery divides into internal carotid for interior of head, external carotid for exterior of head and neck. The internal carotid artery sends branches to the eyes and its appendages, nose, forehead and cerebral arteries to the brain. The external carotid artery supplies the face, front of neck and scalp, with branches to thyroid gland and larynx, tongue and tonsil, face, soft palate and an occipital artery to back of head and neck. After branching off, the external carotid artery passes into the substance of the parotid gland, dividing into temporal and internal maxillary arteries to jawbone.

3. The descending aorta

The aorta arches backwards to the left side, over the root of the left lung. It descends on the left side of the vertebral column, passes through the aortic opening in diaphragm and ends its course by dividing, at the level of the 4th lumbar vertebra, into the right and left common iliac arteries. The descending aorta divides into two parts: the thoracic and the abdominal aorta.

a. The Thoracic aorta: Passing through chest, the thoracic aorta sends branches to heart's covering, bronchi of lungs, diaphragm, glands and fatty tissue of mediastinum (space containing heart and viscera of chest except lungs) and muscles between ribs.

b. The Abdominal aorta: Beginning at diaphragm, the abdominal aorta sends two sets of branches: visceral branches supplying stomach, coeliac axis, liver, spleen, mesentery, kidneys, sperm or ovaries; parietal branches supplying phrenic nerve, lumbar region, sacrum and rectum.

At level of 4th lumbar vertebra, the abdominal aorta, about 2 inches long, divides into right and left common iliac arteries. A few branches are sent to Psoas magnus muscle, ureters and surrounding cellular tissue. The common iliac artery bifurcates into external and internal iliac arteries.

The external iliac artery

About four inches long, the external iliac artery follows the pelvis' brim and at the inguinal ligament, becomes the femoral artery. From the external iliac artery arise two branches of considerable size, distributing blood almost entirely to the lower extremity. They are the deep circumflex iliac artery and the epigastric artery continuing as femoral artery whose branches supply skin and fascia of lower abdomen, external genital organs and all structures at front and sides of thigh.

Femoral artery continues as the popliteal artery running behind knee through popliteal space, supplying knee-joint. Dividing into anterior and posterior tibial arteries, the anterior tibial artery supplies front of leg, becomes the dorsalis pedia, ending between first and second toes. Together with tendons of toe muscles, the anterior tibial passes in front of ankle joint.

The posterior tibial artery supplies back of leg, sole of foot and divides into the medial and lateral plantar arteries for medial and lateral portions of sole or plantar region.

The internal iliac artery: The internal iliac artery passes into pelvis, sends branches supplying parts within and without the pelvic wall, including perineum and all pelvic viscera except ovaries. Branches are sent to the rectum, bladder, uterus and vagina.

The above are the principal arteries connecting all parts of the body.

Circulation of capillaries

From arteries, blood passes through increasingly smaller vessels to end in capillary beds of tissues where oxygen is delivered. Capillaries vary in size according to body tissues. Smallest in brain tissue and intestinal mucous membrane, capillaries are largest in skin and bone marrow.

Network of capillaries are either loose or close. Lungs and eyes' choroid layer have the closest capillary networks. In general, the more active the organ, the closer its capillary network. Some regions have no capillaries: i.e., tendons requiring no further change after full formation. Many tissues and ligaments comparatively inactive in life have wider capillary meshes.

Capillary walls are made of a fine, transparent endothelial layer of irregularly shaped cells, joined edge to edge by an interstitial cement substance. Capillaries are present in nearly all parts of the body except in bone, nails, epidermis, cartilage and cornea of eye. The body's tiny end capillaries cover a combined surface of 1,000 square meters.

After delivering oxygen to body tissues, from tissue metabolism, blood picks up wastes. Loaded with metabolic wastes, blood returns to heart first by small veins, then increasingly larger veins to end in the superior and inferior vena cava emptying into the right auricle.

Veins in general

Veins are of two distinct sets of vessels: pulmonary veins and systemic veins returning blood from the general circulation.

Similar to arteries, practically all body tissues have veins. Following arterioles, beginning as tiny veins, as other veins join in on their way to the heart, they gradually increase in size. Veins are larger and more numerous than arteries thus their capacity is greater than the arterial system.

Similar to arteries, veins have three layers. Perfectly cylindrical, the presence of valves at intervals differentiates veins from arteries. Valves are deduplications of the inner coating, strengthened by connective tissue and elastic fibers, a layer of epithelium covering both sides. Valves are semi-lunar in shape, the convex side attached to the vessel wall, the concave side is free. Veins of body extremities have many valves. No valves are present in small veins and the large vena cava, and those carrying purified blood: hepatic veins, portal veins, renal veins and ovarian veins. Veins have frequent anastomoses both between large trunks and smaller vessels. In cavity of cranium and between veins of neck, anastomoses prevent obstruction, dangerous to the external venous system.

Veins have thinner walls than arteries and contain less elastic and muscular tissues. Superficial veins have thicker coats than deep veins. Veins of lower limbs are thicker than those of upper limbs.

The systemic veins

Systemic veins are divided into three sets. Right under the skin, perforating deeper tissues between layers of superficial connective tissue, superficial veins communicate with deep veins. Enclosed in the same sheath, deep veins accompany arteries. A pair of veins, one on each side accompany smaller arteries: radial, ulnar, brachial, tibial, peroneal arteries. Larger arteries are usually accompanied by one vein: the axillary, subclavian, popliteal, femoral arteries.
Sinuses: found only in the skull, sinuses are venous channels differing from veins both in structure and in mode of distribution. When two layers of dura mater separate, sinuses are formed. Each sinus has an outer coat of fibrous tissue, an inner coat of endothelial layer continuous with lining of veins.
Two groups of systemic veins: 1) Veins of the head, neck, upper extremity and chest terminating in the superior vena cava. 2) Veins of the lower extremity, abdomen and pelvis, terminating in the inferior vena cava.

1. Veins emptying into the superior vena cava

Running on right side of aortic arch, the superior vena cava derives from a union of both innominate veins, one on each side of the aorta. Each innominate vein is the union of subclavian vein from entire upper extremity and internal jugular vein from deep face and cranial cavity.

These are important deep veins of the face and cranial cavity. Superficial veins from scalp, ear and face, empty into the external and anterior jugular veins.

In the forearm, ulnar and radial veins run with similarly named arteries, uniting to form brachial veins. These in turn form the axillary vein which gives rise to the subclavian vein. Blood empties into the internal jugular vein, leading to the superior vena cava. These are deep veins of the upper extremity.

The basilic and cephalic veins are superficial veins of the forearm. Both empty into the axillary vein. In front of the elbow the median vein connects basilic and cephalic.

Mostly on back of hand, hand and finger veins form two plexuses, an inner and an outer plexus. The inner plexus comprises veins from little finger, ring finger and ulnar side of middle finger. They continue into ulnar veins. The outer plexus comprise veins from thumb, index finger and radial side of middle finger. These two plexuses combine on back of hand, forming the superficial arch of veins. The superficial arch of veins from palm of hand forms a plexus in front of wrist to which the median vein is attached.

2. Veins emptying into the inferior vena cava

The inferior vena cava receives blood from all structures below the diaphragm, except from lumbar walls.

From abdominal walls, phrenic and lumbar veins, the right ovarian vein and right spermatic veins open into the inferior vena cava. Left ovarian and left spermatic veins open into left renal vein carrying blood to inferior vena cava. From stomach and intestines, the portal vein brings impure blood to liver. Cleansed in liver cells, hepatic veins bring blood directly to inferior vena cava.

Veins of spinal cord, bodies of vertebrae, etc. empty into inferior vena cava. At about the 4th lumbar vertebra, the inferior vena cava bifurcates, receiving blood from right and left iliac veins. These in turn receive blood from femoral vein of thigh, a continuation of popliteal vein derived from anterior and posterior tibial veins.

The above are deep veins of the lower extremity. Other superficial veins join with deep veins. The reader should now have a small idea of the innumerable vessels in the living body.

CHAPTER 19
A good sexual relationship and a long life

There must be love to have a totally satisfying sexual experience; what is this love that has stirred men and women to impossible deeds? When asked, men have said it was a wonderful feeling that left them alive yet speechless. Love is a yearning, a heart-sickness with loss of appetite, a pang, described another. Some maintain it is a strange, overpowering feeling for the desire of a certain person's presence. From the very first meeting, this feeling must be present.

Love: the different degrees

Without reason or command love manifests in various degrees of feeling and one cannot dispose of it as one pleases. An essential necessity is the sight of the loved one, for love arises through the eyes, but the sense of smell, the sound of a voice, the whistling or singing voice can stir love to a high degree, for how then can we explain the love felt for a blind person?

The deepest feeling of love is felt by abdominal craving pains at the mere thought of the beloved, welling eyes with tears, inciting heartfelt pangs. The feeling of deep love assures perfect sexual compatibility but for a lasting relationship it must accompany a compatible character. Physical attraction is the first requirement, then a partnership of body, mind and spirit. Between man and woman, true love is the desire to share everything and supreme value is granted to the beloved.

Touchstones of true love are self-sacrifice to the partner. Love is life itself, permanent and constant. To Washington Irving, love is the torment of one person, the happiness of two people, the quarrel and enmity of three. Love is a charm with invisible ties uniting two people in intense happiness but when separated, causes great desperation. Some attributes of love are a completely mutual feeling where two persons melt into one, a tie that nothing can undo.

Sexual love is a complex and superior feeling, a pact between two people who must face the difficulties of daily living. To achieve a harmony in living together, in love, two people must learn to share similar pleasures. Only true love can pardon what tears them apart.

In love, man proposes and woman disposes. If a woman refuses, no relationship is possible, but self-improvement may lead to a relationship. Avoid one-sided love affairs, said Robert Storer, for in a Platonic affair, the feeling is analogous to that of a man for a prostitute or of a dog for a bitch. Socrates defined love as the "urge for immortality". Falling in love is nature's indication that with this chosen person one will be able to procreate. In physiology, the chemistry of the blood signifies physical and chemical properties. To fall in love, similar blood properties is essential. Blood is regulated during sleep and the deeper the sleep, the more one stirs the feeling of love in the chosen partner.

Conditions of deep love

While deep sleep is necessary to stir the feeling of love, according to Joseph Barcroft, slight variations in physical and chemical properties of the blood affect the brain. It is possible to fall deeply in love with someone whose thoughts and actions are similar to yours, inciting an at-ease feeling.

As of puberty one searches for a suitable partner. The sex act is the most difficult physiological act, requiring the performance of two people.

Lovemaking is an art more difficult than music. One shuns an unloved one whose caresses do not arouse libidinous sensations. According to Maxine Davis, the latter are absolute prerequisites for mounting during the sex act. Falling in love is nature's way to ensure perfect touch compatibility in order to successfully bring out the libido and reach simultaneous climax. In a sexual relationship, simultaneous orgasmic contraction is the culmination of love.

Seeking deep love. Young people meet in school, college, parties, meetings where people congregate. One may meet the right person. In life, youth is the most sensitive time and the sooner one finds the right partner, the earlier can one begin to procreate and build life together successfully.

Despair in an unrequited love. If love is unrequited do not despair or commit suicide. Creative activity, immersing oneself in books, music, will soon inspire thoughts elsewhere. Distance is a great healer.

Essentials in sexual parts

After falling in love, a couple will engage in sex. In women the clitoris is one of the essential sexual organs. In men, the penis. These organs function only at the end to bring on the climax, as proven by eunuchs of China's imperial courts. These poor castrated men sometimes married. In lovemaking they experienced all the ecstasy of the foreplay but were never able to reach the orgasm. They suffered the worst of tortures.

The clitoris is the female counterpart of the male penis. Nature has endowed women with a diminutive sex organ to preserve the developing embryo from malformations or spontaneous abortion during the sex act. Pregnant women who engaged in sex during the last days of pregnancy experienced uterine contractions lasting 30 minutes. Some had labor pains immediately after the orgasm. Masturbation resulted in yet more powerful uterine contractions. Small sexual parts ensure less blood loss and are an advantage.

A loose, darker skin covers the penis. At the tip it is folded into the foreskin.

Made up of three parts, the penis has an invisible root, a visible body and a tip. A cross section through the penis shows three circular areas, two above and one below. Composed of erectile tissue, the three longitudinal columns are bound together by fibrous tissue.

Also called corpora cavernosa and composed of longitudinal and circular fibers, the two superior columns give off bands forming wide blood spaces, imparting a spongy appearance to erectile tissue. From the penile tip, the two corpora cavernosa are united to about three quarters the length of the penis where it presents a slight enlargement or bulb. Then they separate, forming two powerful fibrous sheaths, each firmly attached to the center bottom of the pelvic girdle (a branch of the ischium). A suspensory ligament attaches upper surface of penile root to center front of pelvic bone (symphysis pubis).

Under the top two corpora cavernosa, the bottom erectile column or corpus spongiosum, lies in a groove. It encloses the urethra through which urine or semen is conveyed to the outside. The corpus spongiosum's enlarged blind end overlaps the corpora cavernosa, forming the glans penis. Close above the bulb, three quarters of the way from penile tip, lie two pea-sized Cowper's glands, its secretions delivered by an inch-long duct onto the floor of the urethra's bulbous region. At the penile tip, a slit of the glans penis' pyramidal zone allows passage of urine or semen. Many fat glands lie at the tip's crown and constricted neck. These sebaceous glands secrete a fatty matter with a peculiar odor, decomposing easily.

The erectile organ in women

The clitoris is one of a woman's erectile organs. Pea-sized, it lies above and immediately outside of the vaginal entrance. In the clitoris lies the glans clitoridis, a small, highly sensitive rounded tubercle. Contrary to the male, the female clitoris has two corpora cavernosa forming an incompletely separated sheath, attaching clitoris to symphysis pubis (front of innominate bones). At vaginal opening there is a mucous layer with erectile tissue. On each side of the vagina lies a reddish yellow oblong body, the size of a horse bean. These are Bartholin's glands. Similar to Cowper's glands in the male, pea-sized Bartholin's glands are active during the sex act. At the sacral region of the spinal cord, parasympathetic ganglia control blood supply to sex organs.

Fall in love and engage in sex

The orgasm is the supreme pleasure man experiences in life. Many believe stimulation of essential sexual parts alone (rape, fornication) provides erotic pleasure. Devoid of prehensile limbs, lower animals alone perform sex rapidly during heat by male penetration. Among humans, neither the size of the erectile organ nor circumcision determine the organ's ability to enable a partner to reach the climax. Only deep love with touch compatibility ensures optimum performance of the sex act. Many sudden disturbances in modern living can prevent a sexual response. To enhance pleasure in lovemaking, some preparation is needed. A dark, warm room with circulating fresh air but without a telelphone, ensure greater pleasure. Body cleanliness, an empty digestive tract and bladder, a good night's sleep are excellent prerequisites.

Enjoy love and sex

Lovemaking always begins by caressing the skin to stimulate Meissner's corpuscles and Krause's end bulbs. Brought to the parasympathetic ganglia the message is relayed to the penis or clitoris, eliciting a flow of blood to the erectile organs' wide blood spaces. As touch stimulation increases, erectile organs gradually fill up with blood. From intense caressing, a measles-like rash spreads over the thighs, buttocks and back. Blood pressure rises to 80 mm. Hg, pulse rate increases 110-180 per minute, perspiration appears on the back, chest wall and thighs, breathing increases to 40 per minute. Sexual tension increases and the pleasure elicited augments in intensity. Lubricated with secretions from Bartholin's glands, the entire vaginal barrel becomes dripping wet.

To receive the enlarged penis, the vaginal barrel expands from a diameter of 5.75 to 6.25 cm. and a length of 9.5 to 10.5 cm. and beyond. Breasts harden, both vagina and penis darken in color. The partners have now reached a point preceding the climax. Women have different sexual rhythms and biorhythms, thus a woman must advise her partner when she is ready for the climax.

In the Chinese novel **Dream in the Red Pavillion**, the mounting movements are described as clouds and rain, circular, then perpendicular motion. When vaginal and penile surfaces are slippery wet from glandular secretions, pelvic thrusts in the male, with accommodation in the female, approach the climax. Penile thrusts change the woman's genital region. Moving forward and sideward, penile thrusts thin out as the vagina's labia majora spread apart. Labia majora comprise the entire region lined by hairs, enclosing all openings except the anus. As the labia minora triple in size, filling up with blood, the vaginal cylinder lengthens, becoming bright red. Labia minora enclose vaginal and urinary openings. Increasing in length and thickness, the glans and the clitoris swell.

The orgasm, the climax

As the penis is withdrawn again and again halfway from the vaginal barrel, pelvic thrusts become involuntary. Thrusts markedly reduce with the impending approach of the explosive orgasmic release. Depending on the intensity of the release, the orgasmic platform may contract 3-15 times.

The external position of the penis allows a man to reach the climax with greater ease. This is not always the case in women who are often obliged to achieve the climax by self-stimulation. Do not despair, for the presence of touch corpuscles on mucous surfaces of breasts, lips, undersurface of skin, can help. Together with pelvic thrusts, nipple or lip stimulation should rapidly bring on the climax. Prior to the explosive orgasm the woman can tighten up the entire abdominal and leg regions, actively forcing blood to internal organs. A series of regular contractions are the climactic sensation.

Normally contractions of the vaginal barrel's outer third recur at 0.8 second intervals from 3-5 up to 10 or 15 times. As time in between lengthens, contractions taper off. Rhythmic contractions last as long as semen flows out, expelling seminal fluid from urethra. Immediately after the climax, blood gorging erectile tissues rapidly disperses.

Simultaneous orgasm increases the harmonious togetherness of both partners who feel marvelously exhausted. After the climax a man loses about half a glass of blood. A woman loses less blood. To maintain the increased metabolism required by the orgasmic release, blood flow increases to erectile organs: blood pressure rises, pulse rate increases, breathing hastens.

The climax—some beneficial after-effects

The sexual orgasm and its after-effects provide the most supreme of physical satisfactions. It has been described as spasms of pleasurable convulsions. After the act, a couple transforms into complete beings; as the couple melts at the highest point there is a togetherness in marriage. Women have described the orgasm as a thrust of intense sensual awareness, a shock, a loss of overall sensory acuity, a sensation of suffusion, of warmth, a pelvic throbbing and an explosive entity.

Sexual intercourse involves one's deepest feelings. It is a profoundly moving experience not something to be taken lightly. Sex is an ever burning, inextinguishable fire, the greatest impulse of life and the main dynamic force wherein the soul finds realization.

The orgasm, some dangerous after-effects

Indulge in this extremely pleasurable endeavor only when in a perfect state of health. After the climax, all other organs return to normal. Overall blood volume lessens; some have experienced muscle contractions throughout the body. Others have felt severe muscle aching of arm and legs, back and abdomen, particularly after several orgasms. Muscle strain may be caused by the climax's unusual physical effort. During the sex act a man is in heavy labor using maximum effort, similar to an athlete. In both men and women contractures of hands and feet have been observed. Contractures are comparable to temporary paralyses or cramps. Rigor mortis is an irreversible cramp. During copulation hemiplegia, stroke or death has taken place.

Masturbation—its dangerous effects

Masturbation may stir a sense of guilt and shame. Severely neurotic and psychotic people masturbate. In self-manipulation sexual parts are not properly lubricated and the highest heart rate has been recorded. Lubrication indicates slow stimulation of sense organs with slow overfilling of penis and clitoris. Normal coitus is more satisfying than the orgasm reached by self-manipulation and women who masturbate are not content with a single orgasm, easily inducing several orgasms until satisfied. This can be dangerous and may lead to a nervous breakdown. In masturbation, the orgasm is obtained in four minutes. With a partner it may take half an hour. Masturbation only satisfies a release, a need for selfish pleasure and becomes harmful when excessive.

Living without sexual intercourse. The study of music, literature, the arts and sciences can stimulate good morality and hard physical work is an excellent outlet for pent-up sexual energies. Imperfect or incomplete accomplishment of the sex act injures one's psychological make-up and may damage the nervous system or other body functions. In **Dream in the Red Pavillion**, a young boy looked into a mirror and masturbated to death.

Disturbance during the sex act. A couple engaged in the act of lovemaking should never be disturbed. History has recorded cases of penis captivum where a woman's vagina suddenly closed tightly on the penis. All efforts to separate the partners were in vain, causing only greater pain. Several hours of relaxation were necessary before the young woman was able to liberate her partner.

Advancing age and sexual activity. If both partners are healthy and careful with their diet, men and women are sexually competent past midlife, until 90 years of age. The only difference is a slower sexual response. Sedatives, narcotics, alcohol, smoking, medication may interfere with sexual responses. With advancing age, women should use some different techniques and oral sex, manual caresses and other forms of body stimulation can better arouse their aging mates. Verbal communication with the partner promotes greater understanding and mutual satisfaction.

For those engaging frequently in intercourse, some general advice

Do not have sex with a full stomach. Morning sex and side positions are recommended. One good sexual experience is superior to several mild sessions. Statistics show that before age 35 no man is impotent but by age 80, 77% of men are affected. When the penis cannot harden or become erect, unable to penetrate to satisfy the partner the man is considered impotent. Frigidity in women is the counterpart.

Impotence is due to rapid performance of the sex act during the course of life.

When large blood spaces fill up rapidly, capillaries tear to pieces and with time, impotence results. Scientific data indicate that there is the least impotence among married people. Slow arousal, petting with foreplay preserves erectile tissues' capillaries and maintains normal sexual function. Other causes of impotence may be anxiety, diminished blood volume, indulgence in alcohol. Even a cold can have adverse effects on sexual function; toxemia and excitement may cause premature ejaculation. Other common causes of impotence are diseases such as arteriosclerosis, diabetes, kidney disease, while drugs, smoking, amphetamines, barbiturates, cannabis, are dangerous to sexual function. Practice moderation in sexual activity. The proper diet preserves sexual powers and with advancing age, isotonic feeding is important.

How to care for the vaginal entrance, the uterus, etc.
Let nature take care of sexual organs and with exception of the male organ nothing external should ever penetrate vaginal surfaces. One woman habitually had her uterus scraped. She eventually developed a tumor while her uterus hung out of the body. She was obliged to undergo hysterectomy.

Upon the slightest uterine inflammation, adopt a semi-liquid diet immediately, then a liquid diet for several days until the condition subsides. Keep the area clean but do not douche yourself with anything. Soon the inflammation will subside.

Older women frequently suffer from prolapsus of the reproductive organs and they fall out of the body. They can either be removed or sewn back.

Some women have had a uterine tumor or fibroids. Do not worry. The condition will rapidly subside upon a light diet. During a lifetime, do not use contraceptives that irritate sexual parts.

TIGHTEN UP THE ENTIRE ABDOMINAL REGION EVER SO OFTEN TO STRENGTHEN MUSCLES

Chapter 20
Alcoholism, smoking, intemperance, violence

Alcoholism

An understanding of the products ingested can deter one from becoming addicted to alcohol.

If honey, fruit, sugar cane, beet-root, milk or starch is converted into sugar, when fermented, alcohol is the result. When this liquid is distilled, it becomes an alcoholic beverage. Zymase, the enzyme in yeast or malt accelerates fermentation, converting sugar into alcohol and carbon dioxide. To distill the liquid, slowly heat it to above 100°. Alcohol vaporizes and re-condenses into a liquid of greater alcoholic strength. Distilled spirits mature best in barrels, casks or puncheons made of seasoned American white oak. A fermented mash of grain distilled and aged in wood produces whiskey. Vodka is a non-aged distilled spirit from a fermented mash of any suitable raw material. In Russia and Poland, vodka is distilled from potatoes then filtered through vegetable charcoal and reduced with water, to potable strength. Rum is any distilled spirit of fermented sugar cane or molasses. Brandy is a potable distilled spirit from wine or a fermented mash of fruit, usually aged in wood.

Alcohol, a product of slow burning or digestion. A product of distillation, alcohol is similar to a product of digestion and rapidly absorbed in the digestive tract. In a short time blood alcohol rises to high level, distributes to all parts of the body and is absorbed until equilibrium between blood alcohol and various organs is reached.

Alcohol rate of absorption. Food in the stomach delays alcohol absorption rate. Milk and meat impede absorption. Slow drinking and dilution impede alcohol absorption. Carbonated drinks increase absorption rate. If taken with barbiturates, alcohol becomes doubly depressant, dangerous to life itself. Alcohol remains for a long time in the body. In a sedentary lifestyle, alcohol can be utilized as food, but due to its slow oxidation (not more than 300 g. can be oxidized in one day yielding 2,100 cal.), does not produce sufficient energy for any physical work. It contains no vitamins or essential amino acids or fatty acids and minerals.

Danger of alcohol to replace food

Reliance on alcohol for calories produces a number of complicating alcoholic diseases. Mentally and physically balanced people drink moderately. Heavy drinkers crave for alcohol and end with early death, risking confinement in asylums. Alcohol shortens life; chronic alcoholism causes kidney disease, degeneration of blood vessels, leading to apoplexy.

Alcohol lowers body defense against infection. Males died in early adulthood affected by testicular wasting away with absence of spermatozoa. Too much alcohol impairs the performance of skilled work and lowers respiratory rate and body temperature.

An alcoholic deprived of alcohol

An addict deprived of alcohol develops an intense craving manifesting tremor, perspiration and great anxiety. A few drinks eliminate the symptoms. More serious are feelings of nausea, fever, rapid heartbeat, convulsions and hallucinations. Delirium tremens includes loss of awareness of the environment and impairment of insight, inflammation of stomach lining and slow digestion. When essential dietary constituents are lost, the alcoholic shows signs of food deficiencies: degeneration of leg muscles with pain and weakness, cirrhosis of liver, darkened skin, jaundice with fluid in abdominal cavity. Headache, nausea, vomiting, infection of inner ear with loss of equilibrium were manifested. Clinics have succeeded in rehabilitating the alcoholic, but the problem is greater.

In the west it is usual to serve steaks or other meats, shrimps in large quantities. Avoid eating large pieces of meat. It may cause loss of sensitivity to dangerous products. In human evolution protein is a most important factor. Meats eaten plain should be sliced paper-thin, or mixed with vegetables. Seafood is concentrated, it should be finely cut and mixed with vegetables.

Origin of tobacco smoking

Tobacco was introduced by Columbus when he saw Indians use tobacco in ceremonials. Indians believed tobacco had medicinal powers. The scientific name for the tobacco plant is Nicotiana, named in honor of Jean Nicot, French ambassador at Lisbon, Portugal, who sent the seeds of the plant to Catherine of Medici, Queen of France. The common name tobacco derives from the word for the tube Indians use to inhale smoke and the cylinder of leaf prepared for smoking.

Tobacco inhalation and its deleterious effects

It is known that tobacco smoking causes disease. After World Wars I & II, it became an alarming signal when deaths from lung cancer and other diseases rose sharply. Cigarette smokers had high death rates. Today, cigarette smoking is associated with lung cancer, coronary artery disease, chronic bronchitis and emphysema. Lip and tongue cancer affects many pipe smokers.

Tobacco: its chemical contents

Tobacco contains nicotine, pyridine and other bases, volatile acids, tars and phenol derivatives, furfural and acroleine; terpine hydrochloride is responsible for its smell. Tobacco leaves are moist because glycerol and glycol are added. The inhaled smoke contains 50-75 micrograms of hydrogen cyanide per 30 milliliters of puff. Suspended particles of smoke contain nicotine, carbon monoxide, carbon dioxide, steam, ammonia and other toxic substances. Tobacco is cut on zinc plates containing lead; therefore there is risk of arsenic and lead poisoning. In small doses, nicotine is a stimulant but in large doses it has paralyzing effects affecting mostly the function of the sympathetic ganglia controlling regulatory organs.

A puff of inhaled smoke forms carbon monoxide. Passing into lungs then into blood, it forms a compound with hemoglobin. This compound is 210 times stronger than oxy-hemoglobin. Combined with carbon monoxide hemoglobin cannot transfer oxygen to the body and allow normal breathing in tissues. Carbon monoxide destroys the source of energy of each cell with the effects of dizziness, headache, heaviness, somnolence, insomnia, nervous excitement, trembling hands and legs, paresthesia, heart discomfort, dyspnea, colic, diarrhea and polyurea.

Dangerous effects of smoke inhalation

A drop of tobacco can kill a dog. One gram of tobacco contains 25 mg. of nicotine. Injected into the bloodstream, 60 mg. of nicotine could kill a man. Smoke produces tar an irritant causing cancerous growths. The smoker's lungs are gray, contracted and scarred, air sacs, distended and torn. In the air tubes of lungs smoke impedes and slows down cilia's sweeping movements. Cancerous cells also develop a persistent cough. Pictures of air sacs' blood vessels indicate a thick coating of deposits with incomplete transference of oxygen to the bloodstream. Smoking reduces circulation in hands and feet and may cause gangrene. Heartbeat increases, depressing the nervous system. Pregnant women have an increased possibility of stillborn infants. The longer one smokes, the greater the decline of sexual activity. Large doses of nicotine can produce grand mal seizures.

To stop smoking, buy some Chinese preserved plums. A few bags of these delectable plums will prevent anyone from desiring another puff of smoke. Ask for bags of Chen Pui Mei at Chinese supermarkets in Chinatown.

A final advice for those insensitive to lethal products such as smoke, alcohol, excess food: wear silk. Fine material brings a message to the brain, stirring the nervous center's sensitivity to dangerous external substances. Gradually one will lose the desire for these products. This is particularly effective for the obese or those who binge.

Intemperance causes

Intemperance is not a part of man's physiology yet it has a greater impact on life than many other environmental factors. Binging, alcoholism, smoking, gambling, are psychological compulsive drives.

Art, music, architecture, painting, emphasize proportion. Modern man lives in small living quarters with huge furniture. Small tables, chairs, sofas should adorn modern apartments. Small pictures artfully hung, a few throw rugs are better than one large rug. No bare bulbs should lighten up the abode and translucent curtains allow daylight to enter. Buy small TV sets and radios and do not adorn walls with large wall hangings.

A warning from 1745

Italian draftsman and etcher Giovanni Battista Piranesi did a series of prints, Carceri d'Invenzione, (Imaginary prisons): a fantastic, visionary architecture of gigantic structures ornated by huge lion heads criss-crossed with tiny staircases where humans climbed, much like ants climbing a tree. Piranesi did not intend this style to be reality, but he foresaw the western world of this century. Today, more and more structures are built like Piranesi's Imaginary Prisons. Perhaps he etched them as a forewarning. We must hearken to his message and avoid erecting huge structures. A city built like a prison camp forces the dweller to acquire prisoner mentality, especially in the U.S. where streets have no twists, turns or circles, only square blocks. Few towns have charm and even parks are square or rectangular.

Huge structures, their effect on man's mind. Massive buildings cause fatigue and incite fear. Fear turns into anger. When angry, meanness will prevail and crimes will ensue. Criminality and insanity can be prevented by a better knowledge of man, by the study of eugenics or man's relationship to his environment, by changes in education and social conditions. In spite of overpopulation, skyscrapers cause loneliness, lassitude, racing, fast walking, intemperance, overeating, compulsive overworking, gossiping, gambling. Family members become alienated where hatred, jealousy and envy are extant. A single nasty word can cause an acquaintance to become a total stranger or enemy. Many neighborhoods have only three skyscrapers and one giant supermarket: these are abnormalities.

Buildings

Buildings should not exceed the height of the tallest tree whose leafy top is soft, gracefully swaying, not tiresome to the beholder. Our eyes are small, and giant skyscrapers weigh on the onlooker, stirring premature aging, fast walking, compulsive drives. Cities should have lanes of houses. Each house should have a garden in front and a backyard creating balance with the height to form an isoceles or right triangle. Walls provide a feeling of possession and safety to the dweller. Cities should not be built like a checkerboard square, instead there should be freedom of form, with an artistic sense.

Man should live in harmony with nature and the Chinese and Spanish have succeeded. Dwellings have a courtyard and garden enclosed by a wall. In Iran, no one will buy a house unless nightingales sing in the garden adorned with decorative trees and multicolored flowers, a running stream, surrounded by birds. An Iranian home greets the visitor with radiant colors, exquisite flowers mingled with perfumes. Walls should be in proportion with the garden and house. Should a wall be in proportion to a skyscraper? No, proof that skyscrapers are abnormal.

A Chinese man who recently arrived in the U. S. said that the U. S. is dreadfully developed. The Caucasian man has succeeded in so many great inventions, radio, television, space program, computers, etc. How about some beautiful cities with parks?

Violence

Violence is a threatening problem. In the U.S. assault victims are admitted to hospitals daily. In 1968 about half a million people were victims of murder and assault. This number exceeds the Vietnam War casualties. Violence is blamed on poverty, discrimination, personal isolation, faulty genetic inheritance, an evil nature and lack of law enforcement, abuse of public news media, radio, newspapers, and magazines. Violence in the world has not been reduced, and the number of victims continues to ravage homes and neighborhoods.

Violent people are considered incurable social or psychopaths. It could be a medical problem, a dysfunction of the brain. An act or state of being is a reflection of the complex circuits of the brain. Experiments have indicated that the limbic brain cells of the hippocampus, are responsible for emotional behavior.

Essentials of normal behavior

Normal behavior depends on the brain's optimum function, and an absolute prerequisite is a ready supply of oxygen. Nothing has been provided to help people maintain blood flow to the brain, yet the brain is the most highly irrigated region of the entire body. Normal behavior depends on normal composition of the blood. Many people indulge in much protein and unlimited amounts of carbohydrates: starch, breads, sugar, soda, etc. Limit the amount of foods consumed.

Factors preventing normal blood flow to the brain

Many factors prevent normal blood flow to the brain. In the U.S. most people work in hermetically sealed buildings where fresh air never penetrates. A continuous flow of fresh air is required in apartments and working quarters. Air-conditioning recycles a room's stale air. Keep windows open in the summer. In cold weather, leave windows open two inches wide to allow fresh air to enter. Schools and libraries must have circulating fresh air, especially when many people sit in a room where carbon dioxide accumulates.

Improper cleansing of the skin and its orifices prevents an optimum blood flow to the brain. Keep the navel, the ear canals and skin very clean.

Chapter 21
Happiness and success contribute to longevity

Happiness: the essentials

Living conditions have gradually improved as time marches on, to ensure a better life for man. The most important requirement is a decent home. At the close of the 20th century there are more homeless people than ever before. In 1987, statistics indicated that the number of homeless approximates figures reached during the depression of the 1930s.

A country cannot be qualified as happy when so many of its citizens have no roof over their heads. The homeless problem is mostly due to lack of solid education with a deeper knowledge of history. A well-educated person has greater resources for happiness or unhappiness, than a poorly educated. Ignorance provides a passive bliss. One can never feel the unspeakable ecstasy of the highest range of happiness or unutterable sadness.

How education affects life and health

In the 4th Century B. C., Aristotle said that the main objective of education is to train for citizenship and personality development. He believed education should be controlled by the state, and democracy would succeed with citizens of a high quality. In his Laws, Plato mentioned that good education produces good men who will act nobly. An improvement in the educational system will eradicate many of the problems ravaging the world.

For five centuries the United States modeled its educational needs after the European system and produced citizens of high quality, noticeable in movies of a generation ago. Since then the study of Ancient history and the history of an old world countriy has been neglected and replaced by American history which spans about 225 years. Mankind has been in existence for thousands of years and written history dates back to 4,000 years and beyond.

In China, the study of Chinese history begins in lower grades whereas Korea and Japan study Chinese history which dates farther back in antiquity than their own. Ancient history helps us interpret the present and provides help in directing our own lives and conduct. When faced with impending disaster, knowledge of history helps us refer to the past. A good example is given by Napoleon who, following the example of Themistocles, handed himself to the British after his second abdication. History exerts a profound influence on the qualities of our conduct, providing the eventual adult with a great depth of feeling, audible in the beautiful voices of European and Asian opera singers, and the depth of feeling of their instrumentalists.

Past generations have lived and toiled to bring us our present mode of living. Man's history distinguishes him from animals who eat, sleep, play, hunt for food, procreate and die. People who have not studied ancient history are like fish swimming in an ocean. Many people prefer to live with their parents, spend their lives alone, some commit suicide to avoid life's problems. Knowledge of ancient history will prevent assassination and killing games.

Man must enhance his personality by bringing out his finest development. Life is less important than the quality of life. By improving his physical and mental formation, man can better solve complex problems. A perfect human will have natural health: a body that functions like a clock which is the highest happiness man can attain, and the greatest fulfillment of life can be within his reach. Happiness as an end in itself is a useless venture for when life succeeds as a whole, then happiness will result as a by-product.

Results of a good education

A good education is more important for an intelligent child. Many people tend to be passive and avoid new sensations. Many remain single, leaving no offspring. There is an inborn fear of raising a family while life itself seems a struggle. This insecurity stems from a lack of history and an educational system leading its graduates to boredom is in dire need of change.

In the event of disaster, endowed with a good education, an adult will direct himself better, for sooner or later a family member will die. Many young people wished for death when their mother died. With a good education, the bereaved will face life with courage and master the pain caused by losses while laughter, happiness, creative activity turn loss into gain. A parent must be a guide for children have a sensitive power of imagination. Parents must offer impressions of life. The primary conditions of happiness are a sense of justice, self-esteem and inner prestige. By witnessing parental strife a child will develop insecure feelings.

The family should provide a feeling of security. Parents must help a child's development and allow him to act freely. They must acquire habits and attitudes, practice skills, develop discipline, and home is the place where one can test oneself before achieving success in life.

Problems facing young people

Young people must go to college. In college, choose courses that can help you prepare what one desires to undertake in life. Avoid snap courses to fulfill requirements. Get acquainted with faculty members, administrative officials and even the dean, and take every chance to get to know them personally. They may be of great help later in life.

After college, continue to read books in philosophy, ancient history, will contribute to a mature individual. A good example is Napoleon who, from an obscure artillery man became First Consul, then Emperor of the French. He confided to his secretary Ménéval that after completing his studies at 16, he had such a thirst for knowledge, he buried himself in the library 16 hours a day, poring over books; today, libraries have preserved 400 pages of his notes. Napoleon never shunned difficulties. As Emperor he continued to read; 600 books accompanied him at each campaign.

Young people must make their own decisions: live with others, face life, understand others, become self-confident to assume responsibility. Thereby security, achievement and love, the three incentives of life will be gained. Other conflicts disturb young adolescents: the power to love and be loved. Teenagers practice rough sports which are dangerous; they can cause gigantism; men may lose sensitivity. Gentle exercises such as yoga, Tai Chi, slow walks are beneficial to mind and body.

Look for the proper mate

Love is the ferment of happiness and if you have never fallen in love you cannot know happiness. Physical attraction is first but a permanent relationship must be based on common interests. Can you still live with this person 10 years hence? When the physical attraction is over, a partnership must grow. A marriage is good only when two people are physically, mentally and emotionally compatible. Loyalty and friendship must be present. A quick marriage can be doomed. A loving relationship between husband and wife, perfect sexual compatibility, are most intense feelings and a person cannot be complete without them.

Raising a family

Early marriage presents economic problems. Money must be carefully budgeted. A woman must prepare a comfortable home for a man who should not do housework after eight hours of toil. Procreate early; young parents are strong and can rear children better. Children from young parents are stronger and may live a longer life.

The greatest happiness in life is peace of mind with a beautiful family. Healthy, beautiful and intelligent children help undertaking difficult tasks. Charlemagne had a happy life with his third wife, Hildegarde; he was benevolent and kind to everyone.
How to acquire personality: The essence of human life, human relations represent 90% of man's happiness. Acquire a good personality toward people; learn to speak in public, influence others, to concentrate, acquire knowledge. Unfortunately eight hours spent daily earning a living provide little leisurely time for self-improvement.

Industry, the number of hours

Before 1895 the work week was 50 hours, then reduced to 48, then 44, and now it is a 40 hours. Illnesses in the past 50 years warrant a six-hour workday. At present, most people are ill-prepared for leisure.

More free time means better self-care, less illness, more jobs for others. Who would not be thrilled with six hours work daily? Life is short, and man should enjoy leisure rather than toil. Life is monotonous routine activities, boring. Great pleasure is to do what one desires and as one wishes.

In search of happiness

Man's drives are organic, determined by education and environment. A person finds his happiness within his framework of reference, his set of values: games, sports, dance, song, creative work, painting, poetry, music. Meaningful and exciting moments bring happiness. Having known great happiness, small ones can also be appreciated: reading a book, basking in the sun, silence, changing seasons, well-groomed, country life, etc. Education contributes to developing new interests.

The years of maturity, are years of acquisition and expansion. A long-lasting relationship is togetherness. Life is worthwhile even if sex has waned; growing old together is a great adventure. Education prepares for maturity years and surmounts barriers without bitterness or fear. Keep a balance, give and take—this is the art of living, enriched and satisfying. Do not use people to your advantage, be generous. Be sensitive and aware of others do not injure others. Maximum personal development is achieved by maximum contribution to society.

"Fortune is a woman," said Machiavelli in **The Prince**. She will smile on those who are young, bold and adventurous. Any goal is within reach through fearlessness and perseverance. Do not retire at 50 or 60 unless ailing. Retirement is the time to appreciate life. City colleges are free for seniors. A discipline can be mastered in three years. Many senior citizens like to gamble. Gambling is a dangerous activity, it increases heartbeat, causes nervous tension and shortens life. Creative work is far better. Learn to sew, knit, paint, play an instrument.

Greater self-consciousness can overcome impotence. Relax. Cleanliness is important; indolence is a sign of decay. Soak in a bath. Dress well; unclean older person is shunned. Personal appearance is self-respect and shows respect.

Be understanding of others, feel responsible, think less of yourself. We wish to inspire seniors to live better, longer and prevent an end in a wheelchair. Bernadotte, king of Sweden told his wife Désirée Clary that we must accept death and resign ourselves to its eventuality. If a person has fulfilled his life, death will not be feared. Reserve your energy and you will survive. Failing strength is a tragedy.

It is important to appear normal, even if ill. The goal in life is to live long and well, without pain and financial worry. To keep finances under control, overhead low, live within your means. A normal life is difficult when too rich or too poor. The best alternative is to have enough and to live the way one wishes.

Proper cooking is important. Death can be prevented with a better knowledge of the living body which can prolong life indefinitely.

CHAPTER 22
PROLONG LIFE WHEN THE END APPROACHES

In the May 2000 issue of Newsweek magazine, Dr. Thomas A. Preston said that most of us need to be prepared for some form of high tech dying. About 75% of Americans die in hospitals where aggressive treatment is given. The majority of dying patients experience severe under-treated pain and nearly 40% spend at least 10 days in intensive care. People are advised to notarize advance directives to avoid desperate do-everything-possible treatments when a cure is no longer possible.

The June 2000 issue of Reader's Digest stated that in hospitals, one out of every 200 patients die of medical mistakes. Medical treatment errors caused 69% of injuries. They lengthen hospitalization or discharge to a disability. Medical professionals are not able to help patients live longer when nearing the end nor are they prepared to deal with degenerative diseases. In 1966, Werner Block wrote **Der Arzt und Der Tod** (The Physician and Death), a collection of pictures spanning six centuries where the physician helplessly stands at the dying patient's bedside, often with death standing in the form of a skeleton. Under a 1491 picture, the caption says: death asks the physician to chase him away but he replies that while many a time he can prolong lives, against death he has no herb. Presently, we are faced with a similar problem. People are sick and dying of AIDS, cancer; Alzheimer has no solution, etc. We resign ourselves to die for no help is available, current methods are powerless.

Great peoples have expressed regret to be obliged to leave this world, to know that in a moment we will be nothing, never to see night and day, the sky, trees, flowers, to feel the sun's warmth. In vain has man searched for the Philosophical Stone. There is no hope for prolonging life, yet among lower organisms, unless killed by heat or poison, many lower animals live long. When life conditions are maintained, lower animals continue to live and carry the potential of unending life. **Conditions for living organisms to live perpetually.** To live perpetually unicellular organisms need a suitable environment: favorable temperature, pH, salt, concentration of toxic substances, essential nutrients: imperative conditions, otherwise they disintegrate into smaller organic compounds. In mammalians, animal tissues have been preserved outside the living organism for a length of time exceeding by far the lifespan of the organism from where they were taken, indicating that unlimited longevity is possible. The mammalian body is made up of tissues of different groups of similar cells, each group with its specialized function.

Normal cellular regeneration: necessary conditions

To function normally, only a fraction of an organ's total number of cells is required, but once a tissue is damaged, the ability to regenerate is lost. Most damaged tissues regenerate, but scar tissue replaces damaged heart and brain tissues. These two tissues never regenerate.

Every day, body tissues die and normally regenerate until something happens to the environment in which tissues are bathed. Both in vivo and in vitro, cells will die if many agents are present in certain concentrations. These agents may be bacteria or viruses, elaborating a toxin inhibiting the action of certain compounds or interfering with cell metabolism. Nutritional deficiencies such as lack of vitamins, essential amino acids, fatty acids, endocrine hormones, can disturb cell metabolism and cause death. Nutritional excesses are equally detrimental: proteins, carbohydrates. Normal blood contains little of these substances. Man consumes large quantities of calcium-rich foods; bread, butter, rice, other starches stack up much poisonous wastes.

In an adult organism the major cause of cell death is aging, responsible for changes in water content of cells, the presence of scar tissue, loss of skin elasticity, accentuation of blood vessels with overall weakness. In arteriosclerosis narrowed vessels decrease oxygen and nutrition. Other factors causing cell death are injurious agents. These substances are either injected into the living body or orally ingested: drugs, pills, medicines, laxatives, antacids. Prepared beverages contain artificial ingredients. In boxed foods, additives stack up in cells and eventually interrupt reserve capacities and synthetic potentialities of a cell, preventing repair and replacement of damaged areas. Young people are beautiful which cannot be said of old people. All foods derive from the earth, older people have ingested excess nutrients.

Help for the dying. The above factors injure cells and prevent self-regulation, the controlling factor in cell repair. In extreme illness do not expose the body to drugs, medicines, X-rays, injections that further disrupt the self-regulatory process, confirming the doctrine presented in the first chapter. Mastery of this axiom can promote longevity. Werner Block's book correctly depicted the helpless physician standing at a dying man's bedside. Once we have reached a point of no return, little can be done. His book is a warning not to reach the point of near death; little help is available for the very ill or dying; the most one can do is give oneself up to a home and let others care for us until the end. No need to despair as we shall see.

Signs to watch out for approaching death

Severe illness is not a hopeless condition; when very ill, there are ways to help oneself. Some internal and external signs indicate approaching death. External changes in appearance are significant: haggard eyes; wrinkled facial skin; wrinkles under the eyes; corners of mouth turned sharply downward, pallid complexion, pinched expression of the face, mouth, icy cold hands and feet, swollen legs, shuffling gait, lack of bladder or rectal control, loose muscles, forgetfulness, unawareness, a scribbled handwriting, etc. These signs may appear singly or grouped.

Some internal signs indicate approaching death: sudden pain here and there, constant pain, needle-like pain all over, difficult breathing, a trickling sensation in legs, hot flashes, popping sounds in the nose, sudden pain under the armpit, constant ringing in the head, prominent veins in arms and legs, constant or intermittent headaches, stinging pain from impacted wax in ear canals or navel.

Abnormal signs of regulatory organs are indicated by a rapid pulse, colorless urine, nail-heads or numerous pimples, a lesion that does not heal, skin tumors, constant fever. Sick digestive organs are indicated by strongly fermented fecal matter, difficult defecation, indigestion, lack of hunger pangs, foul breath. When these signs appear, beware and do something positive.

Importance of a desire to live. The desire to live must be backed by fear of death. Fear of dying means fear of suffering great pain, for death is often preceded by intense pain. Unbearable pain is responsible for the final release. One man's brain burst from the brain case, another man's lungs exploded, another was found kneeling beside his bed, doubled up in pain, his heart had exploded. There is good reason to fear death. We react at the first sign of pain. Pain at death is so powerful we are unable to utter a word. Fear death for it triggers a person into action.

Longevity program

According to the synthetic doctrine in Chapter One, regulation of body fluids can be promoted if less work is given to the remaining five organ-systems: muscles and bones, sense organs, sex organs, reproductive organs and digestive organs.

Muscles and bones are 50% of total body weight. When very ill, abstain from strenuous physical exertion. Avoid sports, running, jogging. Light exercise, walking, bicycling for fun, house cleaning, ping-pong, are harmless. Avoid excessive talking, loud singing. Silence and solitude, early retirement are recommended.

Sense organs are small, but when powerfully stimulated, blood is continuously driven to the brain, disrupting smooth functioning of regulatory organs. Dim all lights and sounds. Lower the radio and TV. Avoid public appearances, crowds, speaking. Seek solitude. Avoid being frightened, robbed, attacked. Avoid excess creative work. Sex organs are usually dormant except during the sex act. When very ill abstain from sex. In a lifetime, digestive organs have worked continuously. Examine teeth for tartar around roots: remove with a scaler. Don't let tartar accumulate. Tartar around roots of gums can cause convulsions, later, death.

Preservation of body heat is important in terminal states. Cotton clothing is good for healthy people but when ill, change clothing material; in summer, wear silk; in autumn, knitted silk and wool preserve body heat well. These are expensive fabrics but excellent for health. Nothing is better than heat radiating from warm shoes. Terminally-ill people must wear booties lined with sheepskin regardless of season. High calf booties enable the terminal ill to walk without a cane, forcing kidneys to function, enhancing digestion. At home, wear a woven wool or down jacket all the

time and leave windows open two inches. Circulating fresh air is most important.
Great scientists' thoughts on death: In 1939, Dr. Alexis Carrel felt that the removal of waste products and proper foods prevent death. Dr. Carrel did not prescribe a program for the terminally ill patient. Dr. Léon Binet recorded the case of a man with acute digestive disorders. An injection of a saline solution arrested his regurgitation. After five hours, vomiting began again and upon injection of saline solution, all vomiting symptoms disappeared, and so on. He mentioned that sea salt is a marvelous medication for pathological cases. Salt should never be injected but ingested through the mouth.
A diet for the terminally ill patient: Because the terminal patient is not well cared for, the following diet is specifically for afflicted people; the ill with endocrine disorders, virulent infections, dysfunctional regulatory organs, etc., can benefit from it. An Asian man eats only foods immersed in a broth. At 70, he looks young. This dish is not difficult to prepare.

1. A one dish meal in broth: Keep bones in a plastic bag in freezer. Place a few bones in a pot, cover with water and simmer. When the aroma is perceptible in the apartment, store broth in a jar in refrigerator. Cook bones again in water to make a second jarful of soup stock. Discard bones. When ready for a dish, remove congealed fat from surface of broth. For variety, a tasty stock may be made with a mixture of seafood. A little shrimp, one crab, a few scallops, conch, clam, oysters, etc. Never discard shrimp shells, crab shells, fish bones. Rinse them quickly in cold water, place them in a pot of water and make a broth.

2. String beans: Use a wok to prevent overcooking. Buy 1/2 lb. of string beans.
Remove both tips from string beans. Wash and cut them in inch-sizes. Cook in a heated wok with a dash of water, add all string beans; stir string beans with spatula. Add a dash of soup stock, half a teaspoon of salt, a pinch of curry powder, mixed seasonings, a dash of wine and soy sauce and a pinch of sugar. Keep stirring the string beans with seasonings, adding several dashes of water as you cook them. String beans must be dry at the end. Cook a platter of string beans in 10-15 minutes.
When cooked, place them in a jar. String beans must be chewable yet dry, firm and green, not limp and lifeless. For the very sick, re-cook vegetables in oven at 325° for 1/2 hour. Vegetables must be tender. Season with breadcrumbs, cheese, etc.

3. Meat in strips: Remove fat and bones from meat. Cut two pork chops into fine pieces. Chop further with knife. Season pieces of meat with: dash of wine, curry powder, mixed seasonings, jam, peanut butter, oyster sauce, bean sauce, a teaspoon of cornstarch. Mix well together. Let stand 15 minutes or overnight.
Brush some lard around the wok; when hot, put pieces of meat in. Cook on one

side a few seconds, then turn around and cook again a few seconds. Turn rapidly around until brown and aroma is perceptible. Store in jar.

Meat in strips may be poached in a broth. When broth is gently boiling, drop the raw pork strips into broth. Let cook until pieces of meat rise to the surface. Serve.

This method is good for shrimps, fish. Seafood requires very little cooking time. Drop seasoned fish slices in simmering broth, turn heat off and let stand till they float to the surface or cook over low heat. This is sufficient for a few meals.

4. Serve a one dish meal: Heat a cup of broth to boiling point. Add two tablespoonfuls of string beans, two tablespoons of meat in strips, a teaspoonful of scallions, sufficient salt, a dash of hot sauce if desired. Cook for one minute over low heat. Serve.

This recipe can vary with different vegetables, similarly cooked. If fish is flaky, it is overcooked. Beat an egg into broth if you like egg-drop soup. This recipe is good for he who has difficulty with daily regularity. It has a cathartic effect, a good reason for a person to thrive on this broth. Meatballs is good with the vegetables.

5. Meatballs • Ingredients: 3 pork chops - 1/4 pound of shrimps - 1 slice of salmon fish - 1 heaping tablespoonful of cornstarch - 1 bunch of scallions - mixed seasonings.

Remove fat and bones from meat. Devein shrimps and rinse quickly. Remove bones and skin from fish. Cut all meat, shrimp and fish into squares and grind in a meat grinder or chop them with a butcher knife. Season with jam, soy sauce, mustard, wine, salt, curry powder and mixed seasonings. Chop scallions and mix with meat. Put cornstarch in 2 tablespoonfuls of water, mix well and pour on the meat. Mix. Make chestnut sized balls. Over very gently boiling water in a steamer, steam four balls at a time for ten minutes. Continue until all are steamed. Store in a jar.

The mixture may be piled above thin strips of fresh bean curd and steamed a few minutes over gently boiling water. They may also be cooked in gently boiling broth and served. Mixtures of foods can be made in croquettes. Only one recipe is here since all sorts of one dish meals and many croquettes recipes are in cookbooks. Learn to make them using very little starch. Lasagna, macaroni and cheese use starch. Cut down on pasta and use more vegetables.

6. Potato and rice balls • Ingredients: 2 large potatoes, 1 cup of rice, 3 pork chops, 1 cup of ham or bacon, 1 cauliflower, 1 bunch of scallions, salt, mixed seasonings.

Over medium heat, cook potatoes in water until a knife pokes through or when aroma is perceptible. Peel and mash them. Set aside.

Place rice in small pot, wash several times with cold water then cover with water one inch above surface of rice. Add a dash of salt, one heaping tablespoonful of sugar. Cook over high flame, turn heat low when boiling; simmer until rice is dry and cooked. **Do not stir**. It is ready to be mashed. Use a pestle and mash it till sticky.

Prepare pork chops as in Recipe 3. They must be partially cooked. Cook bacon till crisp. Cut into tiny pieces. Dice ham into small bits. Cut cauliflower into tiny bits and cook as in Recipe 2. Par boil. Wash scallions and cut into tiny bits.

Place ingredients in a large pot; using half the rice. Add additional seasonings to taste. Handmix shaping into balls 2 inches in diameter. Brush a little lard in two frying pans and place 3 balls in each pan. Use medium heat, brown each ball, turn gently around to brown on all sides. Browning is needed because mixture is cooked. Continue browning balls and store in a jar. For one person, these potato balls can last many days. Children will consume quickly. Excellent if eaten with a salty broth.

One very ill woman only makes mixtures of foods.

Recipe books have similar mixtures or use own ideas. Add mushrooms, water chestnuts, chestnuts, bamboo shoots, Chinese sticky rice, cut up cooked spaghetti, bean noodles, batata, pan-fried plaintains, loose corn and all kinds of vegetables. Such foods given to children will waive the desire for drugs, smoking…. It takes time to prepare but the excellent result takes effort.

7. Delicious fish recipe. Ingredients: A large tail end or head end piece of fish. Fish with scales are superior to fish without scales: Yellow snapper, salmon. <u>Seasonings</u>: salt, wine, soy sauce, garlic powder, peanut butter bean sauce, hoisin sauce, jam or season to taste. Pat fish dry. If fish is two inches thick, cut a diagonal slash on both sides unto bone. Brush a little lard in wok. When fuming hot, place the dry fish in and over high heat, brown about 3 minutes on each side. Brown sides also.

When brown and crispy, place in a baking dish. Add seasonings and half a cup of plain broth. Place in oven for 10 minutes under lowest heat possible. After 10 minutes, test with a sharp knife. If a knife pokes through fish with ease, remove. Remove skin (optional), place in wok and brown over low heat till crisp and serve.

The fish may be served with pan-fried plaintain slices, plain vegetables, or eggplant parmigiana. Fish is protein, do not eat too much. One can vary the cooking:

After browning fish in wok, turn heat to very low, add seasonings and cook, uncovered, until a knife pokes through fish all the way.

Cook fish till it has the consistency of lox, as follows: brush wok with a little lard and when fuming hot, place half a fish in wok and brown the skin for one minute on each side. Quickly remove from wok and place in a pyrex dish. Add seasonings and bake in oven at lowest heat for 1/2 hour. Do not eat too much as it is delicious. Shrimps may be similarly cooked after deveining. The jam in it imparts the wonderful flavor. The following recipe is for a family of five.

8. Pancakes. Ingredients: 1 cup of flour, 2 ripe apples, 2 ripe bananas, 3 eggs, Salt, water and milk. Boil a cup of water mixed with milk, pour it over flour and salt. Mix immediately. The mixture must be thick, not watery. Grate apples and mash bananas.

Add eggs and mix together. Heat a little lard in two pans and make pancakes. Flatten them with a spatula until brown and flat on both sides. Serve with maple syrup or with meat in strips and vegetables. They may be sliced and warmed up later.

9. Pot roast of Pork Neck Bones. Ingredients: a platter of pork neck bones, salt, peanut butter, jam, curry powder, mixed seasonings, soy sauce, wine, ginger. Vary seasonings if desired. Remove spinal cord from neck bones. Place everything in a large pot and do not add water (1/2 cup of broth is enough to dilute sauce). Cook, covered, over low heat until aroma is perceptible, about 2 hours. Turn heat off. Place in refrigerator. When cold, remove all congealed fat from surface and warm up quickly over medium heat, uncovered. Serve with pan-fried plaintains.

This recipe is good for roast beef, pork, ox tail, pigs tail. Reduce seasonings or season to taste. Add an apple and a pear, peeled and diced into inch-size pieces an hour before cooking is done. Add onion and one shitake mushroom for taste, tomatoes or a few cooked chestnuts.

10. Dim Sim Dough. Ingredients: 2 cups of corn starch or wheat starch, 1/8 cup of potato starch, 1 tbsp of lard, 1 cup of boiling water, salt.

Cook lard and water together. When boiling hot, throw it over the mixed starches and form into a dough. Roll it into a long roll. Cut little pieces, roll them out and fill them with any of the following mixtures. Seal them tightly. Steam gently till transparent: 15 minutes.
Beef mixture: 1 lb. ground round. 1 bunch of scallions, 1 pinch of baking soda, 2 mashed plums or other fruit, seasonings.
Shrimp mixture: 1 lb. of shrimp, cleaned and deveined, cut into small pieces, 1 bunch of scallions, 1 can of bamboo shoots cut small, a tablespoon of cornstarch, seasonings and salt. This may be varied with scallops, fish, etc.

11. Gelatin: To cook vegetables and meats without the use of fat, do the following: Cover a platter of pig's feet, hocks or pig's tails with cold water. Season with salt, soy sauce, wine, etc. Cook overnight over very low heat. Pour the gelatin in a jar and place in refrigerator. The next day, remove the congealed fat from surface and place it in a jar for future use. Cover pig's feet with water and cook again. Do this two or three times. When liquid is no longer gelatinous, discard pig's feet. Use some gelatin to cook all vegetables, even meats. Gelatin can be eaten with meats.

12. Desserts: Fruit pie: Make a pie dough as thin as possible. Fruit topped over a bottom layer of cookie crust and a thin layer of Ricotta cheese mixed with a little cream cheese makes an excellent dessert. If the fruit is hard, dice them, add seasonings and cook in wok with constant stirring. When chewable, turn heat off and spread over the cookie crust and cheese layer. Place a glaze over the fruit if desired.

For a regular pie crust, heat the butter or lard and pour on toasted flour and mix till grainy. Add a little cold water so it can be kneaded. Immediately a crust is made. Roll out as thinly as possible before topping it with fruit. Unless the fruit is very ripe, cook apple slices, peach slices, etc. in wok constantly stirring until partially cooked, add seasonings, then pour them above the crust. Cook at 350° or until top crust is brown, then lower to 325° for one hour. Remove and serve.

13. Apple Betty. Ingredients: any fruit: peach, nectarines, pears, plums, etc., bread crumbs, a lemon. Apple Betty is a dessert with little starch. Peel 3 pounds of delicious apples sliced thin. Place in a large pan. Add 8 dashes of mixed cinnamon seasonings, 1 tablespoon honey and 1/4 cup brown sugar, sprinkle salt generously, a grated lemon, with juice. Mix apples well together. On a baking dish alternate layers of apples and breadcrumbs. Cover, cook at 350° for 45 minutes. Remove cover, brown at 400° for ten minutes. Turn heat low and uncover, bake for 3/4 of an hour. Turn heat off and leave in oven. Apple Betty may be eaten with a little ice cream, custard, milk or grated Cheddar or Munster cheese.

14. Mistress or wife's cakes • 1 pound of bacon, 8 ounces of dates, 1 1/2 cups of any nuts, 3 tablespoons of toasted cake flour, 2 tablespoons of honey.
Pie dough made with 2 cups of toasted cake flour, 8 tablespoons of boiling hot lard and a teaspoon of salt, a little cold water. Mix all ingredients well, except water. Add cold water at very end. <u>Filling</u>**:** Cook bacon till fat is rent. Cut crispy bacon into tiny bits. Set aside. Cut dates into tiny pieces. Set aside. Pound nuts in mortar and pestle. Set aside. Cook raw flour over heat, stirring constantly till slightly brown. Mix everything together and add honey. Roll dough very thin and fill round pieces of flat dough with a tablespoon of the filling. Close them up. Brush with egg white. When several are ready, place them on a pan and brown in oven at 350°.

15. Amanda's Chocolate cookies. Ingredients: 1 cup flour, 1 cup oatmeal, 2 tbsp butter, 3 oz cream cheese, 1 egg, 1 cup chocolate morsels, 1 cup mixed nuts, pounded, 2 tsp salt, 1/2 cup of brown sugar. Toast raw flour, pan fry oatmeal about 5 minutes, melt butter, cream cheese. Mix together, roll into small balls flattening out. In oven, cook over low heat till done.

16. Cakes. When baking cakes, look at the amount of sour cream, cream, butter and sugar used in a recipe. Use your judgment and reduce amount of these ingredients. Sugar can be reduced to 1/3 the specified amount. Cream, butter, sour cream, use sparingly: 1 tablespoon of melted butter or lard if desired. A mildly sweet cake is more delightful than a sickeningly sweet cake. Toast flour, melt butter and pour on flour. Do not waste time mixing butter and sugar. Cakes mixed with fruit are better than a plain cake thus the Black Forest cake is an excellent cake. Fruits and nuts are excellent in a cake. The Chinese make a light product by steaming cakes.

17. Custard: Custard may be made with milk or mixed with water.
Ingredients: 4 eggs, 1 cup of milk, 1 cup of water, salt, sugar. (May be steamed)
   In an iron pan, heat 1/4 cup of sugar, hold the handle and swish it around. Over medium high heat, cook until caramelized and brown. Immediately pour it in a pie pan. Let it harden. Beat eggs with a fork, add 5 dashes of salt, 2 tsp. sugar. Add milk and stir well. Pour above the hard caramel. Cook in oven over low heat for an hour, then turn on medium high for ten minutes. Leave in oven till set.

Miscellaneous

Discard overcooked meats falling off bone: they are devoid of nutrients, not fit for animals. When cooking meat over low heat in a covered pot, if fork pokes through, the meat is done. Do not put in all vegetables at once. First cook the hard vegetables, then the softer vegetables. A vegetable that is pale and lifeless is not edible.

Mixtures of foods are easily made with breadcrumbs or finely grated cooked potatoes. Warm them in wok, add meats, fish and prepared vegetables, make them into balls rapidly. They will have the consistency of stuffing.

Restaurants in Chinatown serve fresh Dim Sim daily: some have meat with vegetables; the best are those where meats, vegetables and starches are mixed in a mouthful. Dim Sim originated in China about 2,000 years ago.

Asian cooking uses mixtures of vegetables and meats. There is a tendency to fry foods or use much lard in recipes. Cut down the amount of fat used in various recipes. At the end, dab the product with a paper towel.

To be observed for the rest of your life: if very ill, only eat foods in a broth; light coffee or cocoa, dilute fresh juices and peeled grapes. Eat wet foods with less than 1% starch. Avoid sandwiches, pizza, bread, rice, cookies, cake, very little dry foods; eat heavy foods only in the middle of the day, not at night. When teminally ill, eat only foods that can enhance body regularity. Custards with fruit, yogurt, scrambled eggs and cheese, soups with any mixture of vegetables, pot roasts.

Another alternative to prolong life

Fasting helps remove poisons. On the above diet of wet foods it is easy to begin a fast. Gradually remove all solid foods, confining the diet to light coffee, light juices, clear broth, grapes without skin. Next, remove milk, drink fruit juices and clear, salty, dilute broth. The longer one remains on a liquid diet, the shorter the time needed to achieve desired result. Remain on a juice and broth diet for a month, then fast completely for a few days. When eating is resumed, reverse procedure. If one never achieves the desired result, adopt a diet of wet foods alternating with a liquid diet for the remainder of life. Complete fasting can be done by satiating oneself with one food. Select a few foods of the diet: pot roast of neck bones, pan fried plantains, pistachio nuts, Apple Betty, broth, light coffee or cocoa, orange juice and grapes. Indulge in pot roast and Apple Betty for two weeks till tired of them. Remove from the diet. Continue with the other foods until juices and light broth are left.

A medical annals case: Realizing he was dying, one man began to gradually remove all foods from his diet until he ate one egg the last day, and died. This is not the proper procedure to deal with dying. Sufficient food must be ingested for stool evacuation. It is impossible to do so on one egg. Another older woman said she felt nothing and only hoped to die yet she chain-smoked—a good reason to feel like dying. Finally, she jumped out of her 8th floor apartment window. When neither hunger nor satiation is felt, it is not a reason to die. A liquid diet can help the condition.

If one never recovers from a terminal state, prepare foods carefully and eat a minimal amount of fiber and little fat. Or if you dilute concentrated foods, make custards, aspics, soups, dim sim, light coffee and juices for the remainder of life. Fibrous foods are detrimental. Do babies require fiber? When very ill, the digestive system must be treated as that of a baby.

Daily schedule for a patient with a life-threatening condition or terminally ill

Morning: A cup of coffee, a cup or two of nicely flavored clear broth, a glass of freshly squeezed, diluted juice or some ripe fruit.

Afternoon: Eat any of the above. Avoid starchy foods and deep fried foods. Always eat meals with a drink, alternating each mouthful with soup, coffee or juice.

After 6 PM: A cup of coffee, a cup or two of clear broth, some juice or ripe fruit.

If very ill, eat only foods from organisms high in evolution: pork, a little beef, milk, fruits, cheeses, egg, fowl. Pot roast is excellent.

A terminally ill woman slowly reached a liquid diet and remained on a diet of diluted clear broth and/or clear juices for a month.

If at the absolute end of life, pass fibrous vegetables, fruits, meats through a sieve, pick at foods like birds do, prepare wet foods and increase your liquid intake. The idea is to increase stool evacuation. Three evacuations daily will enable the most terminal patient to survive.

Recipe for the very sick • Ingredients: 2 large eggplants, 1 onion, 2 large tomatoes, 6 mushrooms, 2 hot peppers (optional).

Peel eggplants and cut into cubes, place in wok. Cut onion in small dices. Place tomatoes in boiling water to remove skin. Dice tomatoes. Cut mushrooms in dices. Place everything in wok. Over high heat, cook vegetables with constant stirring for 10 minutes. Add seasonings: jam, shrimp sauce, soy sauce, wine, salt, curry powder, etc. Lower heat and turn vegetables occasionally until soft. Store in jar.

To serve, reheat portions with constant stirring; add grated cheese or shredded meats, fish or soft boiled eggs. Vary with other vegetables: onion, garlic, tomatoes, mushrooms, broccoli, string beans, eggplant, cauliflower. <u>To drink</u>: a pinch of any tea and one level tbsp. Kosher salt in 3 cups of water, boil over low heat.

Vary the recipe by using different vegetables. Cook in wok 10 minutes with constant stirring. Then layer them with cheese and bread crumbs and cook in oven till sizzling.

Clothing for the terminally-ill patient

Dress very warmly: sheepskin-lined boots, wool dress, shawl, hat, a woven jacket in the house. When outside wear a long fur-coat. During sleep, dress up very warmly. Under a down quilt, place a fur blanket above two wool blankets.

Signs of fast-approaching death

On the above diet one may live a few years while terminally ill. When impending death becomes unavoidable, indicated by constant catarrh despite the lightest diet, an oppressive feeling on the head and neck regions. Facial skin very wrinkled, mouth very pinched with dark ringed haggard eyes, etc., with these signs, eat a liquid diet immediately. For a few weeks, light coffee, light cocoa, diluted orange juice, skinless grapes. To get out of a terminal state, only eat breakfast and drink hot water the rest of the day.

One terminally ill woman had trouble lifting her legs when walking. Realizing she approached the end of her days, she began a fasting diet with 12 oranges a day for seven days. She reduced it to one orange every seven days until one orange was eaten for a week, then every other day, every two days, and so forth. She also drank two cups of soup with a teaspoon of reconstituted tomato paste, dilute ginger tea and mint tea. This was kept up for a month and she recovered from her terminal condition.

Chapter 23
Live a long life despite infection with virulent bacteria or viruses

Bacteria and Viruses: a description

Bacteria, some the smallest unicellular living creatures on earth are everywhere: air, soil, water, surviving in organic matter and can digest dead organic material. There are four types: rod-shaped, spherical, spirally twisted and long filamentous, about 1-20 microns long, and 1-2 microns wide. Encased in a gel-like material or capsule of polysaccharides, the cell body has a nucleus, and animal bacteria have no chlorophyll; some have a tail, slashing about when moving.

When living conditions are unsuitable for their metabolism and reproduction only the rod-shaped types form spores. Spores are more resistant to heat, drying, light, disinfectants and other harmful agents. Like all living organisms, bacteria require the usual elements needed for growth: carbon, hydrogen, oxygen, nitrogen, sulfur, phosphorus, potassium, sodium, calcium, magnesium, manganese, iron, copper, cobalt and others. Also needed are vitamins, moisture, optimum temperature and light. It is known that if one essential substance for their livelihood is lacking, their metabolic activity and growth will be limited.

Among the various kinds of bacteria, some are virulent others are not. Bacteria on the skin's surface are not virulent but syphilis, gonorrhea, leprosy, tuberculosis are caused by virulent bacteria. Virulence in bacteria is not due to excessive multiplication in the host's body but specifically caused by the bacterial poisons formed. Virulent bacteria produce two kinds of poisons: endotoxins and exotoxins. Exotoxins are proteins with a molecular weight similar to that of serum globulin, extremely poisonous and $1/30^{th}$ of a mg. is lethal for man. Endotoxins are compounds of fatty substances and carbohydrates and are very poisonous.

Virulent bacteria in the body

Since most remote times scientists have tried to rid the body of killer bacteria. Today scientists know that in vitro, bacteriophages are viruses able to destroy bacteria in the laboratory. When injected into living organisms, however, viruses cannot destroy virulent bacteria.

Antibiotics are used to combat virulent bacteria; these are substances produced by microorganisms, inhibiting growth of other microorganisms. They exert an effect on biochemical activities of certain bacteria. Some antibiotics prevent cell wall formation during cell division; others increase permeability of cell membranes allowing vital substances to leak out of a resting cell, and others interfere with bacteria's intracellular protein synthesis and prevent other metabolic activities of the bacterial cell.

Antibiotics present environmental stresses to enable survival of resistant members of the microbial population. When the entire bacterial population becomes resistant to the antibiotic, the latter becomes ineffective. This has occurred in secondary and tertiary syphilis, advanced gonorrhea, leprosy, tuberculosis, HIV.

A better approach in dealing with virulent bacteria: white blood cells

Bacteria thrive between 5° C. and 38° C. Below 5° C. and above 39° C. bacteria will not grow. With the proper conditions, the living body has the ability to engulf bacteria. To combat invading microorganisms, white blood cells are the body's most important defense mechanism such as neutrophils, monocytes and other macrophages of the reticulo-endothelial system.

White blood cell count increases with strenuous exercise, pregnancy and after adrenaline injection; also in the early stages of fever, at 39° C. When the core body temperature rises from 0.5°-1° C., one begins to sweat. By inducing perspiration, white cells increase to rapidly kill off virulent bacteria.

An acid diet of fruits activates bacterial destruction—acids are unfavorable to bacterial reproduction. In an acid medium of pH 4, bacteria diminish in number. At 60° F. bacteria are present. At a more acidic medium of pH 2-4, and 100° F. body temperature, bacteria are absent. Bacteria can survive in high acidity and low body temperature but cannot survive in both high acidity and high body temperature. Adopt a juice diet and perspire in the hot sun. Salt also helps destroy virulent bacteria. It is said that cholera bacteria were rapidly killed with physiological saline solution. Body regularity is difficult on a juice diet but a tablespoonful of salt in three glasses of hot water or dilute soup will enable proper evacuation of stools.

To cure syphilis, Hippocrates advised three weeks of complete fasting. Can modern man do it? We wonder. A negative Wasserman test will indicate that all the bacteria are destroyed. However a test may not be necessary. The presence of bacteria is usually indicated by sudden cuts on the skin such as a slight cut by a knife. When these signs disappear, no more bacteria are present and you are cured of the disease.

Curing syphilis

Known as the *destroyer of life* syphilis is caused by a delicate, corkscrew-shaped microorganism, a spirochete *Treponema pallidum* having 10-14 clear cut, regular, tightly wound coils. Each microbe is about 5-15 microns long, slightly longer than a red blood cell, visible only in a dark-field microscope. It moves about by a slow undulating rotation on its long axis and by propulsion backwards and forwards. The bacteria invade throughout the body in a few hours after infection. The primary sore is a typical chancre or lesion on the genitals. Primary syphilis lasts 6 weeks. If treated at this point the illness can be entirely eradicated. If untreated, secondary syphilis develops. In secondary syphilis the mucous membrane of eyes, mouth, the skin and nervous system are affected. A mild headache develops with vague pain in joints and bones, a sore throat and a skin rash on palms and soles of feet. If treated at this stage, latent syphilis develops. With the exception of positive serological tests, no outward sign of syphilis is recognizable at this stage.

A latent stage can last a lifetime. In this state one cannot infect anyone directly but the illness can be transmitted to an unborn child and deafness, blindness or some other disorder may affect the offspring. If untreated at the secondary stage one will develop tertiary syphilis where almost any part of the body may be affected. Some disturbances of later syphilis are general paralysis of the insane, the most dreaded of all manifestations of this stage; a gradual change in personality, delusions, loss of memory, apathy, violent rages, incontinence, to end in convulsions and death.

Be aware of external signs on genitals, palms of hands and soles of feet. Go to a hospital for a Wasserman test. Syphilis imitates so many illnesses it is hard to detect. It has been called *the great imitator*. Syphilis can be entirely eradicated by a fruit juice diet and heavy perspiration. It will not be transmitted to an unborn infant.

Curing gonorrhea

Known as the *preventer of life* it is caused by a double bean-shaped microorganism that attacks the mucous membrane of the genito-urinary tract, rectum and eyes. It can also arise from contaminated instruments inserted into the vagina or rectum.

Two to five days after being infected by the germ, men will feel a burning sensation when urinating. After 10-15 days, the infection spreads to the posterior urethra, the prostate, seminal vesicles, causing pain and a feeling of fullness in the scrotum. Women's first symptoms are very mild: a burning sensation with a slight vaginal discharge. The Fallopian tubes and ovaries will then be infected with fever. Some people recover spontaneously. Others are completely cured when treated early with penicillin. In the early stages, one penicillin injection can eradicate the germ. If untreated it will affect a newborn infant. One can become sterile or arthritic. Treat gonorrhea the same way as you would syphilis.

Other venereal diseases are chancroid and granuloma inguinale, affecting mostly the poor, resulting from lack of cleanliness. Chancroid is visible in the swollen lymph nodes, ulcerations, enlargements of genitals, rectal stricture, tender swelling of lymph glands in inguinal region, fever, chills and joint pains. In Granuloma inguinale there is a beefy red ulceration of genitals, leading to fever, pain. When untreated, severe disability results ending in death. In the beginning stages of chancroid, soap and water are important preventives, but sulfa drugs are used to kill the germ. Streptomycin and other antibiotics cure granuloma inguinale.

Curing leprosy

Leprosy is caused by the acid-fast bacillus Mycobacterium Leprae, a slightly curved or straight rod-shaped schizomycete. The bacteria penetrate the body from the skin, mucous membranes of eyes, nose and throat, certain peripheral nerves and the testes. Once it has penetrated the body, the microbe occurs in masses, resembling bundles of sticks. Cuticles of fingers or toes are other vulnerable spots; leave these parts alone and do not push the cuticle down or cut them off.

It is not contagious but some skin to skin contact could transmit the disease. Eating certain foods can cause leprosy; water or soil can too, affecting many people in tropical, damp climates also in subtropical and temperate climates. One young woman ate much corn flakes and developed leprosy, her fingertips turned black and were very painful. Frightened, she fasted completely for a week and all signs disappeared, never to return again. One of the first manifestations of the disease is a marked loss of thermal and tactile sense, as peripheral nervous tissue is destroyed. A leonine appearance of the face with a loss of eyebrows is noticeable. Both signs show a tendency to develop leprosy.

Take care of the illness in the early stages, and some cases of spontaneous recovery are known to have taken place. If not treated early, the illness will progress slowly leading to atrophy and marked deformity of the extremities. Some affectations being claw hand and disfiguring auto-amputation of the extremities. Today, the sulfone drugs are used to combat the disease.

Leprosy is not fatal in itself; a patient dies when another more virulent microorganism overwhelms the weak, afflicted person. Leprosy is prevalent in countries where rice is the main diet. Rice is heavy in starch. To be more rapidly digested, rice should be cooked several times or pounded till sticky. This is one way to allay leprosy; if and when afflicted, remove starches from diet; a good fast at the first sign will rid the body of the disease.

A.I.D.S.

The Human Immunodeficiency Virus (HIV) is transmitted by vaginal and anal intercourse, by inoculation among illicit drug users who share needles, transfusion recipients, hemophiliacs and health care workers. Shortly after the infection, the body begins to produce antibodies to fight the infection.

Chemical make-up of a virus: HIV virus contains nucleoproteins in the form of a nucleic acid core surrounded by a sheath of protein molecules. The outer coat of the virus contains some fatty material and complex carbohydrate.

Viruses: multiplication and effect on the organism

Viruses multiply only in the living cells of a susceptible host—the T-Lymphocytes in the bloodstream, responsible for immune reactions of the body. In the process of immunity, lymphocytes perform an important function, forming globulin, a protein of blood plasma. During an infection, lymphocytes disintegrate and are destroyed in their effort to furnish plasma globulin.

Globulin forms antibodies, with a specific neutralizing or destructive action on the invading microorganism. The adrenal cortex and pituitary gland exert a controlling influence on the dissolution of lymphocytes and the production of globulin, consequently on the production of immune substances (antibodies). When the HIV virus invades the body, lymphocytes lose their ability to furnish plasma globulin. HIV virus changes the DNA of T-Lymphocytes into their own DNA. When sufficient T-lymphocytes are destroyed one is susceptible to infection from other microorganisms. HIV virus later infects blood's macrophages—white blood cells with ameboid movement; they engulf foreign matter. The ability to fight off infections is lost; death ensues in a short time.

The HIV patient and diseases

Widely scattered vascular tumors over the body, tip of nose, penis, vaginal lips, eyes, diseases of the nervous system or A.I.D.S. dementia manifested by minor short term memory loss, meningitis, gastrointestinal diseases, diarrhea, esophagitis, progressive anal herpes or vascular tumors of the digestive tract, enlarged lymph nodes. Fatigue, swollen, hard red lymph nodes, night sweats, weight loss, oral cavity disease, skin disease, sinusitis and allergic rhinitis.

There is no cure for A.I.D.S. Treatment is expensive and unsuccessful, the drug azidothymidine is toxic and others have little effect on the illness. The drug AZT suppresses red blood cell formation and 20% of patients taking it require blood transfusions.

A natural means to suppress A.I.D.S.: In HIV infection, remove all heavy starches from the diet. It will prevent viruses from forming a cell wall, and they will no longer propagate. For survival in all life-threatening diseases adopt a diet to promote daily regularity.

Chapter 24
Live a long life despite Parkinson's, Alzheimer's, Cancer, Muscular Dystrophy, etc.

Parkinson's Disease
This illness is characterized by a stooped posture, slow movement, a fixed facial expression, hand tremors and a tendency to lose balance and fall; but when completely relaxed, no perceptible tremor is noticeable. When obliged to consciously perform an action, tremor is manifested, the greater a conscious effort is required the more pronounced the tremor.

Erratic body movements indicate a sign of diminished total blood volume in the entire circulatory system. In health, five liters of blood are fairly well divided between the functions of the various great systems of the body. In Parkinson's, sufficient blood fills internal organs but in conscious effort, blood must be driven to muscles and bones and total blood volume is insufficient for normal activity, manifesting tremor. Two people affected with Parkinson's disease admitted their daily liquid intake was very small. The problem may be resolved by drinking much liquids.

Alzheimer's: a gradual loss of memory. Alzheimer's is due to the excess intake of carbohydrates: bread, potatoes and beans, flour products, sugar, wine and other alcoholic beverages. Impose a diet on the patient and improvement will be noticeable.

Cancer: Daily, cells die and are replaced by normal cellular regeneration. In extreme stress, overwork, tension, nervousness, the chemistry of body fluids changes. When body temperature increases, sugar turns into alcohol, producing ether. When tissues are bathed in ether, abnormal regeneration of cells will take place, manifested by great pain. Cancer is a life-threatening condition; the reader should know how to deal with this condition.

Muscular dystrophy
Characterized by wasting and enfeeblement of muscles of the trunk and limbs, the illness begins in childhood, progressing over a period of 5-20 or more years. Symptoms are a delay in beginning to walk, frequent falls, a waddling gait, failure to rise from a recumbent position without using hands, clumsiness in walking and running or an inability to lift arms above the head.

This illness indicates extremely poor control of voluntary activity by the brain. Dieting is important to prevent further weakness of muscles and bones. Many diseases such as polio, myasthenia gravis, can be eradicated by a better infant formula or by breast-feeding.

Conclusion

Recently we viewed a documentary on Tibet. At an altitude of 12,000 feet above sea level, this country is located in an atmosphere of rarified oxygen. Tibetans however, expend much energy in their daily living. In classrooms, children read lessons out loud, in unison. Children use up energy when speaking loudly; it is a good cause for illness, poor growth with a detrimental effect on longevity. In religious ceremonies, people use gongs, drums, and chant in unison. Loud instruments destroy many red blood cells and long chants divert blood away from regulatory organs and especially detrimental in cold climates and high altitudes.

Women in general should first be acquainted with the axiom in Chapter One, because they must direct the lives of their children so that in their adulthood they will be more skilled in directing their offspring. The axiom will become part of their daily living, which will later be transmitted to future generations.

Aside from being married and with children some women are not content with one full-time job. Three cases are known where a married woman with children held two full-time jobs. All three women died young. One cannot burn a candle at both ends, and a married woman with children should care for her children first and work part-time if necessary.

Many people are against using animals for laboratory experimentation. Animals are sacrificed to find cures for mankind. It would be more interesting to improve our species by changing food habits during the growth period. Species can be changed by altering food habits during growth which is of short duration in small animals. People should think about building harmonious homes to enhance their living.

Confucius said: do not enter a country where a revolution is imminent, and do not remain in a country where there is confusion.

BIBLIOGRAPHY

Akerblom, Bengt, M.D., Standing and Sitting Posture, Stockholm, Sweden: Nordiska Bokhandeln, 1948.

Airola, Paavo, Health Secrets From Europe, Princeton, New Jersey: Parker Publishing Company 1970.

Alexander, Dan Dale, The Common Cold And Common Sense, Hartford, CT: Witkower Press, 1971.

Arndt, Kenneth A., M.D., Manual of Dermatological Therapeutics with Essentials of Diagnosis, 3rd Edition, Boston, MA: Little, Brown and Company, 1983.

Bach, Christopher, Ions for Breathing Control of the Air. Electrical Climate for Health. Translated and Edited by the Pilcox Consultant Service, 1st English Edition, Oxford, New York, N.Y.: Pergamon Press, 1967.

Barcroft, Joseph, Features In The Architecture Of Physiological Function, New York, NY: Cambridge University Press, 1934.

Barcroft, Joseph, The Brain And Its Environment, Princeton, New Jersey: Yale University Press, 1938.

Barrée, Marie Louise, La Kinesthérapie de la Maladie de Parkinson, Paris, France: Librairie Maloine, 1970.

Bates, William, Better Eyesight Without Glasses, New York, NY: Henry Holt And Company, 1920.

Bauer, A. Julius, The Person Behind the Disease, New York, N Y: Grunne and Stratton, 1956.

Bayrd, Edwin, The Thin Game, New York, NY: Newsweek Books, 1978.

Beaumont, William, M.D., Experiments and Observations on the Gastric Juice and the Physiology of Digestion, Boston, MA: 1929.

Bedichek, Roy, The Sense of Smell, 1st Ed., Garden City, NY: Doubleday, 1960.

Belinkoff, Stanton, Introduction to Inhalation Therapy. Introduction by Meyer Saklad, 1st Edition, Boston, MA.: Little, Brown & Company 1969.

Bennett, Alan, H. Management Of Male Impotence, Baltimore, MD: Williams and Wilkins, 1982.

Berendt, Hans Joseph and M.Green, Patterns of Skin pH from Birth Through Adolescence, Springfield, IL: C.C. Thomas 1971.

Bergstein, N.A.M. Liver and Pregnancy. Excerpta Medica Amsterdam, Holland: 1973.

Bergstein (video recording) produced by BBC Enterprises, Stokie, IL.: Texture Films Inc. 1984.

Best, Charles H. and N.B. Taylor, M.D., The Living Body, London, England: Chapman & Hall Ltd., 1958.

Binet, Léon, Nouveaux Aspects de la Lutte Contre La Mort, Paris, France: Presses Universitaires de France, 1945.

Birren, Faber, Color Psychology and Color Therapy, New York, N.Y.: McGraw Hill 1950.

Birth Reborn (video recording produced by BBC Enterprises, Stokie, IL.: Texture Films, Inc. 1984.

Bishop, C.E., Peripheral Unit for Pain, Journal of Neurophysiology, 1944.

Bisshop and Smith, The American Rocky Mountain Spotted Fever, Circular U.S.

Department of Agriculture No. 478, 1, 1938.

Bonadonna, Telesforo, Attitudine del Maschio Alla Riproduzione e Controllo dello Sperma, Milian, Italy: Collana Tecnico Scientifica, 1944.

Bostwick, Homer, An Inquiry Into The Cause of Death from Old Age, New York, NY: Stringer and Townsend, 1851.

Bonadonna, Telesforo, Attitudine del Maschio Alla Riproduzione e Controllo Dello Sperma, Milan, Italy: Collana Tecnico Scientifica, 1944.

Bouser, Frederick G., The Elementary School Curriculum, New York, NY: Macmillan Co., 1925.

Brain, Sir Walter, Science, Philosophy and Religion, New York, NY: Cambridge University Press, 1959.

Brinton, Selwyn, The Golden Age of the Medici, Boston, Mass. Small, Maynard & Co. 1925.

Brothwell, Don R. and Patricia, Food In Antiquity, London, England: Thames and Hudson, 1969.

Brown, Goodwin, Scientific Nutrition Simplified, a condensed statement and explanation for everybody of the discoveries of Chittendon, Fletcher and others, New York, NY: F.A. Stokes Company, 1908.

Buck, Albert A., M.D., The Mechanism of the Ear, New York, NY: William Wood and Co., 1944.

Budgett, J.B., The Tobacco Question, London, England: Philip & Sons, 1857.

Button, John C., Jr. M.D., Hope and Help in Parkinson's Disease, Norman, OK: The Transcript Press, 1964.

Cabanès, Augustin, M.D. Remèdes d'Autrefois, Paris, France: A. Maloine, 1913.

Cabanès, Augustin, M.D. Remèdes de Bonne Femme, Paris, France: A. Maloine et Barraud, 1907.

Calhoun, Richard, P. Moving Ahead on Your Job, New York, NY: McGraw Hill, 1946.

Calloway, Doris H. and Carpenter, M.D., Nutrition and Health, Phila, PA: Division of Harcourt Brace, Saunders College Publishers, 1981.

Cameron, N.A., Observations on the Patterns of Anxiety, Journal of Psychiatry 101: 36-41, 1944.

Cameron, Stewart, Kidney Disease, the Facts. London, England: Oxford University Press, 1981.

Cannon, Walter B., M.D. Bodily Changes in Pain, Hunger, Fear and Rage, New York, NY: Appleton, 1929.

Cannon, Walter B., M.D. The Wisdom of the Body, New York, NY: Norton, 1939.

Cannon, Walter B., M.D. Some Modern Extensions of Beaumont's Studies on Alexis St. Martin. Reprinted from Journal of Michigan State. Medical Society, Wayne County Medical Society: Detroit, MI, 1933.

Cannon, Walter B., M.D. Organization for Physiological Homeostasis, Physiological Reviews 9, 1929, p. 399-427.

Carrel, Alexis, M.D. Reflexions On Life, New York, NY: Hawthorne Books, 1953.

Cassileth, Barry R. Ph.D., The Cancer Patient, Phila, PA: Lea & Febiger, 1979.

Castera, Constantin, Editeur, Les Aphorismes d'Hippocrate Suivis des Aphorismes

de l'Ecole de Salerne, Paris, France: A l'Enseigne du Pot Cassé, 1945.
Cathcart, Edward P., The Human Factor in Industry, London, England: Oxford University Press, 1928.
Chaplin, Dorothea, Some Aspects of Hindy Medical Treatment, London, England: Luzac and Co., 1930.
Chavany, J.A., Epilepsie, Paris, France: Masson et Cie. Editeurs, 1958.
Chen, James V., M.D. Acupuncture Anesthesia in the People's Republic of China, 1963.
Chenoweth, Lawrence, The American Dream of Success, Boston, MA: The Duxbury Press, 1974.
Choron, Jacques, Modern Man and Immortality, New York, NY: The Macmillan Company, 1969.
Claque, Charles, Oreille Interne, Paris, France: Ed. Maloine 1938.
Cobb, Ivo Geikie, The Glands of Destiny, London, England: W. Heinemann, 1927.
Colavita, Francis B. Sensory Changes in the Elderly, Springfield, IL: C.C. Thomas, 1978.
Cole, Richard Barrett, Essentials of Respiratory Disease, 2nd Edition, Phila, PA: Lippincott, 1975.
Comfort, Alex, Biology of Senescence, New York, NY: Rinehart, 1956.
Committee appointed by Central Control Board, Alcohol: Its Action on the Human Organism, London, England, 1938.
Cowdry, Edmund V. Problems of Aging, Baltimore, MD: Williams and Wilkins, 1942.
Comroe, Julius Hiram, Physiology of Respiration, an Introductory Text, 1st Edition, Chicago, IL: Year Book Publishers, 1965.
Cotes, J.E., Lung Function: Assessment and Application in Medicine, Figures by Cynthia, John and Ann Hall, 3rd Edition, Oxford, England: Blackwell Scientific Publications, 1975.
Cramer, William, Fever, Heat Regulation, Climate and the Thyroid-Adrenal Apparatus, London, England: Longmans Green and Company, 1928.
Cummings, Jeffrey L. and Bruce L. Miller, Edited by, Alzheimer's Disease, Treatment and Long-term Management, New York and Basel: Marcel Dekker Inc., 1960.
Curtis, Glade B., Your pregnancy week by week,,Tucson, Arizona, Fisher Books,1997.
Cyriax, James H., M.D. Deep Massage and Manipulation Illustrated, London, England: Hamilton Hamish, 1945.
Daniels, Victor G., M.D. AIDS, Lancaster, England: MTP Limited, 1985.
Darwin, Charles, On The Expression Of The Emotions In Man And Animals, New York, N.Y., Appleton, 1899.
Davis, Hallowell, Hearing and Deafness, New York, NY: Murray Hill Books, 1947.
Davis, Maxine, Responsability Sexuelle de la Femme, Translated by Jean Cathelin, Paris, France: Buchet-Castel 1957.
Davies, Jack, M.D. Survey of Research in Gestation and the Developmental Sciences, Baltimore, MD.: Williams and Wilkins, 1960.
Dawson, Joseph B and Henry Jellett, A Short Practice of Midwifery for Nurses, 14th Edition, London, England: Churchill, 1948.
Dent, Clinton T. M.D. The Nature and Significance of Pain, London, England: Harrison

and Sons, 1887.
Deseaux, Alfred, Affections de la Chevelure et du Cuir Chevelu, Paris, France: Masson et Cie., 1953.
Detwiler, Samuel R., Vertebrate Photoreceptors, New York, NY: Macmillan and Company, 1943.
Diehl, Harold S. and Willard Dalrymple, Healthful Living, New York, NY: McGraw Hill, 1973.
Diserens, Charles M. The Influence of Music on Behavior, Princeton, NJ: Princeton University Press, 1926.
Ducroquet, Robert, M.D. Walking and Limping, Phila. PA: Lippincott, 1968.
Du Jardins, Terry, Clinical Manifestations of Respiratory Diseases, Chicago, IL: Yearbook Medical Publishers, 1984.
Eagle, Earl T. Edited by, Conference on Studies on Testis, Ovary, Egg and Sperm, Springfield, IL: C.C. Thomas 1952.
Eidson, Ted, AIDS Caregiver's Handbook, New York, NY: St. Martin's Press 1988.
Elgood, Cyril, Safavid Medical Practice, London, England: Luzac and Company 1970.
ELLE Encyclopédie dirigée par Miriam Cendrars, L'Accouchement Sans Douleur, Paris, France: Librarie Arthème Fayard, 1957.
Elsberg, Louis, The Throat and its Functions in Swallowing, Breathing and the Production of the Voice, New York, NY: Putnam's, 1880.
Encyclopedia Britannica, Chicago IL: William Benton, Publisher, 1969.
English Medical Journal, Lancet. October 1, 1870, Dec. 5, 1974.
Engstrom, Hans et al, Structural Patterns of the Organ of Corti, Stockholm, Sweden, Almquist and Wiksell, 1966.
Farber, Martin, M.D., Edited by, Human Sexuality, Psychosexual Effects of Disease, New York, NY: Macmillan Pub. Co., 1985.
Farthing, G.F., S.E. Brown, R.C.D. Slaughton, J.J. Cream, M. Muhlemann, A Color Atlas of AIDS, London, England: Wolfe Medical Publications, 1986.
Fielding, L.Peter, Gastrointestinal Mucosal Blood Flow, New York, NY: Churchill Livinstone, 1980.
Fielding, William J. Sanity in Sex, New York, NY: Dodd, Mead and Co., 1920.
Filliozat, Jean, The Classical Doctrine of Indian Medicine, New Delhi, India: Minshiram Manuharial, 1965.
Fitzgerald, T.K., Nutrition and Anthropology in Action, Assen, Holland: Van Gorcum, 1976.
Fisher, Seymour, The Female Orgasm, New York, NY: Basic Books, 1973.
Fluhmann, Charles F., The Management of Menstrual Disorders, Phila. PA: W.B. Saunders, 1956.
Freeman, Lucy, The Sorrow and the Fury, Englewood Cliffs, NJ: Prentice Hall, 1978.
Fried, Joseph, J., Vasectomy, New York, NY: Saturday Review Press, 1972.
Galiounghi, Paul, The House of Life, Magical and Medical Science in Ancient Egypt, Amsterdam, Holland: B.M. Israel, 1973.
Gallner, Margot, Peter de Sanctis, David G. Bullard, Austin H. Kutscher, Myron S. Roberts, Edited by, Sexuality and Life-threatening Illness, Springfield, IL: C.C.

Thomas, 1984.
Gellhorn, E., Clinical Neurophysiology 10-701, November 1958.
Gilmore, Joseph P. Renal Physiology, Baltimore, MD: Williams and Wilkins, 1972.
Glabman S. and A. Freeze, Your Kidneys, Their Care and Their Cure, New York, NY: Dutton and Company, 1976.
Goldsmith, Lowell A., Edited by, Biochemistry and Physiology of the Skin, New York, NY: Oxford University Press, 1983.
Goldzieher, Maximilian A., The Endocrine Glands, New York NY: Appleton Century Co., 1939.
Goodall-Copestake, Beatrice M., The Theory and Practice of Massage, 2nd Edition, New York, NY: Hoeber, 1919.
Gordon, Hirsch L., M.D., Ph.D. D.H.I. Translated from the original Arabic (Fi Tadbir As-Sihha) by Maimonides and with an introduction by, The Preservation of Youth, New York, NY: the Philosophical Library 1958.
Gray, Henry, F.R.S., Anatomy, New York, NY: Bounty Books, 1977.
Gray, John Stephen, Pulmonary Ventilation and its Physiological Regulation, Springfield, IL: C.C. Thomas, 1950.
Green, Robert Montraville, M.D., A Translation of Galen's Hygiene (Da Sanitate Tuenda), Springfield, IL: C.C. Thomas, 1951.
Gruman, Harris, M.D., New Ways to Better Sight, Harrisburg, PA: Telegraph Press, 1950.
Grutzenhaendler, Joseph, De La Milah, Thèse, Montpellier, France, 1914.
Gorman, Warren, M.D., Flavor, Taste and the Psychology of Smell, Springfield, IL: C.C. Thomas, 1964.
Gumpert, Martin, M.D. The Anatomy of Happiness, New York, NY: McGraw Hill, 1951.
Haldane, John Scott, Respiration, New Haven, CT: Yale University Press, 1922.
Hall, P.F., M.D., Functions of the Endocrine Glands, Phila. PA: W.B. Saunders, 1959.
Hall, W.W. Dr. Sleep or the Hygiene of the Night, New York NY: Hurd and Houghton, 1870.
d'Harcourt, Raoul, La Médecine dans l'Ancien Pérou, Paris, France: Librarie Maloine, 1939.
Hardy, James D., H.G. Wolff and H. Goodell, Pain Sensations and Reactions, Baltimore, MD: Williams and Wilkins, 1952.
Harrer, Gerhart and H. Funkstionsablaufe unter Emotionellen Belastungen, Salzburg, Austria: S. Karger, 1964.
Hartman, Carl G. Science and the Safe Period, Baltimore, MD: Williams and Wilkins, 1962.
Hartman, Ernest, M.D., The Function of Sleep, Princeton, NJ: Yale University Press, 1973.
Hastings, Donald, W., Impotence and Frigidity, Boston, MA: Little, Brown & Company, 1963.
Helming, M.G., Nursing in Respiratory Diseases, New York, NY: National Tuberculosis and Respiratory Disease Association, 1968.
Hiltner, Seward, Rev., Sex Habits of American Men, Edited by A. Deutsch, New

York, NY: Prentice Hall, 1948.
Hippocrates on Air, Waters and Places, London, England: Messrs. Wyman and Sons, 1881.
Hite, Shere, Do Men Really Fall In Love? Reader's Digest, Pleasantville, New York, Feb. 1983.
Hodgson, Jane E., Edited by, Abortion and Sterilization, London, England: Academic Press, 1981.
Hodgkin, John E., E.E. Zorn and G.L. Connors, Pulmonary Rehabilitation: Guidelines to Success, Boston, MA: Butterworth, 1984.
Holmes, W.Gordon, The Science of Voice Production and Voice Preservation for the Use of Singers and Speakers, New York NY: R. Washington, 1880.
Hudlicka O., Muscle Blood Flow, its Relation to Muscle Metabolism and Function, Amsterdam, Holland: Swets and Zeitlinger, 1973.
Humana C. and Wang Wu, The Ying Yang, New York, NY: Avon Publishers, 1971.
Hume, Edward, H., The Chinese Way in Medicine, Baltimore, MD: Johns Hopkins Press, 1946.
Jacobi, Mary Putnam, The Question of Rest for Women During Menstruation, New York, NY: G.P. Putnam, 1877.
Jacobson, Edmund, M.D., The Jealous Child, New York, NY: The Philosophical Library, 1954.
Javert, Carl T., Spontaneous and Habitual Abortion, New York, NY: Blakiston Division, McGraw Hill, 1957.
Jenkins, Richard L. M.D., The Medical Significance of Anxiety, WA: Biological Sciences Foundation, 1955.
Jenson, Lloyd, B. Man's Foods, Champaign, IL: Garrard Press, 1953.
Jerzy-Glass, George B., Introduction to Gastrointestinal Physiology, Englewood Cliffs, NJ: Prentice Hall, 1968.
Johnson, Eric W., Love and Sex In Plain Language, Phila, PA: Lippincott, 1967.
Johnson, Leonard R., Edited by, Gastrointestinal Physiology, St. Louis, MO: C.V. Mosby, 1981.
Jovanovitch, Uros, J., M.D., The Nature of Sleep, Göttingen, Germany, Fischer Verlag, 1973.
Kalmus, Hans & S.J. Hubbard, The Chemical Senses in Health and Disease, Springfield, IL: C.C. Thomas, 1960.
Kellerman, Henry, Sleep Disorders, New York, NY: Brunner Mazel, Pub., 1981.
Kemp, P., Healing Ritual; Studies in the Technique and Tradition of the Southern Slavs, London, England: Faber & Faber, 1935.
King, Lester, S., M.D., The Growth of Medical Thought, Chicago, IL, 1963.
Kinsey, Alfred C., W.B. Pomeroy, E.E. Martin, P.H. Gelhard, Sexual Behavior in the Human Female, Phila, PA: W.B. Saunders, 1953.
Knaus, William A., M.D., Inside Russian Medicine, New York, NY: Everest House Publishers, 1981.
Kohler, Marianne and Jean Chapelle, 101 Recipes for Sound Sleep, New York NY: Walker and Co., 1965.
Kolb, Lawrence, C., Dynamics of Violence, American Medical Association, Editors,

New York, NY: Jan Fawcett, 1971.
Kopetzky, Samuel J., Deafness, Tinnitus and Vertigo, New York, NY: T. Nelson, 1948.
Kostowski, Wlodzimierz, The Habit of Tobacco Smoking, London, England: Staple Press, 1955.
Krueger, Haven C., A.M., M.D., Avicenna's Poem on Medicine, Wichita, KS: C.C. Thomas, 1963.
Lagrange, Fernand, M.D., La Fatigue et le Repos, Publié avec le Concours du Dr. F. de Grandmaison, Paris, France, Librairie F. Alcan, 1912.
Lamb, L.E., What You Need To Know About Food And Cooking For Health, New York, NY: The Viking Press, 1973.
Langston, J. William, Parkinson's Disease and Movement Disorders, Cause of Parkinson's Disease is Unknown, Baltimore, MD: Urban and Schwarzenberg, 1988.
Levitzky, Michael G., Pulmonary Physiology, New York, NY: McGraw HIll, 1982.
Lewis, Jerry, The Pursuit of Happiness, New York, NY: McGraw Hill, 1951.
Lewis, Joseph, In the Name of Humanity, New York, NY: Eugenics Publishing Co., 1949.
Liacre de Saint Firmin, Mme., Médecine et Légendes Buddhiques de l'Inde, Paris, France: E, Leroux, 1916.
Lindsay, Jeanne Warren, MA, CHE, Teens Parenting, Your baby's first year, Buena park, CA, Morning Glory Press, 1991
Llewellyn-Jones, Derek, Every Body, New York, NY: Oxford University Press, 1980.
Love, James K., Deafness and Common Sense, London, England: Frederick Muller,1936.
Luckey, T.D., Edited by, Thymic Hormones, Baltimore, MD: University Park Press, 1973.
Lydston, George F., Impotence and Sterility, Chicago, IL: The Riverton Press, 1917.
Mackie, Rona B., Eczema and Dermatitis, New York, NY: Arco Pub. Co., 1983.
Manacéine, Marie de, Quelques Observations Expérimentales Sur l'Influence de l'Insomnie Absolue, Archives Italiens de Biologie, XXI, 1894, p. 322-325.
Martin, Constance R., Textbook of Endocrinology, Baltimore, MD: Williams and Wilkins, 1976.
Martin, Ernest, Histoire des Monstres Depuis l'Antiquité jusqu'à nos jours, Paris, France: G. Reinwald & Cie, 1880.
Masters, William H. and V.E. Johnson, Human Sexual Response, Boston, MA,: Little, Brown and Company, 1966.
Mayr, Franz X., M.D., Schönheit und Verdauung, München, Germany, Süddeutsche Verlagsanstalt, 1920.
McCollum, Elmer V., E.O. Keiles and A.G. Day, The Newer Knowledge of Nutrition, New York, NY: Macmillan, 1939.
Mckay, Sperlin and Barnes, Growth, Aging and Chronic Disease and Lifespan in the Rat, Archives of Biochemistry, 2, 469, 1952.
Mckenzie, Dan, Aromatics and the Soul, New York, NY: P. Hoeber, 1924.
Medawar, Peter B., An Unsolved Problem in Biology, London, England: H.K. Lewis, 1952.
Melzack, Ronald, M.D., The Puzzle of Pain, New York, NY: Basic Books, 1973.

Menninger, Karl, M.D., Love Against Hate, with the Collaboration of Jeannette Lyle Menninger, New York NY: Harcourt Brace & Co. 1942.
Meader, Clarence, Ph.D. and J.H. Muyske, Sc. D., Handbook of Biolinguistics General Semantics, Toledo, OH: Herbert C. Weller, Part2, 1959.
Mendelson, Curtis, L., Cardiac Disease in Pregnancy, Phila, PA: F.A. Davis Co., 1969.
Millington, P.D. and R. Wilkinson, Skin, New York, NY: Cambridge University Press, 1983.
Mohr, Ulrich, Schmahl and Tomatis, Air Pollution and Cancer in Man, Proceedings of the 2nd Hanover International Carcinogenesis Meeting held in Hanover, October 22-24, 1975. Editors U. Mohr, D. Schmal, L. Tomatis, Technical Editor for IARC W. Davis - Lyons, France: Internaional Agency for Research on Cancer, 1977.
Morton, Dudley J. and P.D. Fuller, Human Locomotion and Body Form, Baltimore, MD: Williams and Wilkins, 1952.
Morton, Rosalie S., M.D., A Doctor's Holiday in Iran, New York, NY: Funk and Wagnalls, 1940.
Montagu, Ashley, Touching, The Human Significance of Your Skin, New York, NY: Columbia University Press, 1971.
Montcrieff, R.W., Odours, New York, NY: Heineman Medical Books, 1970.
Morton, Rosalie S., M.D., A Doctor's Holiday in Iran, New York, NY: Funk and Wagnalls, 1940.
Moses, Bessie L., M.D. Contraception: A Therapeutic Measure, Baltimore, MD: Williams and Wilkins, 1936.
Mosso, Angelo, M.D., Fatigue, Translated by Margaret Drummond and W.B. Drummond, New York, NY: G.P. Putnam's Sons, 2nd Edition, 1906.
Mullins, Lorin, J., Olfaction Annals, New York, NY: New York Academy of Science, 1955.
Munk, William, M.D., Euthanasia or Medical Treatment in Aid of an Easy Death, London, England: Longmans, Green and Co., 1887.
Muyser, Raymond de, L'Amour et La Conception, Paris, France: Eugène Figuière, 1935.
Naficy, Abbas, M.D., La Médecine En Perse, Paris, France: Les Editeurs Vega, 43 Rue Madame, 1953.
Ocksner, Alton, Smoking and Cancer, New York, NY: Mesmer, 1954.
Oldfield, Josiah, The Beauty Aspect of Health and Living, London: E. Chapman and Hall, 1935.
Oliver, Leslie, Parkinson's Disease, Springfield, IL: C.C. Thomas, 1967.
Ortonne, Jean Paul, M.D., D.B. Mosher, M.D. and T.B. Fitzpatrick, M.D., Vitiligo and Other Hypomelanoses of Hair and Skin, New York, NY, Plenum Medical Book Co., 1983.
Pai, Mangalore Narafinha, M.D., Sleeping Without Pills, New York NY, Stein and Day, 1966.
Pallot, D.J., Edited by, Control of Respiration, New York, NY: Oxford University Press, 1983.
Patten, Bradley M., Human Embryology, 3rd Edition, New York, NY: Blakiston Division, McGraw Hill, 1968.

Pattison, E. Mansell, An Interview With A Dying Mother; The Experience of Dying, Englewood Cliffs, NJ: Prentice Hall, 1977.
Parish, Lawrence C., Edited by F. Gshnait, Sexually Transmitted Diseases, New York, NY: Springer Verlag, 1989.
Ramfjord, Sigurd and Major M. Ash, Occlusion, Phila, PA: W.B. Saunders, 1983.
Ribot, Théodule A., Psychology of the Emotions, London, England: Walter Scott Pub., 1903.
Robbins, C.R., Chemical and Physical Behavior of Human Hair, New York, NY: Van Nostrand, Reinhold, 1979.
Rockstein, M. and M.L. Sussman, Edited by, Symposium on Nutrition, Longevity and Aging, New York, NY: Academic Press 1976.
Roger, Joseph L., Traité des Effets de la Musique sur le Corps Humain, Traduit du latin et augmenté de notes par Etienne Sainte-Marie, Préface, Paris, France: Chez Brunot, 1803.
Rose, F. Clifford, M.D., Editor, Amyotrophic Lateral Sclerosis, Progress in Clinical Neurological Trials, New York, NY: Demos Publications, 1990.
Routh, Joseph I., Ph.D., Fundamentals of Inorganic, Organic and Biological Chemistry, 3rd Edition, Illustrated, Phila., PA: W.B. Saunders Co. 1954.
Rubin, Isadore, Sexual Life after Sixty, New York, NY: Basic Books, 1965.
Savill, Agnes, The Hair and Scalp, London, England: B. Arnold, 1935.
Saxon, Sue V. & M.J. Elton, Physical Change and Aging, New York, NY: Teresias Press, 1978.
Schendel, Gordon, Medicine in Mexico, Austin, TX: University of Texas Press, 1968.
Schmidt, Rudolf, M.D., Pain, its Causation and Diagnostic Significance in Internal Disease, Translated & edited from the 2nd edition and revised German edition by Karl M. Vogel and Hans Zinsser, 2nd Ed. Phila, PA: J.B. Lippincott, 1911.
Schmidt, Robert F. and G. Thews, Ph.D., Human Physiology, Translated from the German by Marguerite A. Biedeman-Thorson, Berlin - Heidelberg, Germany: Springer Verlag, 1983.
Schulian, Dorothy and Max Schoen, Edited by, Music and Medicine, New York, NY: Henry Schuman Inc. 1948.
Schwartz, Louis and S.M. Peck, M.D., Cosmetics and Dermatitis, New York, NY: E.B. Hoeber, Inc. 1946.
Scuderi and del Bo, La Vascularizzazione del Labirinto Umano, Arch. Ital. Otolar. Supplement 11, p. 1-90, 1952.
Semka, Thomas J. Eugene D. Jacobson, Gastrointestinal Physiolobgy, The Essentials, Baltimore, MD: Williams and Wilkins, 1983.
Setchell, B.P. The Mammalian Testis, Ithaca, NY: Cornell University Press, 1978.
Shepard, Mary E., Nursing Care of Patients with Ear, Eye, Nose and Throat Disorders, New York, NY: Macmillan Co., 1958.
Shepard, Roy J., M.D. Alive Man, the Physiology of Physical Activity, Springfield, IL: C.C. Thomas, 1972.
Shepard, Roy J., M.D., Physical Activity and Aging, New York, NY: Year Book Publishers, 1978.
Shimizu, Koichi and Kazuyoshi Ujje M.D., Structure of Ocular Vessels, Tokyo, Japan:

Igaku-Shoin, 1978.
Shuster, Sam, Dermatology in Internal Medicine, New York, NY: Oxford University Press, 1978.
Silverman, Sylvia S. Clothing and Appearance, New York, NY: Teachers College Columbia University, 1945.
Silverstein, Alvin, M.D. & V.B. Silverstein, Sleep and Dreams, Phila., PA: Lippincott Co., 1974.
Simmons, William A. H. & Lewis, Jennifer M..Premature Babies, St. Louis, Missouri, C.V.Mosby Co. 1985.
Sinski, James T., Dermatophytes in Human Skin, Springfield, IL: .C. Thomas, 1974.
Sloan, Archibald W., Man in Extreme Environments, Springfield, IL: C.C. Thomas, 1979.
Slonim, N. Balfour & Lyle H. Hamilton, Respiratory Physiologby, 4th Edition, St. Louis, MO: C.V. Mosby, 1981.
Sobel, Harry J. and Wendy K., Behavior Therapy in Terminal Care; a Humanistic Approach, Cambridge, MA: Ballinger, 1981.
Spencer, W.G., Translated by, Celsius de Medicina, with an English Translation, Cambidge MA: Harvard University Press, 1935.
Sperber, Perry A., Treatment of the Aging Skin and Dermal Defects, Springfield, IL: C.C. Thomas, 1965.
Squire, John, Edited by, Structural Basis of Muscular Contraction, New York, NY: Plenum Press, 1981.
Storer, Robert V. Maladjustments of Sex, London, England: John Bale & Sons, 1935.
Steinhaus, Arthur H. & F.M. Grunderman, Tobacco and Health: Some Factors about Smoking, 2nd Edition, New York, NY: Association Press, 1942.
Strelcyn, Stefan, Médicine et Plantes d'Ethiopie, Warszawa, Poland: Panstwowe Wydawnictwo Naukowe, 1958.
Sundeman, Frederick W. & Frederick Boemer, Normal Values in Clinical Medicine, Phila., PA: W.B. Saunders, 1949.
Szass, Thomas S., M.D., Pain and Pleasure, London, England: Tavistock Publications, 1957.
Tamar, Henry, Principles of Sensory Physiology, Springfield, MA: C.C., Thomas, 1972.
Thakkur, Chandrashekhar G., Ayurveda - Indian Medicine, Bombay, India: The Times of India Press, 1965.
Thompson, M.R., Recent Advances in the Medical Aspects of Smoking, Lansing, MI: The Matthew Publishing Co., 1964.
Thompson, W.A.R., A Change of Air, New York, NY: Scribner's, 1979.
Topley, Williams Whiteman C. General Editor, Sir Graham Wilson, Sir Ashley Miles, M.T. Parker, Principles of Bacteriology, Virology and Immunity, 7th Edition, Baltimore, MD: Williams and Wilkins, 1983-1984.
Travers, Gayle A., Respiratory Nursing, New York, NY: J. Wiley, 1982.
Velard, Joseph, T. Essentials of Human Reproduction, New York, NY: Oxford University Press, 1958.
Veith, Ilza, Translated by, The Yellow Emperor's Classic of Internal Medicine, With

an introductory note by Ilza Veith, Berkeley & Los Angeles, CA: University of California Press, 1966.

Velten, Carl, Sitten und Gebrauche der Swahili, Goettingen, Germany: Dandehoek and Ruprecht, 1903.

Walker, John, Folk Medicine in Modern Egypt, London, England: Luzac and Co., 1934.

Wallerstein, Edward L., Circumcision, An American Fallacy, New York, NY: Springer Publishing Company 1980.

Wellcome, Sir Henry, Spanish Influence on the Progress of Medical Science, Madrid, Spain: The Wellcome Foundation Limited, London, England, 1935.

Weschke, Charles, Ph.D., Overcoming Sleeplessness, Minn: The Book Masters, 1935.

Wikler, Simon J., Your Feet are Killing You, New York, NY: Frederick Fell, 1953.

Wilkinson, Darrell S., The Nursing and Management of Skin Diseases, London, England: Faber and Faber, 1958.

Williams, A. Roy, Ultrasound, Biological Effects and Potential Hazards, New York, N.Y. Academic Press, 1983

Williams, Edward R., Work and Rhythm, Food and Fatigue, London, England: G. Allen and Unwin, 1936.

Wolberg, Lewis Robert, M.D., The Psychology of Eating, New York, NY: Robert M. McBride and Company, 1936.

Wolff, Eugene, M.D., Anatomy of the Eye and Orbit, 6th Ed., Phila, PA: W.B. Saunders, 1968.

Wolff, Harold G. and S. Wolff, Pain, 2nd Edition, Springfield, IL: C.C. Thomas, 1958.

Wolstenholme, G.E. and Maeve O'Connor, Editors, Pain and Itch Mechanisms, Ciba Foundation Study Group No. 1, London, England: Little, Brown and Co., 1959.

Wyburn, George, R.W. Pickford, R.J. Hirst, Human Senses and Perception, Edinburgh, England: Oliver and Boyd, 1964.

Zimmermann, Jack M., M.D., Hospice: Complete Care for the Terminally Ill, Baltimore, MD: Urban and Schwarzenburg, 1986.

Index

A medical annals case 222
Abdominal aorta 193
Abducent nerve 61
Abnormal white cell count 186
Abort 11
Absorption 119,
Acne pustules 37
Active fatigue 87
Activities to avoid in pregnancy 11
Acute infection 93
Adrenals, function, secretions 175
Adrenal gland 174
Adenohypophysis 170
Adenoids 37
Adrenals 120
Adrenal gland 174
Advice for poor sleepers 102
Advice for having frequent sex 202
Age and sense of smell 83
Aging and sense of smell 83
Aging process 104,
  combat aging 105, aging skin 161
Air, passage of 143
Alcmeon 98
Alcohol 204
Alcohol content of certain foods 141
Alpha cells of pancreas 173
Alternative to prolong life 221
Alzheimer's 229
Amines, structural formula 81
Amniocentesis 12
Ampulla 78
Anal canal 121
Anesthesia at labor 16
Anterior lobe of pituitary 170
Anxiety 88
Aortic arch 192
Apnea 22
Appendicitis 94

Appendix 122
Appetite 107
Approaching death 214, 67
Aqueduct of Sylvius 58
Aqueous humor 72
Arachnoid 59
Arteries 191
Artificial stimuli at evacuation 127
Ascending aorta 192
Ascending colon 122
Asphyxia 82
Auditory nerve 61
Audubon, J.J. 42
Audubon's Birds of America 40
Autism 29
Author's feeding method 25
Author's grandson 24
A.I.D.S. 227
Awakening, healthful 101
Axiom 1-6

Baby, form a beautiful 22
Back pain 92
Bacteria 224
Bacterial growth in feces 123
Balinese dance 48
Barcroft, J. 8, 13, 66
Basilar membrane 75
Bath, daily 32, 73
Beaumont, William, Dr. 130
Beetle Phengodes, 5
Beneficial effects—touch massage 85
Beneficial effects of climax 201
Bernard, Claude 25, 131
Best lighting 73
Beta cells 173
Bicycling 43
Bile 118, 120, gallstones 128
Bilirubin 119

Binet, Leon Dr. 216
Birthmarks 30
Blind hamsters 7
Blind spot 72, 73
Blinking 70
Block, Werner, Dr. 213
Blood 177-179
Bloodflow through skin 84
Blood fluctuation in pregnancy 13
Blood pH test 16
Blood platelets 186
Blood poisoning 93
Blood pressure 150
Blood supply, large intestine 121
Body heat 153
Body odor 82
Bowman's capsule 151
Brain fissures, gray/white matter 56
Brain size 66, development
Brainstem 58, ventricles, foramens
Breasts 27
Breastfeeding method 25
Breath odor 82
Breathing, preserve 144,
  rate changes 142, oxygen 66
Buildings 207
Bulging eyes 166
Burn, sudden 91
By-pass surgery, longevity in 149

Caecum 120
Caesarian section 16
Calcium 126, absorption 168,
  safe level 168
Calcium ions and pacemaker 149, 167
Calcitonin 169
Calisthenics 43
Caloric, expenditure 43,
  intake for women, men 46
Caloric value, alcoholic beverages 141
Cancer 229

Cannon, Walter 99, 107
Capillaries 194
Capsule of Tenon 71
Carbohydrates 132, 133, 134, 140
Care for vagina, uterus 203
Cell regeneration, abnormal 96
Cells, blood 182
Cellular structure, olfactory
  epithelium 81
Cerebrospinal fluid 59
Cervical spinal nerves 62
Cervix 8
Chancroid 226
Cheiro 159
Chemical composition of tooth 109,
  of skin 157, of lymph 189
Chewing 110
Child, form beatiful 31
Childbirth without pain 15
Choroid 71
Cholesterol and liver cells 119
Chyle 117
Chyme 115
Circulation in digestive tract 125
Circulation through heart 191
Circumcision 19
Circumvallate papilla 79
Cleansing 32
Climbing 43
Clothing 33,
  synthetics for terminal patient 223
Clotting, blood 187
Cochlea 75
Coccyx 59
Cold floor 106
Cold spots 84
Colitis 22
Colon 122
Color and eyesight 74
Coma 103
Combat fatigue 87

Comfort, Alex Dr. 103
Components of skin 155
Conception, natural 7, prevent 11
Conditions for deep love 198
Conduction, nerve impulse 64
Constipation 125
Contrejean, C. 116
Cooking criteria 41
Copper 138
Copulation 11
Cord, umbilical 19
Corpora cavernosa 198
Corpus luteum 8
Corpus striatum 57
Corti, organ of 76
Cortical region, adrenal gland 174
Coughing 45
Cowper's glands 9, 199
Cramp 97
Cranial nerves 60
Creative activity 43
Crying 53
Cut 91

Daily bath 32
Daily exercise 48
Daily schedule for terminal patient 222
Danger of alcohol 204
Danger of odours 82, of powerful emotions 88
Dangerous after effects of orgasm 201
Dangerous effects of masturbation 202
Dark curly hair 158
Dartos 9
Death, agony, sudden 67
Deep bruise 90
Deep love, conditions 198
Defecation 123
Deficiency of thyroxine 165
Dent, Clinton Dr 90
Dentine 34

Dentures 109
Deoxycholic acid 119
Dermis 155
Descending aorta 193
Descnding colon 122
Desire to live 215
Determinism 40
Develop infant feeding method 25-27
Diabetes 174
Diet for premature babies 22
Diet for terminal patient 216
Dieting 153
Digestion, good conditions 115, 116
Direct sunlight 31
Disease and taste perception 80
Displasia 22
Disturbance during sex act 202
Drugs and hearing 74
Drugs in pregnancy 14
Duodenal ulcer 116
Duodenum 116
Dura mater 59
Dwarf uterus 15
Dying explained 66-67
Dying nerve 35

Ear 75
Earpick 37
Earwax 36
Eccrine sweat glands 160
Ectopic pregnancy 13
Education 209
Egg, human 8, implantation 10
Ejaculatory duct 10
Elastin 155
Elimination tips for good, 125, 126
Emotion 14, 53, 87
Endolymph 78
Enlarged cervical expansion 59
Epidermis 155
Epididymus 10

Epidural block 16
Epilepsy 29
Episiotomy 17
Equilibrium sense 78
Erythropoietin 152
Essential amino acids 135-136
Esophagus 113
Eustachian tube 75
Excrescences 162
Excruciating headache 96
Exercise, effect on heart 149, excess 45, for fitness 47
External iliac artery 193
Extreme terminal state 68
Eyeball 71
Eyebrows 70
Eyes 70, 71
Eyesight, tips for perfect 74

Facial nerve 61
Factors, causing fatigue 187, prevent thyroxine formation 166
Falling in love 199
Fallopian tubes 7
Fat and absorption 119
Fat soluble vitamins 138-139
Fatigue 44, 86
Fats 133, best 41
Faulty nutrition and vision 73
Fear 54, of death 88
Fecal impact 96
Feces 123, 124
Feeding author's infants 25-27
Feet as support basis 47
Fertilization, ensure 10
Fermentation 121
Fever and taste buds 90
Fila olfactoria 61
Filiform papillae 79
Filtration rate, kidney 152
Filum terminale 59

Fimbria 7
Fissures, brain 56
Fluorine 138
Food digestion 114, 130
Food selection criteria 39-40
Food swallowing 113
Foods activating a goiter 166
Footgear 34
Foramen magnum 59
Forceps delivery 16
Free nerve endings 84
Function of sleep 98
Function of thyroxine 165, 166
Fungiform papillae 79

Galactina method 26
Gallbladder 117
Gallstones 119
Ganglia, spinal nerve 61
Gases in plasma 180
Gastric glands 114
Gavage tube 22
Giant pyramidal cell of Betz 37
Gigantism 171
Glasses, danger of 74
Glaucoma 73
Glossopharyngeal nerve 61
Glucagon 174
Glycogen 128
Goiters 166
Goldsheider A, 106
Gonadotrophic hormones 172
Gonorrhea 226
Gowland Hopkins F, Sir 138
Grand mal seizures 29
Granulocytes 184, 185
Granuloma inguinale 226
Great scientists on death 216
Grief 54
Growth 23
Growth processes, ensure 171
Guinea pig, transverse sections 2

Hair 157, formation, loss 158, grooming 32, 33
Hand insertions, at labor 17
Happiness 209, 212
Head and neck arteries 192
Head blow 92
Headache 96
Healthful awakening 101
Healthy people 2000 42
Heart attack 146
Heartbeat changes 145, 146
Heart, circulation 191, 192
Heart description 146-148
Heart size and weight increase 44
Heartbeat monitoring 16
Heat, body 223
Help for the dying 214
Heme 183
Hemoglobin 183
Hemolysis or laking of blood 187
Henle's loop 151
Hiccuping 53
High blood, calcium 169, pressure 149
Hippocrates 11, 85
Holes in skin 38
Home delivery 17-18
Homeostasis 181
Hormones of pituitary 170
Horse's tail 59
Hours of industry 211
Human behavior 65
Human egg 8
H I V patient's diseases 228
Humming 54
Hunger 107, loss of pangs
Hypersecretion, parathormone 169
Huxley, Aldous 27
HCl formation 116
Hypo and hyperthyroidism 166
Hypodermis 156
Hypoglossal nerve 61
Hypothalamus 58

Ileo-caecal valve 120
Ileum 116
Illness and voice 52
Immediate eye loss, action to take 73
Importance of sleep 99
Improve premature growth 23
Immortality 215
Immunization shots 38 prepare for
Implantation 11
Importance of sleep 99
Impotence 203
Improve premature growth 23
Incus 75
Induced labor 15
Industry, hours of 211
Infant feeding method 25-27
Infants' stools 28
Infectious diseases 37
Inflammation, tonsils, adenoids 37
Inguinal canal 9
Injections & kidney filtration rate 153
Inorganic blood constituents 179
Insomnia 99-100
Insulin 173
Intelligence 66
Intemperance 206
Internal capsule 57
Internal iliac artery 194
Internal secretions in blood 180
Intracranial pressure 59
Intravenous feeding 22
Irving, Washington 197
Iodine 165, 166
Iron 137
Islets of Langerhans 173
Isotonic feeding 116
Itch 36, 89

Jaundice 119, 128
Jealousy and envy 89
Jejunum 116
Jewelry 38
Jogging 42
Johnson L.R. 118

Kanner, Leo Dr 29
Keloid scars 38
Ketone bodies 128, 173
Kidneys 150-152, disease 153
Krause's end bulbs 83

Labor pain 16
Labyrinth, ear 75
Lachrymal gland 71
Language, spoken 51
Large intestine 120, 121
Larynx 51
Laughter 53
Laxatives 127
Layers of eyeball 71
Lens 71
Leprosy 227
Lewis, J. 21
Lewis, Sir Thomas 89
Life span 149
Lifespan of taste buds 80
Lifting weights 47
Light 14
Lighting for close work 73
Lipid in fats 141
Lithocholic acid 119
Liver, 127
Living without sex 202
Local pain 89
Long section through tooth 209
Longevity program 215
Loss of teeth 35, of eye 73
Loud speech 14
Love 197

Love and sex 200
Lumbar spinal nerves 62
Lumbo-sacral expansion 59
Lymph nodes or glands 189
Lymph vessels 188
Lymphatic system 188
Lymphocytes 185
Lymphoid tissue 37

Macula 72
Macular organs 78
Magnesium 117
Male puberty 10
Male reproductive organs 9
Malleus 75
Mantegazza, Paolo 20
Masculinity 9
Massage 88
Masters & Johnson 149
Masturbation 202
Maturity, years of 212
Maxine Davis 198
Medication and hearing 74
Medulla, adrenal 174
Meissner's corpuscles 83
Melanin 155
Melanocytes 156
Melatonin 176
Membrane potential 63
Menstrual cycle 8
Menstruation 8
Merkl's disks 83
Mesmerizing tub 77
Milk formation 28
Miscellaneous, for cooking 221
Modiolus 75
Moles 162
Montagu, Ashley 85
Motor oculi 60
Mouth, appearance of 110
Monocytes 185

Moxibustion 126
Muscular dystrophy 229
Music, effect of 17, 88
Myelin sheath 64
Myxedema 166

Nailheads 161
Nails 159
Natural pain reduction at labor 17
Navel 37
Necrotizing enterocolitis 22
Nerve conduction, conditions 63
Nerve fiber 60
Nerves, spinal 61, cranial 60
Nervous breakdown 103
Noise 74
Normal behavior 208
Normal blood composition 96, 177
Normal composition of body 97
Number of brain cells 63

Obesity 34
Object perception 72
Odors distinguished 81
Olfactory nerve 60
Optic chiasma 58
Optic nerve 60
Optic thalamus 57
Orbital muscle 72
Organ of Corti 76
Organic constituents of blood 180
Organs of equilibrium 77
Orgasm 10, 200
Otolith 78
Ovaries 7
Oval window 76
Oversecretion, thyroxine 166
Ovulation 8
Oxygen deficiency and absorption 119

Pacemaker, natural 148

Pacini corpuscles 83
Pain 89-96
Painful toenails 159
Pancreas 128, 173
Pancreatic juice 118, 129
Parasympathetic ganglia 65
Parathormone, effect on Calcium 169
Parathyroids 167
Parathyroid insufficiency 169
Parkinson's 229
Pascal's Principle 2
Pavlov 66
Pearly butterfly 3
Pelvic examination 17
Penile lumen 10
Perfect, infant 29, growth 31
Perilymph 78
Peristalsis 115
Perpetual life, conditions 213, 214
Perspiration 153
Petit mal 29
Petrous bone 75
Pharynx 112
Phosphate in blood 167
Phosphorus 137
Physical fitness 48
Pia mater 59
Pineal gland 176
Piranesi, G. B. 207
Pituitary 7, 170
Plasma 177-180
Plexuses 62
Pneumogastric nerve 61
Poison: immediate action 80
Poisons, remove rapidly 68
Poisons in feces 123, 180
Posterior common ligament 59
Potassium 137, pacemaker effect 148
Powerful emotion 87-88
Pregnancy 15, activities to avoid
Premature infant 22

Prenatal conditions, improve 12
Preparation and tooth growth 109
Preserve, hearing 77, energy 42-48
Preston, Th. Dr. 213
Problems of intravenous feeding 22
Processing information 63
Prolactin 28
Prolong life 106
Prostate gland 9
Prostration 44
Protect eyes 74
Protein 135
Prostate gland 9
Puberty, changes in 172, female 8
Pulse and breathing rate 142
Putrefaction 122
Pyorrhea 35

Raising a family 211
Recipes 216-218, for very sick 223
Rectum 122
Red blood cell 183
Reduce labor pains 15
Reflected light 73
Reflex action 62
Regeneration, normal 214
Regulatory organs 2
Reissner's membrane 76
Renin 152
Reproduction, enhance 172
Reproductive hormones 171
Required hours of sleep 103
Respiratory gases in blood 180
Retina 71
Rods and cones 72
Rolando's fissure 57
Round window 75
Running 42
Ruffini's corpuscles 83

Sacculi 78

Sacral spinal nerves 62
Saliva 111
Salivary glands 111
Salt, effect on pacemaker 148
Salts in plasma 179
Scala, vestibuli 75, media, tympani 75
Schwann's or glial cells 63
Schwann's sheath 60
Sclera 71
Scrotal sac 9
Seated position 46
Search of a mate 210
Sebacious glands 159
Secretion, adrenal gland 174
Selection, foods 40
Sella turcica 170, 7
Selye's theory 106
Semen 10
Semicircular canals 75
Seminal vesicles 9
Sense of smell 81
Sense organs 70
Sex and advancing age 202
Sexual activity and aging 202
Sexual orgasm and pregnancy 13
Sexual parts, essential 198
Shepard, Roy Dr. 41
Siamese twins 14
Sieved blood, path of 151
Sigmoid flexure 122
Signs of fast approaching death 223
Singing voice 52
Skating 43
Skiing 43
Skill acquisition 66
Skin, cleanliness 23, holes 38, playing with 38, functions 163, sense organs 85, cells 155, components 155
Sleep 99, ensure 100-101, importance
Sleeping limb 48
Small intestine 116

Smell sense 81
Smoke inhalatiion, danger of 206
Snake, moving 4
Snoring 145
Soft palate 112
Solitary glands 121
Speech 51
Speed of nerve impulse 63
Spermatic cord 9
Spermatozoa 10
Sphincter vagina 8
Spinal accessory nerve 61
Spinal cord 57
Spinal nerve 59, 61
Spleen 187
Splenic flexure 122
Spoken language 51
Spontaneous abortion 10, copulation 17
Standing position 46
Stapes 75
Sterilization 10
Stimulation of sense organs 84
Stimulus 63
Stomach 114
Stone, kidney 153
Stool evacuation 124
Storer, Robert 197
Substances excreted from blood 180
Sunlight exposure 31
Surgery, thyroid and parathyroid 170
Suspensory ligament 71
Swallowing 112
Sweat glands 160-162
Swimming 43
Sympathetic ganglia 64
Symptoms of parathyroid hypersecretion 169
Synthetic fabrics 82
Syphilis 225
Synapses 63

Tai Chi or Shadow Boxing 43
Taste, buds 79, sensation 80
Teeth 108-109, 34, care of, loss of, pyorrhea 35
Terminal illness 222-223
Testes 9
Testosterone 172
Tests during pregnancy 12
Tests on infants at delivery 16
Thirst 107
Thoracic, aorta 193, spinal nerves 62
Thoughts on death 216
Thymus gland 54, involution 55
Thyroid 164, thyroxine
Tips to eliminate 125, 126
Tobacco, chemical contents 205
Tonsils 37
Touch, organs 83
Touch transmission, massage 84
Trachea 80
Transplant 149
Transverse colon 122
Trifacial nerve 60
Trochlear nerve 60
Tumors 91
Two-point discrimination 84

Ultrasound 12
Umbilical cord 19
Urethra 10
Uterus 7
Utricle 78

Vacuum extractor 16
Vagina 8
Vaginal examination 13
Vas deferens 10
Vagus nerve 61
Vegetable oils 41
Veins 194, systemic 195,
    emptying into vena cava 195, 196

Vena cava 195, 196
Video deliveries 18
Vigorous exercise 44
Violence 208
Virulent bacteria 224
Viruses 224-225
Vision dependence 72
Vital force 68
Vital parameters 47
Vitamin D 32
Vitamins 138-140
Vitreous humor or body 72
Vocal activity and longevity 50-53
Voice 50, box 52

Walking 42, baby 31
Warm spots 84
Warts 162
Wastes in blood 184
Water 136
Weak kidneys, external signs 152
Weeping 54
Wens 162
Whistling 54
White cells 184, 225
White matter 60
Williams, A.R. 12
Wisdom of the Body 99
Women's erectile organs 199
Work and pregnancy 12
Working, children 39
Wrinkles 162

In 15th century Florence, philosophers at the court of Lorenzo the Magnificent discussed philosophy, religion and science. They quoted the Greek philosopher Gemistos Plethon who prophesied that some day the whole world would receive one and the same creed with one spirit, one mind, one preaching... where the perfect truth would stream into every shore of this globe and prove the divinity of man's soul. The renowned Marsilio Ficino beseeched man to give his whole strength to free holy religion from the detestable condition of contented ignorance.

His message passed away, unheeded, crushed and drowned by centuries of war and bloodshed. Five centuries have passed since Lorenzo's time. It is now the correct time for new ideas to heal the wound between Christianity and scientific thought and enrich man's spiritual and intellectual life.

In the 1800s the great French physiologist Claude Bernard was convinced that after extensive analyses of vital phenomena, one must perform a synthesis to see the reunited action of the parts.

Research director of a non-profit medical organization, Ms. Ho is the author of 16 other books on the living body. The present volume is an expanded, updated and modernized version of her 10th book written between 1981 and 1989, without notes. A copy of the 10th book is deposited at the Library of Congress. A synthesis of the most important information from all disciplines of the living body, this book allows man to solve every living problem, waiving doubt, ignorance, fear and despair, providing the power to conquer every vital function and control life and death, fulfilling the dream of the Renaissance.

The synthetic axiom in Chapter 1 is the 15th version of a synthetic theme from the author's third book.

For a lifetime's dedication to her work, Ms. Ho has received the following honors and awards: Royal Patronage for Life, awarded by Prince Kevin, Principality of Hutt River Province, Queensland, Australia. The 20th Century Award for Achievement. Honorary appointment to the Research Board of Advisors, ABI. Life Member of Order of International Fellowship. Induction into 5th Edition of ABI's International Book of Honor, Hall of Fame. Certificate of Merit, Dictionary of International Biography, Dedication of Volume XXVI. The International Order of Merit. The Order of Biographical Excellence.

ISBN 1-884-99601-9

USA $25.00
Canada $33.00